Multimodality Therapy
in Gynecologic Oncology

Multimodality Therapy in Gynecologic Oncology

Edited by

Bernd-Uwe Sevin

Professor and Chairman
Department of Obstetrics
and Gynecology
Mayo Clinic Jacksonville,
USA

Paul. G. Knapstein

Professor and Chairman
University Gynecologic
Oncology
Johannes Gutenberg Universität
of Mainz, Germany

Ossi R. Köchli

Division of Gynecology
and Gynecologic
Oncology
Department of
Obstetrics
and Gynecology
University of Zürich,
Switzerland

With contributions by

R. Angioli
H. E. Averette
N. F. Hacker
M. Höckel
P. G. Knapstein
O. R. Köchli

R. Kreienberg
V. Schneider
B.-U. Sevin
J. T. Soper
G. V. Wain

29 illustrations
64 tables

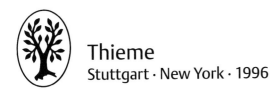

Thieme
Stuttgart · New York · 1996

Library of Congress Cataloging-in-Publication Data

Multimodality therapy in gynecologic oncology / edited by B.-U. Sevin, P. G. Knapstein, O. R. Köchli ; with contributions by R. Angioli ... [et al.].
   p.   cm.
Includes bibliographical references and index.
ISBN 3-13-101241-2 (GTV). -- ISBN 0-86577-588-5 (TMP)
1. Generative organs. Female--Cancer--Adjuvant treatment.
2. Breast--Cancer--Adjuvant treatment.   I. Sevin, B.-U.
II. Knapstein, Paul Georg.   III. Köchli, O. R.
IV. Angioli, R.
[DNLM: 1. Genital Neoplasms, Female--therapy. 2. Combined Modality Therapy. 3. Breast Neoplasms--therapy.
WP 145 M961 1996]
RC280.G5M85   1996
616.99′465--dc20
DNLM/DLC
for Library of Congress   96-14486
                                                    CIP

Cover drawing by Renate Stockinger

Important Note: Medicine is an ever-changing science undergoing continual development. Research and clinical experience are continually expanding our knowledge, in particular our knowledge of proper treatment and drug therapy. Insofar as this book mentions any dosage or application, readers may rest assured that the authors, editors and publishers have made every effort to ensure that such references are in accordance **with the state of knowledge at the time of production of the book.**

Nevertheless this does not involve, imply, or express any guarantee or responsibility on the part of the publishers in respect of any dosage instructions and forms of application stated in the book. **Every user is requested to** examine carefully the manufacturers' leaflets accompanying each drug and to check, if necessary in consultation with a physician or specialist, whether the dosage schedules mentioned therein or the contraindications stated by the manufacturers differ from the statements made in the present book. Such examination is particularly important with drugs that are either rarely used or have been newly released on the market. **Every dosage schedule or every form of application used is entirely at the user's own risk and responsibility.** The authors and publishers request every user to report to the publishers any discrepancies or inaccuracies noticed.

© 1996 Georg Thieme Verlag, Rüdigerstraße 14, 70469 Stuttgart, Germany
Thieme Medical Publishers, Inc., 381 Park Avenue South, New York, NY 10016

Typesetting by Fotosatz-Service Köhler OHG, D-97084 Würzburg (Apple Macintosh/Linotype SQ 230)

Printed in Germany by Gulde-Druck, D-72070 Tübingen

ISBN 3-13-101241-2 (GTV, Stuttgart)
ISBN 0-86577-588-5 (TMP, New York)   1 2 3 4 5 6

Preface

This book was written to provide the clinician with a practical overview of multimodal therapy for gynecologic malignancies, including breast cancer. Emphasis is placed on nonsurgical treatment modalities. Diagnostic and surgical procedures are discussed in concept only, without going into detail, as deemed necessary to define their role within the framework of multimodal therapy.

In each chapter the currently available treatment options for each organ site are discussed, always following the same format. After a short historical review of the development from single modality treatment (usually surgery or radiation), the author discusses the development and practice of currently accepted multimodality treatment concepts, supported by data from the medical literature. An attempt is made to differentiate between accepted treatment regimens, based on scientific data, and methods that are either still considered experimental or lack sufficient scientific support. Literature reviews of reported data will be compiled to summarize available data.

For each disease site, treatment options utilizing radiation, chemotherapy, or other modalities are separately addressed for primary and recurrent diseases. Combinations of multiple treatment modalities (e.g., radiation and chemotherapy) are discussed in individual segments of each chapter (e.g., "Radiation Therapy"), as deemed appropriate by the author. Schematic flow charts will aid the reader in visualizing complex diagnostic, therapeutic, and follow-up procedures used in multimodality treatment concepts. Chapter 3 includes a general discussion of the different forms of radiation therapy used in the mangement of endometrial cancer. However, these basic aspects of radiotherapy also apply (with some modification) to radiotherapy of other pelvic malignancies and therefore will not be repeated in other chapters. A short general discussion of the management of radiation-related complications is presented in the section on current Treatment Strategies in Chapter 3.

The emphasis of this book is on clinical management, combining various treatment modalities. The book will provide the reader with a summary on the standards in clinical practice of gynecologic malignancies, including breast cancer. For further details in specific areas, the reader is referred to other textbooks in this and in related fields.

Since the philosophy and clinical application of multimodal therapy is relatively new, recently completed and ongoing studies are used to discuss past, current, and future aspects of care in more detail. Laboratory research is included in the discussion, as it may lead to new treatment options in the near future.

Miami, Spring 1996   B.-U. Sevin, M.D., Ph.D.

Addresses

R. Angioli, M.D.
Sylvester Compr. Cancer Center
University of Miami
1475 NW 12th Avenue (D-52)
Miami, FL 33136, USA

H.E. Averette, M.D.
Professor and Chief
Division of Gynecologic Oncology
Sylvester Compr. Cancer Center
University of Miami
1475 NW 12th Avenue (D-52)
Miami, FL 33136, USA

N.F. Hacker, M.D.
Director of Gynecologic Oncology
Royal Hospital for Women
188 Oxford Street
Paddington, NSW 2021, Australia

M. Höckel, M.D., Ph.D.
Professor
Johannes Gutenberg University
Medical Center
Department of Obstetrics and Gynecology
Langenbeckstr. 1
55131 Mainz, Germany

P.G. Knapstein, M.D.
Professor and Director
University Gynecologic Clinic
Johannes Gutenberg University of Mainz
Langenbeckstr. 1
55131 Mainz, Germany

O.R. Köchli, M.D.
Division of Gynecology and Gynecologic Oncology
Department of Obstetrics and Gynecology
University of Zürich
Frauenklinikstr. 10
8091 Zürich, Switzerland

R. Kreienberg, M.D.
Professor and Director
University Gynecologic Clinic
Prittwitzstr. 43
89075 Ulm, Germany

V. Schneider, M.D.
Laboratory for Cytodiagnostics
Burgunderstr. 1
79104 Freiburg, Germany

B.-U. Sevin, M.D., Ph.D.
Professor and Chairman
Department of Obstetrics and Gynecology
Mayo Clinic Jacksonville
4500 San Pablo Road
Jacksonville, FL 32224, USA

J.T. Soper, M.D.
Department of Obstetrics and Gynecology
Duke University Medical Center
Box 3079
Durham, NC 27710, USA

G.V. Wain, M.D.
Director of Gynecologic Oncology
Westmead Hospital
Westmead, NSW 2145, Australia

Contents

R. Kreienberg and V. Schneider

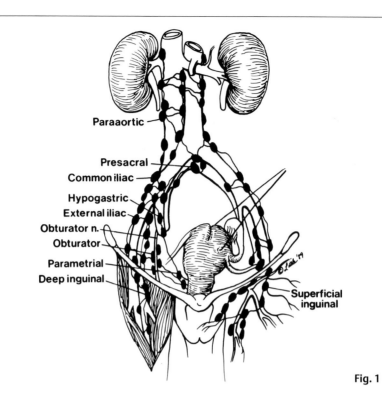

Fig. 1

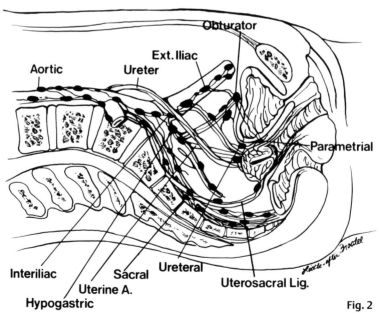

Fig. 2

Lymphatic spread patterns (frontal and lateral view).
Text see page 2.

1 Introduction

B.-U. Sevin and H. E. Averette

History of Multimodality Therapy

Gynecologic Onology is a subspecialty of Obstetrics and Gynecology that focuses on the diagnosis and treatment of women with gynecological malignancies. In the United States, the development of this field started in the early 1960s, and was formalized with the foundation of the Society of Gynecologic Oncologists (SGO) on Key Biscayne, Fl. in January 1969. During this meeting, the founding members defined the nature of a Gynecologic Oncology Service, as well as the objectives of the society.[1] "A qualified tumor service must offer complete cancer care. To do so requires adequate facilities, trained personnel, and sufficient numbers of cancer patients to maintain the professional skills of the staff. Complete cancer care requires the equipment for implantation and external radiation therapy, as well as facilities for radical pelvic surgery and the supporting services it requires. Complete cancer care requires the services of individuals trained in radiotherapy, chemotherapy, and radical pelvic surgery. Such persons should be organized as a gynecologic oncology team, hold regular meetings, and have a Tumor Registry as part of their activities." The objectives of the society were as follows: "To identify those principles, knowledge, and skills related to gynecological malignancy. To guide the development of a subspeciality devoted to this field of interest. To promote the training and certification of specialists in gynecological malignancy, and to promote research, education, and practice of this subspeciality." In 1973, the American Board of Obstetrics and Gynecology recognized gynecologic oncology as a defined subspecialty of obstetrics and gynecology, with its own 2 to 4 years advanced training program, followed by written and oral exams. The first textbook in gynecologic oncology was published in 1975 by DiSaia, Morrow, and Townsend and was followed by many more.[6, 7, 9, 10, 12, 14, 19, 22] In addition, many textbooks were published addressing special topics related to gynecologic oncology.[4, 5, 8, 13, 16, 17, 18, 20, 23, 24, 25]

The gynecologic oncologist is a specialist, who by virtue of education and training, is prepared to provide *comprehensive* management of patients, including radical pelvic surgery, radiation therapy, chemotherapy, and the management of all treatment or cancer associated complications. This was, and still is, the only field in oncology that *combines* different treatment modalities for the management of a limited group of malignancies. In contrast, all other oncologic specialties remain monotherapeutic entities, such as surgical, medical, and radiation oncology, whereby training in one treatment modality is applied to a larger group of malignancies. In this environment, multimodal therapy is rendered by a multidisciplinary team approach, in which specialists from surgical, medical, and radiation oncology work closely together to provide care for the patient with cancer.

Parallel to the development of the educational program in gynecologic oncology, a multi-institutionial clinical research organization, the Gynecologic Oncology Group (GOG), was formed to study multimodality therapy in a prospective, controlled fashion. Multimodality therapy, combining different treatment modalities, must modify standard treatment plans and dosages (e.g., in radiotherapy) that were developed as monotherapeutic concepts to optimize treatment results, while avoiding complications.

One of the first objectives of the GOG was to determine disease extent in each patient through surgical staging with the goal of individualizing adjunctive, postoperative therapy. These efforts resulted in clinical data, which to a large extent, resulted in the current standards of therapy discussed below.

Because of its origin in pelvic surgery, gynecologic oncology in the United States did not include the therapy of breast cancer, which remained the primary domain of surgical oncologists. However, over the last 30 years, it has become quite obvious that surgical monotherapy is insufficient for curing patients with breast cancer, unless the disease is very early and clearly confined to local tumor growth. The historical development of current breast cancer therapy is a reflection of the changes that have occurred in the past, based on good prospective clinical studies, which have resulted in a better understanding of the biology of the disease. It also illustrates the successful development of multimodality treatment concepts in an environment in which different specialists work together on the same disease. Most countries do not offer subspecialty training in multimodal therapy like gynecologic oncology, and the treatment of patients with gynecological cancer is rendered with this multidisciplinary team approach including gynecologists, surgical, medical, and radiation oncologists. In either case, most patients are now treated with more than one modality. Therapeutic goals should not only include improvement in cure rates, but also avoidance of treatment-related complications. Quality of life, and eradication of disease have become the important goals of modern multimodal cancer therapy.

Surgery is, in almost all cases, the first step in treating patients with gynecological malignancies. The objective of these operations is twofold: the resection of the primary and possibly metastatic tumor and the accurate determination of the extent of tumor spread. Metastatic spread to pelvic and para-aortic lymph nodes is particularly important in cancer of the cervix, corpus, and ovary (Figs. **1** and **2**, see page X). According to the International Federation of Gynecology and Obstetrics (FIGO), most gynecological malignancies are staged clinically and/or by surgical exploration (ovary, breast, endometrium). Even if only staged clinically (cervix, vulva), tumor tissue needs to be obtained to make the histological diagnosis of cancer, and many of these neoplasms are treated primarily with surgery. In the early stages of primary disease, local and/or regional treatment, such as surgery or radiation, may suffice to cure the patient. However, once the malignancy has spread to regional or distant sites, systemic therapy with potent cytotoxic agents (chemotherapy), hormones, and/or biological response modifiers are necessary to control metastatic tumor growth. The current basic treatment concepts for primary and recurrent disease are discussed in each chapter of this book.

It has become obvious that multimodality therapy has become standard for all patients with gynecological cancer, except for those with early disease. Not all neoplasms are treated equally, and individualized therapy, based on maximal knowledge in regard to tumor biology and disease extent in each patient, offers the best hope for cure. Surgical staging is currently the only way to accurately define disease extent. It also provides tissue from primary and metastatic sites for special studies that may aid in the treatment selection of an individual patient. While hormone receptors are good predictors for response to progestin therapy, no method was available in the past to predict response to chemotherapy. Histology certainly does *not* provide information in regard to chemotherapy response. More recent studies, such as ploidy, proliferative cell fraction, or oncogene studies provide general prognostic information, but so far have shown no correlation with chemotherapy response. The clinician can only empirically select chemotherapy for an individual patient based on clinical trials in which a large number of patients were treated with fixed treatment regimen. The same holds true for radiation therapy and treatment combinations. However, every clinician has experiences that clearly demonstrate significant inter-patient variations in response to therapy. Tumor heterogeneity between tumors of identical morphology has become one of the most challenging concerns in oncology. In addition, intratumor heterogeneity may be an added challenge. Most gynecological neoplasms can easily provide fresh and sterile tissue from primary and metastatic sites, since most patients undergo surgery as the first step in the path of multimodal therapy. Since the patients who are found to have disease spread beyond the local site of origin will most likely benefit from multimodal therapy, the need to study differences between primary and metastatic disease is obvious. Genetics and molecular biology have become the most promising areas of cancer research in recent years. The coming years will yield more information regarding carcinogenesis, functional cancer biology, and mechanisms of the different treatment modalities employed. Laboratory studies need to be applied to individual tumor tissues. In vitro chemosensitivity testing may aid individualized chemotherapy selection.[20] Biologic engineering will play a larger role in medicine. The gynecological oncologist will need to think and practice more and more as a tumor biologist, incorporating past experiences and new data into daily clinical practice.

Specialization and subspecialization seem to be unavoidable for developing the necessary expertise. Applying the acquired skills, including the daily practice of advanced cancer surgery, are necessary to maintain these skills, which require sufficiently large patient numbers. Centralization of care, possibly in "cancer centers," may be the best way to provide optimal and cost-efficient multimodality therapy in the future.

Training Programs

Specialty education in obsterics and gynecology was first formalized with the formation of the American Board of Obstetrics and Gynecology (ABOG) in 1930.[15] Criteria for residency training programs were established including broad teaching in both obstetrics and gynecology. However, a number of pelvic surgeons felt that the large field of obstetrics and gynecology did not provide sufficient training in gynecological surgery. This was clearly expressed in a lecture by Alexander Brunschwig, presented to the New York Gynecological Society in 1968, entitled "Whither Gynecology?".[2] Brunschwig felt the specialty field of gynecological surgery should include the management of all gynecological surgical problems, benign and malignant, of the female pelvic organs, related urinary and gastro-intestinal tract, and breast. In 1969, the president of the ABOG, Dr. A. Marchetti, appointed a committee to discuss subspecialization in obstetrics and gynecology. A conference on Specialization in Obstetrics and Gynecology was held in December 1969. The committee determined that advanced training beyond the residency would promote improvement in women's health care. Three subspecialty divisions, gynecologic oncology, maternal–fetal medicine, and reproductive endocrinology were established in 1972, and approved by the American Board of Medical Specialties in March 1973. The objectives and educational requirements for subspecialization were initially defined by an ad hoc committee under the chairmanship of Dr. John L. Lewis Jr. These have been modified over the years and will continue to change in the future.[21] Currently, the educational program requires at least 3 years of training in an approved graduate education program (fellowship) in gynecologic oncology, as outlined in the yearly BULLETIN of the ABOG.[3] Certification by the subspecialty board requires satisfactory completion of the minimum of 2 years of

clinical training, 1 year of research, a graduate course in statistics, and passage of the written and oral examinations. The subjects covered in the written examination are outlined in the "Guide to Learning in Gynecologic Oncology" developed by the ABOG and include diagnostic techniques, pathology, physiology, carcinogenics, genetics, statistics, immunology, chemotherapy, pharmacology, radiation therapy, therapeutic principles, technical procedures, and research.[11] After passing the written examination and after a minimum of 2 years of clinical practice that should consist of more than 50% patient care in gynecologic oncology, and presentation of a case list of all patients cared for, the candidate can apply to take the required oral examination. Other requirements for the oral exam include that the candidate is a certified "Diplomate" of the ABOG, has an unrestricted medical license, full and unrestricted hospital privileges, and a good moral and ethical character. In addition, he/she has to present and defend an adequate "thesis," which must be a clinical or basic research publication in press or published in a peer review journal in the area of gynecologic oncology. After fulfilling all requirements and passing the oral examination, the candidate may receive specialty certification by the ABOG. So far, more than 600 physicians have been certified in gynecologic oncology.

Cooperative Clinical Research Programs

The evolution of clinical trial groups offered a large realm of research activities, combining patient care and advancement of knowledge. In the past, medical practice was largely defined by clinical experiences of individual physicians or institutions. Especially in Europe, the philosophy and reality of clinical care was frequently defined by "schools," that is, disciples of influential clinicians, usually professors of leading academic institutions. The "dogma" of such schools was helpful in establishing certain procedural and philosophical standards of care in an era when progress was defined by these individuals, who forcefully publicized their own theories and treatment concepts. Since these were usually based on extensive personal and institutional experience, quality of care was assured. However, such "schools" also produced a restrictive element, which at times did not permit the development of new thoughts and concepts. In the worst scenario, personal preferences defined clinical practice, even in the absence of sound clinical experience. The classic statement of the professor to his disciples to enforce his authority, "From my clinical experience, …" has been sarcastically modified to "From my clinical experience of one example, the best treatment is … ," which expressed the flaws of this approach to medicine of that era.

With the era of modern medicine came the demand for reproducible clinical data to guide clinical practice. The GOG and other cooperative groups provided the data from which many of our current management plans for pelvic malignancies evolved. For breast cancer, a variety of large clinical trials from Europe and the United States (e. g., the Milan group under the leadership of U. Veronesi, the National Surgical Adjuvant Breast Cancer Project (NSABP) under B. Fisher) redefined the standards of care for breast cancer in regard to optimal surgery, as well as adjuvant hormone- and chemotherapy. Partially as a result of these studies, came a new and better understanding of the biology of cancer. From the theory of tumor growth as being primarily a local–regional event, which can be cured with appropriate radical surgery or radiation, evolved the current understanding that neoplasms may metastasize, via the lymphatic and/or hematogenous route, to distant sites even when the primary tumor is still relatively small. Invasive and metastatic potential, as an inherent characteristic of individual neoplasms, became the focus of clinical and laboratory investigations and are thought to be the primary determinant for prognosis. Therapeutic efforts shifted from local–regional monotherapy to multimodal regional–systemic treatment regimen to prevent or treat metastatic tumor gowth. A significant aspect of current cancer research focuses on the identification of prognostic parameters of individual tumors to aid the clinician in selecting patients who could benefit from systemic therapy after individually tailored local–regional treatment for primary disease.

The Role of Basic Laboratory Research in Gynecologic Oncology

Ever since the beginning, physicians were involved, if not the driving force in studying the anatomy and function of the normal human body and its pathological alterations. With the development of more sophisticated experimental tools and methods, going beyond what the eye can see (with or without the light microscope), the clinician was faced with the conflict between commitments to patient care and research. The rapidly evolving specialty of biomedical research, which was dominated by bright full-time basic science Ph.D.s, created a competitive environment in which the clinicians found themselves quickly outnumbered and outfunded. The description of the double helix structure of DNA by Francis Crick and James Watson in 1953 (Nature), based on X-ray crystallography pictures, can be seen as a huge real and symbolic milestone in this development. The ability to study and better understand subcellular structures and function also resulted in incredible progress in clinical diagnostics and therapeutics. The clinician scientist became more and more a follower and applier of scientific knowledge than a leader and originator. Applied clinical research became the major research tool, while bench research became more and more the domain of nonclinicians. This development should not be seen as a negative one. Realizing the complexities of biological systems, understanding mechanisms of the multitude of pathological changes, and considering the large armamentarium of therapeutics should lead us all to develop a realistic degree of humility. We need to accept the limitations of our capacity to know about what is currently known and to stay abreast of the rapidly growing body of new knowledge. Subspecialization was the answer to the mushrooming of clinical know-how. In basic research we are faced with a similar problem. Individual areas of research have become increasingly focused and separated. The gap between the clinician and basic scientist must be bridged. The team approach offers the best chance to succeed. However, because of the divergent backgrounds and objectives, prolonged cooperation has not always been successful between the patient-oriented physician and the laboratory oriented Ph.D. Mutual *understanding* and *communication* are two important pillars of such cooperation. The laboratory scientist needs to become aware of clinical diseases and clinical research to effectively collaborate. On the other side, the clinician must experience the life of a laboratory scientist, appreciate the excitement and frustrations of research endeavors, learn to speak their language, and understand their needs for funding. This is one of the major objectives of the 1 year of research required by the subspecialty board of the ABOG (see above). The experience, even though limited in time and scope, should enable the clinical oncologist to understand the nature and limitations of laboratory research. In addition, the clinician will develop skills in one of the fields of laboratory research, learn the basic aspects of study design, background research, trials and tribulations of study execution, data analysis, interpretation, and publication. Participation in all aspects of daily laboratory activities, care of equipment, timely procurement of supplies, and the many discussions with other researchers are invaluable experiences. Understanding time and cost issues for laboratory projects, the need for funding, and the limitations in delivering publishable results in a fixed time frame, will hopefully prepare the clinician to realistically collaborate on joint clinical-laboratory research endeavors. The needs of the clinician are continually defined by their clinical practice. These needs have to be translated into research projects together with the basic science researcher. This is where the the clinician can again take the initiative and become the driving force for projects that best fulfill the clinical needs. *Clinically guided basic research* will thus produce *preclinical* data that can be tested in *clinical* trials. Small pilot studies can be done in individual institutions and then finally evaluated with larger numbers in multicenter study groups like the GOG.

References

1. Averette HEA. Presentation at the 25th. Anniversary Meeting of the Society of Gynecologic Oncologists. 1994: Orlando, Florida, February 19, 1994.
2. Brunschwig A. Whither gynecology? Am J Obstet Gynecol 1968; 100 : 122 – 127.
3. BULLETIN for 1995 – 1996, The Divisions of Gynecologic Oncology, maternal-fetal medicine, reproductive endocrinology: The American Board of Obstetrics and Gynecology, Inc., 2915 Vine Street, Dallas, Texas 75204-1069.
4. Burghardt E, Monaghan JM, eds. Volume 2 (4): operative treatment of cervical cancer. In: Bailliere's clinical obstetrics and gynaecology. London: Balliere Tindall; 1988.
5. Burghardt E, Monaghan JM, eds. Volume 3 (2): Operative treatment of ovarian cancer. In: Balliere's clinical obstetrics and gynecology. London: Bailliere Tindall; 1989.
6. Burghardt E, Webb MJ, Monaghan JM, Kindermann G eds. Surgical gynecologic oncology. Stuttgart: Georg Thieme Verlag; 1993.
7. Coppelson M, ed. Volume 1 – 2. In: Gynecologic oncology. New York: Churchill Livingstone; 1981.
8. Deppe G ed. Chemotherapy of gynecologic cancer. 2nd. ed. New York: Alan R. Liss; 1990.
9. DiSaia P, Morrow CP, Townsend DE, eds. Synopsis of gynecologic oncology, 1st ed. New York: Wiley & Sons; 1975.
10. DiSaia PJ, Creasman WT, eds. Clinical gynecologic oncology, 4th ed. St. Louis: CV Mosby; 1995.
11. Guide to Learning in Gynecologic Oncology, The Division of Gynecologic Oncology. The American Board of Obstetrics and Gynecology, Inc., 2915 Vine Street, Dallas, Texas 75204-1069, 1991.
12. Gusberg SB, Shingleton HM, Deppe G, eds. Female genital cancer. New York: Churchill Livingstone; 1988.
13. Hepp H, Scheidel P, Monaghan JM, eds. Lymphonodektomie in der gynäkologischen Onkologie. München: Urban & Schwarzenberg; 1988.
14. Hoskins WJ, Perez CA, Young RC, eds. Principles and practice of gynecologic oncology. Philadelphia: JB Lippincott; 1992.
15. Isaacs JH. The evolution of gynecologic oncology as a surgical specialty, ACS Bulletin 74, 21 – 24, 1989.
16. Kaufmann M, Kübli F, Drings P, Burkert H, eds. Medikamentöse Therapie des Genital- und Mammakarzinoms. Basel: S. Karger AG; 1989.
17. Knapstein PG, di Re F, DiSaia P, Haller U, Sevin B-U, eds. Malignancies of the vulva. Stuttgart: Georg Thieme Verlag; 1991.
18. Knapstein PG, Friedberg V, Sevin B-U, eds. Reconstructive surgery in gynecology. Stuttgart: Georg Thieme Verlag; 1990.
19. Köchli OR, Sevin B-U, Benz J, Petru E, Haller U, eds. Gynäkologische Onkologie. Heidelberg: Springer Verlag; 1991.
20. Köchli OR, Sevin BU, Haller U. Chemosensitivity testing in gynecologic malignancies and breast cancer. Basel: S. Karger AG; 1994.
21. Lewis JL. An account of the early developments of the Division of Gynecologic Oncology. Conference proceedings, The American Board of Obstetrics and Gynecology, Inc. Conference on the impact of subspecialization on residency training and practice of Obstetrics and Gynecology. The American Board of Obstetrics and Gynecology, Inc., 2915 Vine Street, Dallas, Texas 75204-1069.
22. Morrow CP, Curtin JP, Townsend DE, eds. Synopsis of gynecologic oncology. 4th ed. New York: Wiley & Sons; 1993.
23. Perez CA, Brady LW eds. Principles and practice of radiation oncology. 2nd ed. Philadelphia: JB Lippincott; 1992.
24. Perry MC, ed. The chemotherapy source book. Baltimore: Williams + Wilkins; 1992.
25. Zander J, Graeff H. Kirschnesche allgemeine und spezielle Operationslehre: Gynäkologische Operationen, Berlin: Springer Verlag; 1991.

2 Vulva and Vagina

G. V. Wain and N. F. Hacker

Introduction and Historical Overview

Historically, surgical therapy has been regarded as the treatment of choice for cancer of the vulva, and radiation therapy has been the preferred option for patients with vaginal cancer. Several factors, including the unique anatomic features of these tumors, the poor radiation tolerance of the vulva, the relative infrequency of cases, and the generally successful results of therapy have combined to reinforce these prejudices. Consequently, multimodality approaches have been investigated much later than has been the case for either cervical or endometrial cancer. In recent times, however, as the limitations of singel-modality therapy have been more widely appreciated, interest in combining modalities has increased.

The role of radical surgical therapy for vulvar cancer was pioneered by Taussig[97] and Way,[108] who established en bloc radical vulvectomy and inguino-femoral lymphadenectomy, with or without pelvic node dissection, as the treatment of choice for invasive squamous cell carcinoma of the vulva. With the more complete dissection of the primary tumor and regional lymph nodes achieved by these surgical procedures, overall survival for vulvar cancer improved from about 25% to about 65%.

During the past 15 years, concern has been expressed about the physical and psychological morbidity associated with these radical operations, and the identification of risk factors for local recurrence and lymph node metastases has allowed more conservative operations to be performed on selected patients with early disease.

For patients with more advanced disease, the limitations of surgery in relation to both survival and morbidity have led to the successful integration of both chemotherapy and radiation into the primary management of vulvar cancer.

Vaginal cancer is one of the rarest gynecological cancers, representing approximately 1% of female genital malignancies. Due to the the rela-

tive infrequency of the lesion, no individual practitioner or institution is able to build up a large contemporary experience. Most reports on vaginal cancer span several decades and involve a number of different management techniques. Furthermore, the unique anatomic features of the vagina and the variation in lymphatic drainage at the site of the lesion, mean that each reported series contains a fairly heterogenous group of tumors, thus making interpretations of the data difficult.

Until the advent of radium therapy, surgical treatment for vaginal cancer was utilized with very poor results. Taussig stated in 1934 that "primary cancer of the vagina is very rare and almost universally fatal. We acknowledge our total inability to do anything (surgically) effective to treat the disease."[98] He proposed the use of radiation therapy for these cancers. Since then, treatment regimes have integrated external beam radiation therapy with brachytherapy, and results of treatment have improved substantially. In most institutions, vaginal cancers are now treated primarily with radiation. The integration of multimodality therapy is usually applied on an individualized basis.

Primary Disease

▓ Vulvar Cancer

The vulva includes the mons veneris, the labia majora and minora, the clitoris, and the vulvar vestibule, which contains the urethral meatus and vaginal orifice. Lymphatics from the vulva course anteriorly toward the mons veneris, turning laterally at the mons to terminate mainly in the inguinal lymph nodes, which are situated along the line of the inguinal ligament and along the saphenous vein. They lie above the fascia lata and cribriform fascia and below Camper's (superficial) fascia (Fig. **1**). Beneath the cribriform fascia are the femoral nodes, which lie along and medial to the femoral vein.[78] The femoral nodes receive efferents from the inguinal nodes, but may

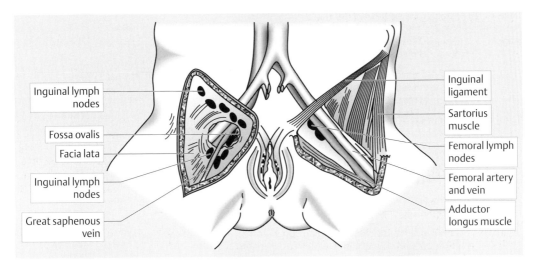

Fig. **1**   Lymphatic drainage of the vulva

also receive some direct channels from the vulva through the cribriform fascia. From the femoral nodes, efferent lymphatics pass to the external iliac nodes particularly the medial group. Iversen demonstrated a significant degree of uptake of radioactive colloid by the contralateral pelvic lymph nodes when the colloid was injected into the anterior labia minora.[46] This suggests a degree of decussation of lymphatic channels from this area of the vulva.

Histologically, vulvar cancers are predominantly squamous cell carcinomas (90%), with melanomas (2–4%), basal cell carcinomas (2–3%), and adenocarcinomas comprising most of the remainders. Basal cell carcinomas do not metastasize and can be treated by local excision. There is no current evidence to suggest that squamous cell carcinomas should be treated differently from adenocarcinomas, except when the latter are associated with Paget disease of the vulva, in which case wider excisional margins are usually required. Sarcomas of the vulva are extremely rare (less than 1%) and the available literature on these tumors suggests that they should be treated with wide excision.[99] Melanomas of the vulva and vagina will be discussed below in a separate section.

Vulvar cancer spreads by the following routes:

1. Direct extension, involving adjacent structures, such as the urethra, vagina, and anus.

2. Lymphatic embolization to regional lymph nodes.
3. Hematogenous spread to distant sites, including the lungs, liver and bones.

While lymphatic metastases may occur early in the disease, hematogenous spread usually occurs late and is very rare in the absence of lymph node metastases.

Modern treatment of vulvar cancer must be individualized. Optimal management of the individual patient requires careful consideration of the most appropriate surgical procedure for both the vulva and the groins and the appropriate integration of surgery and radiation therapy. With careful patient selection, a more conservative approach can frequently be offered without compromising survival.

Staging and Diagnostic Procedures

Until 1988, staging of vulvar cancer, as agreed upon by the International Federation of Gynecology and Obstetrics (FIGO), followed the traditional TNM classification of the UICC (International Union Against Cancer). This involved assessment of the size of the primary tumor, clinical status of the regional lymph nodes, and the presence or absence of clinically detected metastases. At its meeting in October 1988, the Gynecology Oncology Committee of FIGO changed some of the rules for the staging of vulvar cancer.[24] The

Table **1**   FIGO staging vulvar cancer (1995)

Stage I	Lesions 2 cm or less in size confined to the vulva or perineum. No nodal metastasis
Stage I A	Lesions 2 cm or less in size confined to the vulva or perineum and with stromal invasion no greater than 1.0 mm.* No nodal metastasis
Stage I B	Lesions 2 cm or less in size confined to the vulva or perineum and with stromal invasion greater than 1.0 mm.* No nodal metastasis
Stage II	Tumor confined to the vulva and/or perineum or more than 2 cm in the greatest dimension, with no nodal metastasis
Stage III	Tumor of any size width: (a) Adjacent spread to the lower urethra and/or (b) unilateral regional lymph node metastasis
Stage IV A	Tumor invades any of the following upper urethra, bladder mucosa, rectal mucosa, pelvic bone, and/or bilateral regional node metastasis
Stage IV B	Any distant metastasis including pelvic lymph nodes

* The depth of invasion is defined as the measurement of the tumor from the epithelial–stromal junction of the adjacent most superficial dermal papilla to the deepest point of invasion

revised FIGO staging now takes into account the prognostic significance of the histopathological status of the lymph nodes rather than their clinical assessment (Table **1**), but there are still major deficiencies. In a paper applying the new FIGO staging criteria to patients with vulvar cancer entered on several Gynecologic Oncology Group (GOG) protocols, Homesley et al.[42] observed very little difference in survival between stages I and II, while within stage III, there were different subgroups with survivals ranging from 34% to 100%. They suggested a modification based on the number of positive lymph nodes and a refinement of the tumor dimension factor.

The inadequacy of clinical assessment of the lymph nodes has been well established: Iversen[45] found lymph node metastases in 100 patients in his series of 258 cases of vulvar cancer. These were clinically detected in only 64 cases. Furthermore, while involvement was clinically suspected in 40 other cases, this could not be confirmed histologically. Management decisions about the lymph nodes and vulvar cancer should not be based on clinical assessment alone.

The GOG have analyzed detailed surgicopathologic characteristics of 588 patients with vulvar cancer and related them to survival.[42] The presence of lymph node involvement, the number of lymph nodes involved, and the diameter of the tumor were predictive of survival.

Surgical Management

Until relatively recently, the standard treatment for virtually all vulvar cancers was radical vulvectomy and bilateral inguinofemoral lymph node dissection. Improved understanding of risk factors for local and regional recurrence has allowed significant modifications of the standard surgical management of this disease. Appreciation of the fact that the local benefits of surgery are limited by the closest resection margin, rather than by the extent of organ removal, has allowed vulvar conservation for small lesions when the vulva is otherwise normal.[37] Conversely, when the lesion is larger and/or close to the anus or urethra, the standard radical vulvectomy is insufficient to resect the lesion with adequate margins. For lesions involving the anal canal, rectovaginal septum, or proximal urethra, ultraradical surgery has been the standard approach, combining radical vulvectomy with some type of pelvic extenteration. With the current understanding of this disease, however, the use of individualized multimodality therapy to optimize, cure, and minimize morbidity has become more important.

Table **2** Vulvar Cancer Stage, and Actuarial Survival—cases treated between 1982 and 1986 (FIGO Annual Report, 1990)

Stage *	No. of Cases (%)	Five-Year Survival (%)
I	762 (29.3)	272 (71.9)
II	786 (30.3)	201 (54.3)
III	766 (29.5)	124 (36.6)
IV	273 (10.5)	25 (21.0)
Not Staged	11 (0.4)	0
Total	2598	622 (52.3)

* Note: old FIGO staging

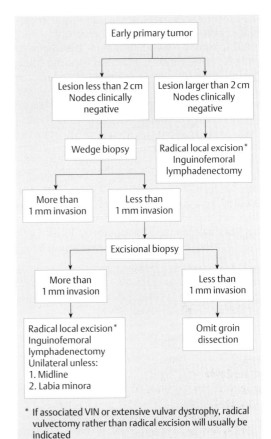

* If associated VIN or extensive vulvar dystrophy, radical vulvectomy rather than radical excision will usually be indicated

Fig. **2** Management of early vulvar vancer

Early (T$_{1-2}$,N$_{0-1}$) Vulvar Cancer

The results of treatment of early stage vulvar cancer are generally favorable (Table **2**), with excellent results reported within favorable subgroups.[42] The emphasis on treatment of these favorable subgroups should be toward reduction of morbidity rather than improvement in survival rates.

With regard to specific surgical management, the patient with a "small" vulvar cancer and clinically negative lymph nodes will be considered first. A brief summary of the management of these patients is shown in Figure **2**. The condition of the remainder of the vulva is important. If the remainder of the vulva is healthy, these lesions can be managed by radical local excision. The resection should be to the level of the inferior fascia of the urogenital diaphragm, so that the lateral and deep margins adjacent to the tumor will be the same for a radical vulvectomy as for a radical local excision.

If the vulvar cancer arises amid widespread vulvar intraepithelial neoplasia (VIN) or vulvar dystrophy, treatment is often influenced by the patient's age. In elderly women, radical vulvectomy is often the best approach, as this provides symptomatic relief from the distressing itchiness and excoriation. In younger patients, however, better cosmetic results can be obtained using radical local excision for the invasive component and superficial excision for the VIN.

Treatment of such cancers with radical local excision, rather than with radical vulvectomy, is supported by an analysis of the available litera-

ture, which indicates that the incidence of local invasive recurrence after radical local excision is no higher than that after radical vulvectomy.[34] The accumulated data from ten series of vulvar cancers less than 2 cm in diameter (old FIGO stage I) showed that the local recurrence rate of 165 patients treated with radical local excision was 7.2 % (12 patients) compared to a rate of 6.3 % (23 of 365 patients) in patients treated with radical vulvectomy (Table **3**). If local recurrence does occur, it can usually be successfully treated by further resection, with or without radiation therapy. In the GOG study of early stage I vulvar cancers treated with "modified radical vulvectomy," there were ten vulvar recurrences in 121 evaluable patients.[93] Seven of the lesions were in areas remote from the initial neoplasm and were thought to represent new primary cancers rather than recurrences. Eight of the ten vulvar recurrences were salvaged by further resection.

The second consideration in treatment of patients with vulvar cancer involves the groin lymph nodes (Fig. **2**). Attempts to introduce the concept of "microinvasive" carcinoma of the vulva led to several reports of treatment failure due to groin recurrence in undissected lymph nodes. This resulted in the statement from the International Society for the Study of Vulvar Disease that the term "microinvasion was misleading and dangerous and should be dropped".[55] This society recommended that a substage "Ia" be adopted for a single lesion that is 2 cm or less in diameter, with 1 mm or less of stromal invasion, but this has not been adopted by FIGO. Such classification depends on the whole lesion being

adequately excised and histopathologically assessed. If there is no involvement of capillary-lymphatic spaces and the inguinal nodes are clinically uninvolved, the risk of inguinal node involvement in such patients is less than 1%.[87] Although groin metastases have been documented in occasional patient with less than 1 mm stromal invasion,[105] the incidence is so low that it is of no practical significance. Such lesions can be adequately treated with radical local excision only, providing that the margins of excision are greater than 8 mm on the final pathology specimen.[37]

When there is invasion greater than 1 mm, the lesion is larger than 2 cm in diameter, or there are multiple foci of invasion, the inguinal and femoral nodes need to be assessed (Fig. **2**). This obviously implies that if the entire lesion is less than 2 cm in diameter, it should be entirely excised and histologically assessed before any final decision about the lymph nodes is made. If the lesion is well lateralized and involves only the labia majora, it would appear adequate to perform an ipsilateral inguinofemoral groin node dissection, as the incidence of contralateral nodal involvement in the presence of negative ipsilateral nodes with this sort of tumor is less than 1% (Table **4**).

The need for a complete inguinofemoral dissection rather than the so-called "suerficial inguinal lymphadenectomy" has been confirmed by the GOG study:[93] In this study of 121 patients with early vulvar cancers, six of nine patients

Table **3**   Local recurrence rate after radical local excision versus radical vulvectomy *

	Number	Recurrence	DOD
Radical local excision	165	12 (7.2%)	1 (0.6%)
Radical vulvectomy	365	23 (6.3%)	2 (0.6%)

* Data accumulated from Refs. 9, 12, 13, 14, 15, 16, 17, 18, 19, 20
(From Cancer, 1992—In Press) [11]. Reproduced with permission from the publishers)

Table **4**   Incidence of positive contralateral nodes with negative ipsilateral nodes in patients with unilateral stage I cancer

Author	Unilateral lesions	Contralateral nodes positive	Percent
Wharton et al., 1974 (25)	25	0	0
Parker et al., 1975 (12)	41	0	0
Magrina et al., 1974 (25)	77	2	2.6
Kneale et al., 1974 (25)	66	0	0
Iversen et al., 1974 (25)	112	0	0
Buscema et al., 1974 (25)	38	0	0
Hoffman et al., 1974 (25)	70	0	0
Hacker et al., 1974 (25)	60	0	0
Total	448	2	0.4

* Information not contained in the paper but obtained from personal communication
(Reproduced with permission from Berek JS and Hacker NF, Practical Gynecologic Oncology Baltimore: Williams and Wilkins, 1989)

with groin recurrence had the recurrence in the operated (ipsilateral) node-negative groin. This incidence of groin recurrence compared unfavorably to historical controls of patients who underwent complete inguinofemoral node dissection: In this latter group there were no groin recurrences.

Lesions of the clitoris, perineum, or those obviously crossing the midline require dissection of both groins. In view of the evidence for decussation of lymphatics from the anterior labia minora, it is also recommended that bilateral groin node dissection be performed for patients with tumors involving these structures. It is worth noting that the two patients in Magrina's series with contralateral positive nodes both had lesions involving the labia minora.[61]

Clitoral lesions in younger patients present a unique problem. Resection of the clitoris has major psychosexual sequelae. In addition, wide dissection of this area interrupts the lymphatic channels passing forward in the labia, often causing marked edema of the posterior vulva, which may ultimately require completion of the vulvectomy for relief. The only cosmetically acceptable option for treating clitoral lesions in young women is the use of radiation therapy. This will be discussed in a later section.

Advanced Vulvar Cancer

The results of treatment for patients with advanced vulvar cancer are not as good as those with earlier stage disease (Table **1**). Looking at the results reported to FIGO for 1039 patients with stage III or IV disease (old FIGO staging) treated at 80 institutions between 1982 and 1986, the overall actuarial survival was 36.6 and 21.0 percent for each respective stage. By allocating patients in the GOG series to the new surgicopathologic FIGO stages III and IV, the GOG reported a 5-year survival of 74% and 31% respectively.[42] Patients may be considered to have advanced vulvar cancer either because of characteristics related to the primary tumor, with involvement of neighboring structures such as the anus, urethra, vagina, or pubic bone or because of clinically obvious groin node involvement. The occasional patient will of course present with both problems, namely extensive local disease in association with clinical groin node involvement. Both situations represent different therapeutic challenges, and both represent situations that are unlikely to be

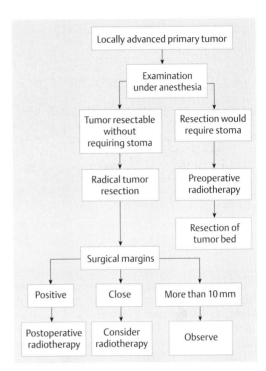

Fig. **3** Management of advanced primary tumor

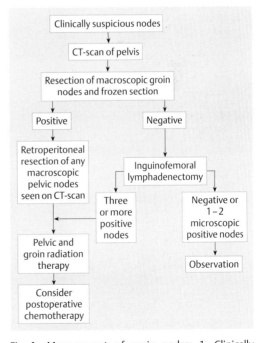

Fig. **4** Management of groin nodes: 1. Clinically suspicious nodes

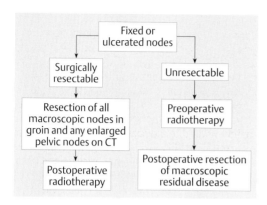

Fig. **5** Management of groin nodes: 2. Clinically obvious nodes

cured by surgery alone. An outline of our approach to the primary tumor and to the lymph nodes is summarized in Figures **3–5**. Each of these clinical situations will be considered in turn.

Management of the Locally Advanced Primary Lesion

In general, therapeutic approaches to locally advanced vulvar cancer have followed two diffe-rent pathways. The first approach has been to extend the radicality of the procedure with exenterative type surgery, and the second has been to combine radiation therapy with surgery, to allow a reduction in the radicality of the surgery. This latter option will be considered in more detail in the next section.

When the primary lesion involves the anus, vagina, or urethra, the standard radical vulvectomy cannot (by definition) encompass such extensive disease with surgical margins adequate to ensure local control: Surgical attempts to encompass such gross disease with radical vulvectomy have been associated with a high local failure rate.[62] Early local recurrences after surgical resection of T$_3$ lesions are usually due to a reluctance to resect the lesion with adequate margins by resecting a part of the distal urethra or vagina. It is quite feasible to surgically resect the distal half of the urethra or the vagina and still retain urinary continence, or vaginal function, respectively.

Cavanagh and Shepherd[14] reported the results of pelvic exenteration in combination with vulvectomy in ten patients with locally advanced vulvar cancer. They reported a 50% 5-year survival: Interestingly, all of the survivors had negative inguinal nodes, while all patients who died of the disease had positive nodes.

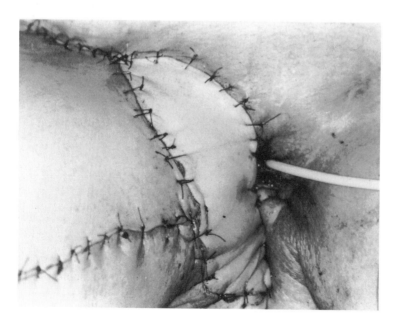

Fig. **6** Gracilis myocutaneous graft for groin defect after resection of vulvar cancer recurrent in the groin

Adding their patients to other series reported in the literature, they found a combined 5-year survival of 47% (25 of 53) for such treatment.

Various modifications of such radical surgical therapy have also been reported. Grimshaw et al.[29] used the technique of radical anoproctectomy combined with vulvectomy (with permanent sigmoid end-colostomy) in 23 patients when the tumor involved the anus or perineum. They reported a 5-year survival rate of 62.1%, and 80% of the survivors (12 of 15) had negative nodes. If the primary tumor is fixed to the pubic bone, partial resection of the pubic bone with the tumor has also been utilized: This approach may be more appropriate for recurrent disease after radiotherapy. Using this technique, King et al.[52] reported a 50% survival for six patients with primary tumors and an 83% survival in six patients with recurrent tumors.

Occasionally, the primary tumor can be resected. However, the patient is then left with a large defect, requiring plastic reconstruction of the vulva or vagina. Various types of grafts have been utilized in vulval reconstruction, including the gracilis-myocutaneous graft (Fig. **6**)[64] and grafts using other fibromuscular tissue such as tensor fascia lata, rectus abdominus, or glutaeus maximus.[53]

Management of Involved Lymph Nodes

Vulvar cancer should also be regarded as advanced if there are multiple lymph nodes involved or if this lymph node involvement is macroscopic. This represents a separate component of assessment and treatment of a patient with vulvar cancer. As suggested by the results obtained in the above reports, single modality management of involved inguinal lymph nodes is not usually curative. The surgical excision of a single microscopically involved node is usually sufficient. However, if there are multiple nodes involved, macroscopic nodal involvement, capsular penetration, or extranodal disease, surgical excision alone is not usually curative, and adjuvant postoperative radiation therapy should be considered.

A more detailed discussion of the place of radiation and positive nodes will be included in the following section on radiotherapy, but an important GOG randomized study of vulvar cancer has provided information on the role of radiation therapy in the management of patients with positive nodes.[41] In this study, patients with positive groin nodes were randomized between ipsilateral pelvic lymphadenectomy versus bilateral groin and pelvic radiation. There was a statistically significant survival advantage at 2 years for the group with positive nodes receiving radiation therapy. This advantage was mainly related to a decreased incidence of groin recurrence in this group. The groin recurrence rate in patients who did not receive radiation therapy was 23.6% (13 of 55) compared to 5.1% (3 of 59) in those who received postoperative groin irradiation. In relation to pelvic control, however, patients treated with pelvic lymphadenectomy instead of pelvic radiation therapy had a lower rate of pelvic recurrence (1.8% vs. 6.8%). However, this difference was not statistically significant. Some of the patients treated with radiation alone would have had macroscopic pelvic lymph node metastases, and radiation therapy at standard dosage is unlikely to sterilize such nodal disease. Currently, postoperative radiation to the pelvis and groin area is recommended for most patients with positive nodes after groin node dissection, and there may be a further improvement in survival if bulky pelvic lymph nodes are resected prior to radiation.

Although postoperative pelvic and groin irradiation is beneficial in terms of survival, chronic morbidity may be high because of gross leg edema. Therefore, we have recently tried to limit this morbidity by removing only grossly enlarged nodes rather than performing a complete groin node dissection, relying on radiation to sterilize any microscopic nodal metastases. Our approach to patients with clinically suspicious inguinal lymph nodes is to obtain a preoperative CT or ultrasonic scan of the pelvis to determine whether or not there are any enlarged pelvic nodes (Fig. **4**). Any palpably enlarged nodes in the groin are removed through a separate incision and are sent away for frozen section diagnosis. If the presence of metastases is confirmed, a full lymphadenectomy is not carried out, but palpably enlarged nodes are resected. If the frozen section reveals no metastatic disease in the resected nodes, a full formal inguino-femoral lymph node dissection is performed. Any enlarged pelvic nodes appearing on the CT scan are removed via an extraperitoneal approach, but in the absence of any nodes on the CT scan, a pelvic dissection is not performed.

Radiotherapy

Early reports of severe local reactions, ulceration, necrosis and fibrosis, failure to control local or groin disease, and poor survival rates after treatment of patients with vulvar cancers using radiotherapy,[6, 95, 103] have resulted in the historical view that radiotherapy has little role in the curative management of these patients. Not surprisingly, radiation therapy was previously only utilized for patients who were either medically compromised or whose tumors were significantly advanced, with little anticipation of a successful outcome. More recently, however, the usefulness of radiation therapy in improving locoregional tumor control and in decreasing the extent and morbidity of curative surgery has become increasingly appreciated.

The study of Stoeckel from 1930,[95] reporting a 5-year survival rate of 12%, has been a much quoted example of the lack of effectiveness of radiation therapy. His material was collected from 126 cases treated by radiation therapy at different institutions employing different types of equipment and techniques, usually carried out on patients regarded as unsuitable for surgery. More contemporary studies from Europe, using more modern treatment techniques, have revealed a more favorable outcome. Frischbier and colleagues[28] reported a 70% 5-year cure among 33 patients with stage I and II disease and a 33% 5-year salvage among 85 patients with stage III and IV.

From the extrapolation of data from squamous cell carcinomas in other sites of the body, particularly in head and neck cancers, considerable information is now available about dose control requirements for such cancers. A radiation dose of 4500 cGy over 5 weeks will sterilize over 90% of subclinical nodal metastases, and a total dose of 6500 cGy will sterilize tumor masses up to 3 cm in diameter.[26] All evidence would suggest that these dose-control data probably apply to epidermoid cancers regardless of the organ of origin.

Various radiation treatment techniques have been described, depending on whether the vulva, groins, pelvis, or indeed all three sites, need to be treated. One approach for treating all three sites is to treat with an anterior field that encompasses the inguinal regions, lower pelvic nodes, and vulva and a narrower posterior field that encompasses the lower pelvic nodes and vulva, but excludes the majority of the femoral heads. If the fields are evenly weighted to the midplane of the pelvis using 6 MV photons, the contribution of the anterior field to the groin nodes (at 3–5 cm depth) will generally be 60–80% of the dose to the midpelvis.[33] The difference may be made up by supplementing the dose to the groins with anterior electron fields of appropriate energy. Kalnicki et al. have described another technique, in which a partial transmission block that also reduces the dose to the femoral heads is utilized.[48] Gross disease in the groins or vulva may be boosted with en face electron fields. In some cases, interstitial implants may be used to boost the dose to the primary site.

Acute radiation reactions are brisk, and doses of 3500 to 4500 cGy routinely induce confluent moist desquamation. However, with adequate local care, this acute reaction generally heals within 3–4 weeks. Sitz baths, steroid cream, and treatment of possible superimposed candidal infection all help to minimize the discomfort. If the patient is sufficiently flexible, she may be placed in a frog-leg position[70] during treatment, allowing the skin of the inguinal crease to be spread evenly, thus allowing some skin-sparing effect and reducing the skin reaction on the medial thigh. If the vulva is to be treated with more than 4500 cGy, a break in treatment is usually required.

The use of preoperative radiation therapy has been proposed by several authors over the last two decades. Boronow reviewed the results of exenterative surgery in 1973 and suggested a therapeutic alternative; the utilization of an integrated radiosurgical treatment plan, individualized for each patient on the basis of the initial clinical extent of disease and occasionally on the patient's age and general medical condition. Subsequently, he reported an actuarial 5-year survival of 72% when using this technique for 48 cases of advanced or recurrent vulvovaginal tumors.[9] Although the published experience of preoperative radiation therapy is small, several additional investigators have reported excellent responses and high local control rates for advanced tumors after relatively modest doses of radiotherapy (Table **5**). The complete pathological response documented in many of the cases described in these reports (ranging from 36% to 100%) gives additional evidence for the radioresponsiveness of these lesions.

Table **5**   Preoperative radiotherapy in carcinoma of the vulva

Author	Year	No. of Patients	Complete Response	Ref.
Acosta	1978	14	5 (36%)	46
Jafari	1981	4	4 (100%)	49
Fairey	1985	7	?	47
Hacker	1984	8	4 (50%)	48
Boronow	1987	40	17 (42,5%)	45

In relation to the primary lesion, there are a number of theoretical advantages to using preoperative radiation therapy for patients with advanced vulvar carcinomas. These include:

1. Less radical resection of the vulva may be necessary to achieve local control after radiation therapy has sterilized peripheral microscopic disease.
2. Tumor regression during radiotherapy may permit adequate surgical margins to be obtained, without sacrificing such important structures such as the urethra, anus, and clitoris.

The results from the few series reported so far suggest that these theoretical advantages are likely to be confirmed in clinical practice, and it is currently our preference to use such a technique instead of primary exenterative surgery (Fig. **3**). Papers reporting on the use of preoperative radiation therapy reveal that the incidence of serious complications from therapy is usually quite low. Universal, moist desquamation of the vulva is present during radiation treatment, and this may necessitate cessation of therapy for 1–2 weeks. It invariably settles spontaneously when radiotherapy is discontinued. Subsequent problems with wound healing, strictures, or fistulae after surgical resection appear to be minimal.

An alternative approach to integrated therapy has been to use postoperative radiation therapy as an adjuvant treatment when surgical margins have been less than satisfactory. The incidence of recurrence after tumor resection is highest when the pathological resection margin is less than 8 mm.[37] If such a margin is not achieved surgically, either because of anatomic limitations or because of unrecognized microscopic extension, postoperative radiation therapy is likely to improve local control, although this has not been studied to date. Our preference is to operate

primarily if the disease can be removed with clear surgical margins and without need for stoma formation (Fig. **3**). We have succesfull employed postoperative radiation therapy for close surgical margins (less than 5 mm) in a limited number of patients, usually with no significant morbidity.

Radiation therapy may also play a specific role in the management of patients with fixed or ulcerating nodal disease (Fig. **5**). Single modality therapy alone, whether it be surgery or radiation, is unlikely to provide adequate control in these patients. Preoperative therapy may shrink fixed and matted nodes, facilitating subsequent surgical excision. If preoperative radiation therapy is used, resection of any residual macroscopic disease after completion of radiation therapy is recommended.

While the role of integrated or adjuvant radiation therapy for patients with multiple or macroscopically positive groin nodes seems clear, its place in the management of clinically uninvolved inguinal lymph nodes is less evident. Radiation treatment of clinically uninvolved inguinal nodes may obviate the need for radical inguinal lymph node dissection. Depending on the primary tumor characteristics, approximately 20% to 30% of patients with nonsuspicious groin nodes would be expected to have histological evidence of metastases. On the basis of theoretical dose control data, it would seem likely that standard doses of radiation (e.g.) 4500–5000 cGy) would control these subclinical metastases.[26]

Several papers from the literature provide indirect evidence that this may be so. Frankendal[27] treated 29 patients, who had clinically negative groins with radical vulvectomy, without inguinal node dissection. Twelve of these patients received elective inguinal nodal irradiation with doses varying between 3000 and 6000 cGy. None developed nodal recurrence.

Seventeen other patients received no radiation therapy and three developed inguinal failure. Daly and Million treated six patients with elective inguinal and pelvic nodal radiation therapy in doses of 4500 to 5500 cGy; none developed nodal failure.[19] In a later paper from the same institution, Henderson et al.[39] reviewed 91 patients whose cancers drained primarily to the inguinal nodes and were treated electively with radiation therapy to the inguinal nodes. This series included 13 patients with vulvar cancer. Of the 49 patients evaluable for regional failure, the authors observed only two inguinal failures after treatment with 4500–5000 cGy in 5 weeks, and both of these were outside of the treatment fields. Of note, is that one of the failures occurred in one of the 13 patients with vulvar cancer.

A significant caution, however, must be attached to this approach at present. A recent randomized study was reported by the GOG in which patients with N_0 or N_1 nodes were randomized between groin dissection and groin irradiation.[94] Patients treated with radiation received 5000 cGy at 3 cms using anterior fields. Fine-needle aspiration cytology for N_1 nodes was encouraged. The study was terminated early when patients in the radiation group developed an increased groin recurrence rate. In the groin dissection trial, there were five patients with positive nodes out of 23 (21.7%), none of whom relapsed in the groin. In the radiation trial, five of 26 (19.2%) patients developed groin recurrences and died. The precise explanation for this is not yet clear, but it possibly reflects the difficulty in clinically assessing groin node status. The authors comment that two of the groin node positive patients in the dissection group had centimeter volume disease in the resected nodes, and that the dose of radiation prescribed may have been inadequate for control. Our surgical experience has convinced us that nodes that are obviously involved at the time of dissection have sometimes not been palpable prior to opening the skin. It is possible that although the nodes were not clinically involved, they were still macroscopically involved, and thus not amenable to sterilization with the dose of radiation administered. Further information about this study is awaited (particularly an analysis of the failures) to determine whether or not there were any physical or technical problems that could have contributed to the outcome. Being the only randomized prospective study of groin irradia-tion, the GOG experience would certainly suggest that at this stage, radiation alone cannot replace groin-node dissection in patients with clinically nonsuspicious nodes.

The incidence of lower extremity edema after inguinal radiotherapy is negligible,[39, 91] but the addition of radiation therapy after full groin dissection is likely to result in a very high incidence of lymphedema. The GOG study[41] of groin and pelvic radiation therapy after inguinofemoral lymphadenectomy did not show any difference between those who did or did not receive radiation in relation to lymphedema. However, the authors point out that evaluation of lymphedema was not a major consideration in the study, and the true incidence may have been underreported. Femoral head fractures have been reported in patients treated with radiation therapy to the inguinal nodes. Therefore, techniques limiting the dose to the femoral heads should be utilized. The long-term cosmesis and function of the radiated vulva has not been studied extensively. Despite these side effects, the addition of post-operative radiation for histologically proven lymph node metastases is recommended because of the proven survival benefit.[41]

Numerous factors may add to the short and long-term morbidity of radiation treatment in patients with vulvar carcinoma. Patients with advanced vulvar carcinomas are often treated with radiation after radical surgery, which may compromise vascularity and lymphatic drainage. Large, ulcerative, cutaneous lesions frequently have superimposed infection. Patients are frequently elderly and may have complicating medical diseases, such as diabetes, heart disease, and osteoporosis. The altered lymphatic drainage may make patients unusually sensitive to cellulitic infections: One of our patients died from septicemia secondary to streptococcal cellulitis during postoperative radiation therapy to the groins.

Chemotherapy

Because vulvar cancer is traditionally treated surgically (with or without radiation therapy) and it occurs predominantly in an older population generally thought to be unsuitable for aggressive toxic chemotherapy, there is very little data in the literature on the use of primary chemotherapy for this disease. Most reports have employed chemotherapy only as salvage therapy, and the true

Table **6** Single agent cytotoxic chemotherapy in squamous carcinoma of the vulva

Drug	Dose and Schedule	No. Entered	CR	PR	Ref.
Adriamycin	45 mg/m² i. v. Q3 weeks	6	0	4	(52)
Bleomycin	15 mg i. m. twice weekly	11	2	3	(53)
Cisplatin	50 mg/m² i. v. Q3 weeks	22	0	0	(54)
Piperazinedione	9 mg/m² i. v. Q3 weeks	13	0	0	(54)
Mitoxantrone	12 mg/m² i. v. Q3 weeks	19	0	0	(55)
Etoposide	100 mg/m² i. v. days 1, 3, 5	18	0	0	(56)

activity of a particular chemotherapeutic agent may be reduced by prior radiation therapy. The use of chemotherapy in combination with radiation therapy has recently been reported more frequently.

Squamous cell carcinoma accounts for the vast majority of vulvar malignancies, and it is only in this cell type that any numerically significant series have been reported. Several drugs have undergone phase II testing, and the results of these studies are summarized in Table **6**. Only Adriamycin and bleomycin appear to have any significant activity as single agents. Cisplatin, a drug that has displayed significant activity in a range of gynecological malignancies, was shown to have very disappointing results in the GOG phase II study.[101] Of 22 evaluable patients, none demonstrated an objective response, 10 demonstrated stable disease and 12 progressed on treatment. The dose of cisplatin used in this study was only 50 mg/m², and 17 of the patients had received prior radiation therapy. Given the better responses seen in other gynecologic squamous cell cancers, a better response could have been anticipated in patients who had not been pretreated.

Several drug combinations have been tested with squamous cell carcinoma of the vulva. The EORTC used a combination of bleomycin, methotrexate, and lomustine (CCNU) for patients with locally advanced, inoperable disease, to assess response rates and operability after chemotherapy.[21] Of 28 evaluable patients, 18 (64%) showed a response, three of them being complete, and 15 partial. Response rates for primary and recurrent tumors were similar. After chemotherapy, eight patients were found to have resectable disease and seven underwent surgery. However, the level of toxicity in this regime was high. Two toxic deaths occured, including one case of fatal pulmonary fibrosis and one patient

who died as a result of complications of severe myelosuppression. Nine patients stopped treatment because of severe toxicity. The authors commented that although the patients in this study were elderly (mean age 71.9 years), they were of reasonable performance status and had no severe impairment of renal or pulmonary function: They thought that the excessive toxicity was related to the frequent low doses of methotrexate and have modified the schedule in subsequent studies.

In another case report, where a combination of bleomycin, vincristine, mitomycin C, and cisplatin was utilized, a patient with a large tumor involving the labia and vagina and extensive nodal disease was shown to have a complete clinical response after three cycles of treatment.[89] The subsequent vulvectomy specimen showed only a small focus of tumor, and the patient was alive and free of disease 20 months after completing therapy.

Impressive results and responses have recently been reported using combination therapy with retinoic acid and interferon in the treatment of squamous carcinomas of the cervix and of the skin.[59, 60] It has been suggested that these agents are important in the prevention of such cancers when intraepithelial lesions at these sites are present. To date there have been no reports of such treatment in vulvar cancer, but it is possible that the excellent responses reported in skin and cervical cancer may be replicated with such therapy. The results of phase II studies (currently underway with this relatively nontoxic therapy) are awaited.

Chemotherapy has been used more extensively in the rarer tumors that occur in the vulva. In childhood rhabdomyosarcomas, which were treated in the intergroup rhabdomyosarcoma study protocols,[36] eight of nine patients treated with various combinations of local excision, vincristine, actinomycin, and cyclophosphamide were alive and free of disease after 4 years. The last patient was alive with disease at 2.5 years. In France, four patients treated with a similar protocol, had a similarly successful outcome.[25] There do not appear to be any reports on the use of chemotherapy in adult vulvar sarcomas.

Several authors have extrapolated from the excellent results reported with chemoradiation for carcinoma of the anus the possibility to explore the use of similar treatment (with or without subsequent local excision) for locally advanced vulvar tumors.[25, 49, 57, 102] In the largest series by Thomas et al.,[102] 33 patients with advanced or recurrent tumors were treated with 5-fluorouracil (5-FU) infusion with or without mitomycin C. Of nine patients receiving chemoradiation as primary treatment, six had an initial complete response, however, three of these six subsequently relapsed in the vulva. Five of these six patients had salvage surgery performed, consisting of local excision in four, and a radical vulvectomy in one. This latter patient died of pneumonia postoperatively. Thus, seven of nine patients had their vulvar carcinoma controlled with chemoradiation alone or with the addition of local excision of residual disease. The inguinal region was included in the radiation field in seven of the ninen patients, and none of the patients developed overt nodal or distant disease.

A further report from the United Kingdom also reported the use of chemoradiation in patients with advanced vulvar cancer.[88] Of 29 patients treated with 5-FU and mitomycin C, one patient died as a result of the treatment. The stated complete pathological response to the treatment (35%) was less than that reported from a previous study using radiation alone,[30] although the latter report included only eight patients.

Because the use of radiation alone is uncommon in advanced vulvar carcinoma, it is difficult to precisely assess how much the addition of chemotherapy contributes to the outcome of patients treated with combined chemoradiation. Concurrent infusional 5-FU is theoretically attractive in this disease setting, as it may have synergistic or additive effects with the radiation. However, it appears to add morbidity to the treatment. Moist desquamative vulvitis is severe and universal, and frequently necessitates a break in treatment for 1 to 2 weeks. Despite the wide use of such a technique in anal carcinoma, the benefits of adding chemotherapy to radiation

in this disease setting have not been proven in any prospective randomized study. At this stage, we prefer to use radiation therapy alone, particularly in older patients, as we have seen impressive responses with tolerable morbidity. Given the variety of anatomical combinations available with advanced disease and the relative rarity of such a presentation, meaningful, large, comparative trials would require international collaboration.

Prognosis

Survival and cure rates for those patients with negative nodes have been excellent, ranging from approximately 70% to 90%. Treatment results of patients with involved nodes are much worse, with 5-year survivals ranging from 12% to 41% when treated with surgery alone.[16, 31] Survival for all patients in the GOG study[42] was related to the number of positive groin nodes present and to the diameter of the primary tumor. After adjusting for these major prognostic variables, other factors such as clinical stage, histological grade, depth of tumor invasion, tumor diameter, lesion location, and age of patient were analyzed and determined to have no independent effect upon survival. However, they had an independent predictive relationship to the presence of disease within the lymph nodes. Five-year survival was worse with increasing number of nodes involved. The patients with more than three positive groin nodes had a 5-year survival ranging from 36.1% to 0%, depending on the actual number of nodes involved.

▪ Vaginal Cancer

Overview and History

The vagina is formed from an inpouching of the primitive urogenital sinus, which joins with the caudal ends of the müllerian ducts. The vaginal wall consists of three histological layers; mucosa, muscularis, and adventitia. The adventitia consists of connective tissue, which is abundantly supplied with elastic fiebers and venous and lymphatic plexuses. The vagina is supported by external fibrous and muscular tissue, the central parts of which coalesce to blend with the pelvic floor musculature. The thin vaginal wall and lack of a dense fascial investitute predispose the vagina to early local spread. The close apposition of the vagina to the bladder and rectum limits treatment options and leads to a high rate of treatment-related complications in these organs. Because of these unique anatomic features, adequate surgical margins cannot usually be obtained by standard techniques without sacrificing the neighboring organs, such as the bladder or rectum.

Cancer of the vagina spreads primarily by local invasion and lymphatic permeation with embolization, as do cancers of the cervix and vulva. Although there are rich anastomotic lymphatic channels around the vagina, the basic pathways of lymphatic drainage have been defined[78]: The lymphatics of the vault drain to the lateral and posterior pelvic nodes, the central portion of the vagina to the lateral nodes, the anterior part into the paravescial lymphatics, and the posterior wall into the deep pelvic nodes. The part of the distal vagina caudal to the levator ani muscle drains into the nodes of the inguinal region. Many variations of this system have been reported, and once the established routes of drainage become obstructed with tumor, the extensive anastomotic channels allow alternative drainage to occur. This means that treatment fields for vaginal cancer must take generous account of the likely variations that may occur with individual tumors.

Staging and Diagnostic Procedures

The FIGO staging of vaginal cancer is detailed in Table 7. Perez proposed a modification of this staging; dividing Stage II into II A and II B on the basis of submucosal infiltration, and parametrial involvement, respectively.[73] This subdivision is often quoted in the literature but the clinical distinction between the two substages is poorly defined and subjective. The FIGO staging rules for vaginal cancer specifically state that there must be no involvement of either the external os of the cervix or the vulva when allocating a case as vaginal cancer. If either of these organs are involved, the case is designated as either a cervical, or a vulvar tumor, respectively. The result of this convention is that the true incidence of vaginal cancers is probably underestimated. There are inadequacies in the clinical staging of vaginal cancer, as the staging system only acknowledges palpable invasion and clinically detected metastases or neighboring organ involvement. It fails to take into account the size of

Table **7**   FIGO staging for vaginal cancer (1988)

Stage I	The carcinoma is limited to the vaginal wall
Stage II	The carcinoma has involved the subvaginal tissue but has not extended to the pelvic wall
Stage III	The carcinoma has extended to the pelvic wall
Stage IV	The carcinoma has extended beyond the true pelvis or has clinically involved the mucosa of the bladder or rectum. Bullous edema, as such, does not permit a case to be allotted to stage IV
Stage IV A	Spread of the growth to adjacent organs and/or direct extension beyond the true pelvis
Stage IV B	Spread to distant organs

the lesion, which is likely to effect prognosis. The distinction between stage I and II can be very slight, and tumors with microscopic or subclinical involvement of the bladder or rectal muscle (but not the mucosa) may be officially staged as stage II but have clinical consequences similar to those of a stage IV tumor. In treatment terms, the two most important factors are the size and site of the lesion.[44]

Pretreatment assessment of vaginal cancers should include careful examination under anesthesia to define the extent of the lesion, with cystoscopy and proctosigmoidoscopy to exclude bladder or rectal mucosal involvement. Imaging techniques, utilizing CT-scanning, ultrasound, or MRI, should be used to assess the regional lymph nodes, particularly for evidence of macroscopic pelvic or inguinal nodal metastases. Although there are no data in the literature on the place of surgical resection of enlarged lymph nodes prior to instituting radiation therapy in vaginal cancer, it seems reasonable to extrapolate dose-control data from other sites[26] and assume that such macroscopic nodal disease will not be controlled with standard single-modality therapy. We therefore recommend surgical resection of enlarged lymph nodes prior to radiation therapy.

Surgical Management

Due to the anatomic features of the vagina, surgery is the appropriate primary treatment for only a small number of vaginal cancers.

Depending on the site and stage of the lesion, a variety of surgical procedures have been utilized; usually incorporating radical hysterectomy, pelvic lymphadenectomy, and partial vaginectomy for vault or forniceal lesions, radical vulvectomy and bilateral groin dissection with partial vaginectomy for distal lesions, or exenterative type procedures for advanced central lesions, particularly if a recto- or vesicovaginal fistula is present.

Several series have reported good results from the surgical treatment of highly selected patients, particularly for those whose lesions involved the vaginal vault or fornix. In the series of Rubin et al.,[86] seven of eight patients who underwent such procedures were cured with no major complications. Many series report the occasional survivor, and this suggests that surgical therapy may be considered for the occasional and well-selected patient. The obvious problem is that with a significant resection of the vagina, the patient is usually left with a very short vagina postoperatively, unless the tumor is very high and small or a neovagina is constructed.

If a surgical approach is selected for advanced vaginal cancer, exenterative type surgery involving radical excision of the vagina in association with the bladder and/or rectum is usually re-quired. If the lower third of the vagina is involved, the procedure needs to combine exenteration with bilateral groin node dissection. Partial vulvar resection may also be needed to achieve clear margins. This approach has been used in some series for highly selected patients, but results have been relatively poor: In Rubin's series[86] there were seven patients treated by primary exenteration but only one of these survived for 5 years. This probably relates to the high incidence of nodal involvement with such advanced lesions, which makes this single modality approach of limited value.

Treatment of the primary lesion usually requires a radiotherapeutic approach as detailed below, but occasionally a combined approach is indicated. The use of combined modality therapy needs to be individuaized. The patient shown in Figure **7**, with a complete vaginal prolapse, had a stage II squamous-cell carcinoma of the vagina. After radiation therapy, she had persistent disease on biopsy of the vaginal lesion, despite ensuring that the prolapse was replaced into the pelvis and the lesion was kept within the treatment field during therapy. Subsequent post-radiation hysterectomy and vaginectomy removed the residual tumor with adequate surgical margins. Another patient with multifocal invasive, but relatively superficial adenocarcinoma

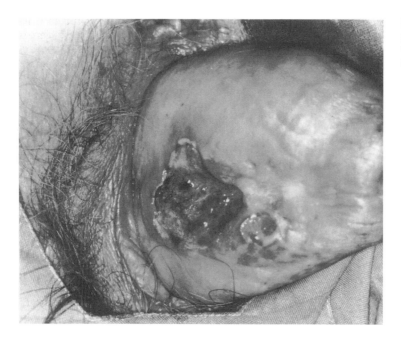

Fig. **7**   81-year-old patient presenting with stage II vaginal cancer with complete vaginal prolapse

Fig. **8** Operative specimen of radical hysterectomy and complete vaginectomy

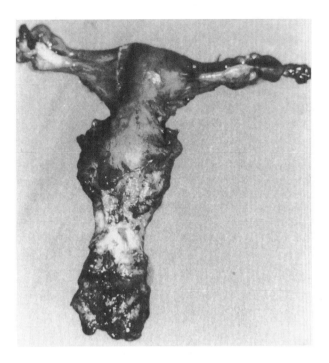

of the vagina, was initially treated with radiation therapy, but the lesions persisted after treatment. She underwent a radical hysterectomy and complete vaginectomy (Fig. **8**) with good surgical margins. Her vagina was reconstructed using split-thickness skin grafts over an omental pedicle graft to the vaginal vault.

Radiation Therapy

Radiotherapy is the most frequently used modality, and several authors have advocated that it is the treatment of choice for carcinoma of the vagina, "since it provides good tumor control and satisfactory functional results".[74] Successful treatment with radiation depends on the techniques used and the dose of radiation delivered to the tumor. The unqiue anatomy of the vagina allows high doses of radiation to be delivered directly to the tumor, thus improving local control. Reviewing their experience with 149 invasive vaginal cancers treated over 31 years at the Mallinckrodt Institute of Radiology, Perez et al.[74] concluded that tumor control in stage I disease is adequate with brachytherapy alone, and that the addition of external irradiation did not improve the probability of local tumor control or survival. In stage I disease, seven of

50 patients (14%) failed in the pelvis, three of them in combination with distant metastases.

While detailed surgicopathologic data on lymph node metastases in vaginal cancer have never been published, this incidence of pelvic failure for stage I tumors when external beam therapy is omitted suggests that the true incidence of positive nodes is roughly equivalent to that of stage I cervical cancer, that is, approximately 15%. In a more recent communication, Perez et al.[75] advise that the use of external beam irradiation in stage I disease should be reserved for more aggressive lesions that are "more invasive, infiltrating, or poorly differentiated," on the assumption that these ill-defined criteria will identify those patients most at risk for nodal metastasis.

In more advanced stage lesions, Perez et al. found improved local tumor control rates in patients receiving combined brachytherapy and external beam irradiation, compared to patients receiving either technique alone.[74] They looked at their data in relation to the likelihood of local failure and correlated this to the dose of radiation delivered. They suggested that doses in the range of 7000 to 7500 cGy to the medial parametrium or the primary tumor volume were necessary to achieve tumor control. Of the 13 patients receiving doses greater than 7500 cGy, there was only one failure in a patient with a stage IIA Tumor, who received about 8000 cGy. No failures were noted with higher doses, whereas with doses below 5000 cGy, the failure rate in various stages was in the range of 35 %.

A variety of brachytherapy techniques have been described and used in the treatment of vaginal cancers. Standard tandem and ovoid techniques may be suitable for small lesions in the vaginal fornices. However, if the lesion invades to any significant depth, delivery of an adequate dose to the tumor is impossible with standard intracavitary treatment alone.

Puthawala et al. reported 23 patients treated with a combination of external beam therapy and interstitial iridium-192, applied using Syed-Neblett template, and four other patients who received interstitial therapy alone.[81] They were able to deliver a total minimum tumor dose of 8000 cGy to patients with stage I and IIA disease and 10000 cGy to patients with more advanced disease. The implants were individualized (as to number and depth of insertion of guide needles) depending upon the site and extent of disease, as well as upon the presence or absence of the uterus. If the uterus was present, the Fletcher-Suit uterine tandem was also used in conjunction with the template. Eighty-five percent of the patients (23 of 27) experienced local tumor control. Fifteen patients (56%) remained alive for a minimum period of 40 months after treatment, ten (37%) died of distant metastases and two died of intercurrent disease with no evidence of local or distal disease. These results appear to be, both in terms of local control and survival better than in series in which the brachytherapy used was intracavitary rather than interstitial.

Surgery can also be usefully integrated into the accurate placement of interstitial radiation. We have successfully treated a patient with a bulky stage III vaginal cancer by implanting iridium needles as an open procedure after a course of external beam therapy: A laparotomy was performed at the completion of the external beam therapy, and the iridium needles were placed directly into the tumor under visual guidance, allowing excellent distribution across an anatomically irregular lesion. As an additional advantage, the small bowel was able to be suspended above the pelvis using a polyglycolic acid-absorbable mesh sling,[51] giving the small bowel additional protection from radiation injury.

Complications related to radiotherapy relate to both the stage of the disease and the dose of radiation received. Patients at highest risk for complications include those who have had a previous hysterectomy and those who have a history of pelvic inflammatory disease or endometriosis. Following radiotherapy for small lesions, the complications usually consist of scarring and shortening of the vagina. When larger lesions are treated by radiotherapy, a moderate degree of vaginal dryness, stenosis, and scarring is inevitable, as are proctitis and cystitis. Major complications such as necrosis of the rectum, bladder, or urethra with fistula formation are reported in 7% to 13% of cases.[56, 86, 74,]

Radiation therapy must also encompass the area of nodal drainage. For cancers of the middle and upper vagina, the pelvic lymph nodes must be included in the treatment field, whereas for tumors involving the lower vagina, the inguinal nodes must also be included. In the series of Perez et al.,[74] seven patients received irradiation to clinically negative inguinal lymph nodes: Only one of these patients, who had a large lesion involving the whole vagina, developed an inguinal lymph node recurrence after 5000 cGy to the groin. There were no groin recurrences in the 100 patients with primary tumors in the upper and middle third of the vagina who did not receive elective inguinal irradiation. In contrast, three of 29 patients with lower third primaries, and one of 20 patients with tumors involving the entire length of the vagina, developed groin nodal metastases. The authors concluded that elective irradiation of the inguinal lymph nodes should be carried out in patients with primary tumors of the lower third of the vagina or if the lesion involves the entire organ. Our policy, if radiation is to be the primary treatment, is to perform a pretreatment CT-scan of the pelvis and remove any detectable macroscopic lymph nodes by retroperitoneal resection prior to radiation.

Chemotherapy

With tumors that are so uncommon as those found in vaginal cancer, there is nothing more than anecdotal experience in the literature of the use of chemotherapy. Out of 16 patients treated with a wide variety of chemotherapeutic and hormonal therapies at the University of Michigan, three complete responses were seen in four patients treated with combination cisplatinum and dichloromethotrexate.[76] Another patient, treated by Katib et al., had a complete response when treated with a combination of bleomycin, methotrexate, and cisplatinum.[50] The GOG experience with the use of platinum for advanced or recurrent vaginal cancer revealed one complete response among 16 patients, and the duration of response was 3 months.[100] As with vulvar vancer, several recent studies of the use of combined chemoradiation, particularly with 5-fluorouracil, have suggested that complete responses using this combined therapy are achievable;[22] obviously, there are no randomized studies available to compare this approach with standard therapy. The established success of this treatment with anal cancers probably justifies its use in advanced vaginal cancers, but vigilance should be maintained for any apparent increase in morbidity with this approach.

Melanomas of the Vulva and the Vagina

Vaginal melanoma is extremely rare, with approximately 140 cases reported in the literature. Vulvar melanoma is more frequent and is the second most common vulvar cancer. The 5-year survival for vaginal melanoma is only 7%, with 12 reported cases alive at 5 years.[10] The 5-year survival reported for vulvar melanomas ranges from 36% to 54%.[4, 66, 79] Often, these melanomas arise at the vulvovaginal junction, and it is often difficult to determine the precise organ of origin.

Staging and Diagnostic Procedures

The FIGO Staging system used for staging squamous cell carcinomas is not applicable for melanomas because these lesions are usually much smaller, and prognosis is related to the depth of penetration of the tumor. The leveling system proposed by Clark and co-workers[15] for cutaneous melanomas is less applicable for vulvovaginal melanomas, as the papillary dermis is not well defined in vulvar skin. Chung and colleagues proposed a modification of Clark's system, which retained levels I and V but arbitrarily defined levels II, III and IV using measurements in millimeters.[18] Breslow measured the thickest portion of the melanoma from the surface of the intact epithelium to the deepest point of invasion.[11] These systems are compared in Table **8**. In 48 patients treated at the Mayo Clinic and reported by Podratz et al.,[79] the 10-year surival rates were 100, 83, 65, and 23 percent for Clark's levels II, III, IV, and V. These authors concluded that overall survival rates, treatment failures, regional extension, and patterns of recurrence demonstrated the applicability of the microstaging system as a prognostic index for vulvar melanoma in a manner similar to the established role of this method for melanomas at other, nongenital, sites.

Surgical Management

The ideal surgical management of melanomas of the vulva or vagina, without clinical evidence of regional or distant metastasis, remains controversial. A similar controversy exists in the management of cutaneous melanomas, namely the extent of excisional surgery required and the value of prophylactic excision of the regional lymph nodes. The high rate of recurrence and the propensity for these lesions to widely metastasize make data interpretation on these questions difficult. As most patients who die from this disease will do so with at least a

Table **8**   Microstaging of vulvar melanomas

	Clark's levels (1989)	Chung (1990)	Breslow (1991)
I	Intraepithelial	Intraepethelial	<0.76 mm
II	Into papillary dermis	<1 mm from granular layer	0.76–1.50 mm
III	Filling dermal papillae	>1–2 mm from granular layer	1.51–2.25 mm
IV	Into reticular dermis	>2 mm from granular layer	2.26–3.0 mm
V	Into subcutaneous fat	Into subcutaneous fat	>3 mm

significant component of distant metastases, the degree of radicality of the primary surgery is clearly only one component of the question. Improved understanding of the microstaging system and stratification of the risk of metastasis has allowed some individualization of surgical management.

The recent trend towards more conservative surgery for vulvar melanomas is congruent that of other cutaneous melanomas, where recent cooperative studies have demonstrated that less radical local resection is equally as effective as traditional radical approaches.[2, 107] In a large multicenter study of cutaneous melanomas (no thicker than 2 mm) by the World Health Organization Melanoma Group, Veronesi et al.[107] reported no difference in disease-free survival or overall survival rates between the group of 305 patients treated with narrow excision margins (at least 1 cm margin), compared to 307 patients treated with wide excision margins (greater than 3 cm). Although the numbers of vulvar melanomas reported are much smaller, there is some evidence that this information can be safely extrapolated to vulvar lesions. Rose and colleagues[83] described eight patients with vulvar melanoma with less than 2 mm of invasion. Radical local excision with 2 cm margins, rather than radical vulvectomy, produced a disease-free survival rate of 75%. Lesions with less than 1 mm of invasion may be treated with wide local excision of the primary lesion,[18, 77] as nodal metastases in these patients are rare.

For more deeply invasive lesions on the vulva, en bloc resection of the primary lesion and regional nodes is indicated. This approach should remove embolized melanoma cells and eliminate bridge recurrences. The effectiveness of this approach was demonstrated in the Mayo Clinic experience,[79] where subsequent recurrent groin disease developed in only 1 of 44 patients treated with en bloc dissection of the inguinal lymphatics at the time of vulvar resection. Although radical vulvectomy has been widely advocated for vulvar melanomas, this procedure usually results in inadequate vaginal margins, as most of the lesions occur either at the clitoris, the labia minora, or close to the urethra. To overcome this problem, exenterative surgery has been advocated for lesions involving the vaginal or urethral mucosa,[67] but the poor survival of patients with such lesions (due to their distant metastases) makes it difficult to support these recommendations.

The value of elective regional lymphadenectomy for cutaneous melanomas remains uncertain, despite the results of large cooperative studies. The large WHO collaborative study[106] showed that immediate or elective node dissection in stage I melanomas of the distal two-thirds of the extremities did not improve the prognosis over dissection at the time of disease appearing in the nodes. This is in contrast to other studies that have shown a significantly higher surival rate after immediate nodal dissection.[90, 3] It is probable that any benefit from this dissection is outweighted by the high incidence of distant metastases with more deeply invasive lesions and the fact that the node dissection for these lesions is not performed as an en bloc dissection. Unlike tumors of the lower extremities, the location of vulvar melanomas makes en bloc dissection of the primary tumor and the regional nodes more feasible, and because of the theoretical advantage of removing "in transit" tumor cells, it is best performed for these lesions.

Radiation Therapy

Traditionally, melanomas have been regarded as radioresistant tumors. Thus, experience with primary treatment of these lesions using radiation has been limited. However, the widely reported poor results after radical surgery have recently created an increased interest in the use of radiation therapy for these lesions. Higher rates of partial and complete regressions of cutaneous lesions have been seen with the use of high-dose individual treatments (greater than or equal to 400 cGy per fraction) compared to conventional dose treatments (180 cGy per fraction.[38, 69] There are several anecdotal reports in the literature of complete responses of vaginal melanomas to radiation treatment, usually given as palliative treatment.[8, 58, 82] We have treated three patients with vaginal melanomas with a combination of wide local excision and radiation therapy. All three achieved local control: two patients died of systemic disease at 11 and 16 months, and the third patient is disease free at 29 months. The preservation of major viscera and the minimal morbidity of this approach have encouraged us to continue this approach rather than apply ultraradical surgery.

Chemotherapy and Immunotherapy

Chemotherapy and immunotherapy have been disappointing with melanomas, despite extensive clinical trials. Many responses to therapy are partial, and duration is frequently limited to weeks. Estrogen receptors have been reported in human melanomas, and responses to tamoxifen have been reported.[58]

Recurrent Disease

▦ Vulvar Cancer

The problem of recurrent vulvar cancer should be considered separately for each of the possible anatomic sites of recurrence, namely vulva, groin, or distant, as each represents a different therapeutic problem and challenge. Treatment of recurrent vulvar cancer obviously depends on the previous treatment modalities already applied and the condition of the patient.

Local Recurrence

Most local recurrences can be successfully treated with further wide surgical excision, which may require a myocutaneous graft to cover the resultant defect. In the GOG series of early stage I vulvar cancers with negative groin lymph nodes,[93] eight of ten patients with vulvar recurrence alone were salvaged by further surgical resection. Hopkins et al.[43] reported on the surgical management of 34 patients with recurrent vulvar cancer. All patients underwent surgical excision, with the type of surgery tailored to location and extent of recurrence. Surgery included wide radical excision in 25, with 14 (56%) patients remaining free of disease; radical vulvectomy in five, with four (80%) remaining free of disease; and exenteration in four with one (25%) remaining free of disease. Provided there is no nodal involvement, either initially or at the time of recurrence, locally recurrent vulvar cancer can usually be successfully treated. Alternatively, radiotherapy alone or in combination with surgery, may be successful, and several complete responses in this situation have been documented.[9, 23, 80]

Groin Recurrence

Groin recurrence of vulvar cancer is much more difficult to treat, as most of these patients develop distant disease or disseminated skin metastases. If the patient recurs in the groin, she is unlikely to be salvaged by any combination of therapy and usually dies from systemic disease. In the series of the University of Michigan,[43] of 34 patients with recurrent vulvar cancer, ten had metastatic disease of the groin lymph nodes at the time of recurrence: All of these patients died of their disease. In Boronow's series, two patients with groin recurrence were treated.[9] The first patient who had N_2 nodes, was treated with preoperative radiation but relapsed in the groin with associated disseminated disease. A second patient, also with N_2 nodes in the groin, was treated with radiation after surgical resection, but subsequently recurrend again in the groin with associated systemic disease. In Prempree's series,[80] three patients with recurrences in the groin were treated with radiation but only one showed a short period of local control. The use of chemoradiation in this context was reported by Thomas, who described its use in three patients with inguinal recurrence: None had a complete response and all died from the disease, two having developed lung metastases.[107] These poor results all emphasize the importance of appropriate management of the groins at the initial presentation, including the use of adjuvant therapy, as outlined above.

Distant Metastases

Salvage of patients with metastatic disease seems unlikely on the basis of the currently available data on chemotherapy for vulvar cancers (see above discussion for primary disease). Despite the paucity of data, our approach to a patient with metastatic disease is to offer a therapeutic trial of single-agent cisplatinum, as occasional responses have been observed. The patient with a response is also likely to gain some benefit in terms of survival duration and symptom control.

▦ Vaginal Cancer

Recurrence of vaginal cancer carries a grave prognosis. Of the 33 patients that recurred in the series of Rubin et al.,[86] 30 died of their disease. Average survival from recurrence was 8 months.

Eighteen patients recurred with pelvic disease and 15 with extrapelvic disease. The average time to pelvic recurrence was 12 months, with a range of 2 to 40 months. The average time to extra-pelvic recurrence was 14.6 months, with a range of 3 to 37 months. In stage I disease, three out of three recurrences were local. In contrast, in stages II, III, and IV, recurrences were distant in 9 of 13, 3 of 6, and 4 of 11 cases, respectively.

As with the treatment of primary disease, the therapeutic approach to recurrent disease clearly must be individualized. If surgery has not been utilized, and if the patient is medically fit, exen-terative surgery may be appropriate for central (vaginal) recurrence. Even if surgery is not curative in intent, many patients obtain a pal-liative benefit from a surgical maneuver to divert or symptomatically treat fistulae, whether they be from the bladder or the rectum.

Ongoing Research

The major mortality in vulvar cancer is in relation to positive nodes. The indications and the need for adequate primary management of the regional lymph nodes are well established. Improvement in the survival of patients with involved nodes is the area most likely to improve overall survival. Macroscopic lymph nodes ap-parently cannot be treated adequately with single modality therapy. Also awaited, is con-firmation that pretreatment resection of macro-scopic nodes in association with postoperative radiation therapy will improve survival. Circum-stantial evidence from the GOG study of pelvic radiation for positive inguinal nodes, and pre-liminary data from our own institution[35] suggest that this is so.

Systemic disease with vulvar cancer is usual-ly consequent to involved lymph nodes. The absence of active chemotherapeutic agents for this disease limits the treatment of advanced disease. While agents such as cisplatin have not been shown to be useful in the treatment of advanced or recurrent disease, there appears to be some anecdotal evidence of their usefulness in other adjuvant settings. The use of radiosensiti-zers (such as 5-FU in association with radiation therapy) has become widespread, but the bene-fits when compared to radiotherapy alone have not been proven. It is still unclear whether they add to response or survival, or merely to

morbidity when used in conjunction with other modalities. The small number of patients eligible for such studies makes meaningful results almost impossible to achieve.

The identification of patients at high risk of local recurrence after surgical resection has been accurately defined in relation to the surgical margins obtained.[37] Further evaluation is needed to determine whether this risk can be further reduced with the addition of postoperative radiation therapy. The morbidity associated with such additional treatment also needs further investigation.

In relation to vaginal cancer, the relative infrequency of such lesions is likely to impede meaningful research. Surgicopathologic data are unlikely to be obtained in a disease so rarely treated with surgery. Clinical parameters must be relied upon to identify high-risk patients who may benefit from multimodality therapy. Ex-perience with multimodality therapy in other disease sites is likely to be extrapolated and incorporated into the routine management of patients with vaginal lesions. The future direction of research into this site of disease is likely to reflect other research directions, in-cluding the improvement of brachytherapy techniques, the integration of surgical pro-cedures, the resection of macroscopic lymph nodes prior to radiotherapy, and the search for more effective chemotherapeutic agents.

Further information regarding the tumor biology of vulvar neoplasms may provide in-formation regarding specific risks of nodal metastases of recurrence. Preliminary reports have suggested two different types of vulvar intraepithelial lesions on the basis of clinical, pathologic, and viral profiles.[71] Verification of the clinical significance of this information is awaited. Another report, suggesting that smoking is a major risk factor for the development of vulvar cancer,[12] suggests that the emergence of such risk factors may clarify the etiology of this disease.

Follow-Up

Patients who have completed treatment for vul-var cancer should remain under medical supervi-sion, as they remain at risk for the development of local recurrence, regardless of the nature of the primary treatment. As already detailed, such local recurrences are frequently well treated.

Recurrence in either the groin or in distant sites is less amenable to treatment, and aggressive attempts to document asymptomatic recurrences in these sites are less justifiable. Patients with vulvar cancers are at a significantly increased risk for contracting other lower genital tract malignancies, in particular cervical malignancies.[12] Therefore, cervical cancer screening with Pap smears and colposcopy is indicated. Due to the high incidence of smoking in this population and because of the association between smoking, other malignancies, and several other medical conditions, the patient should be encouraged to stop smoking.

References

1. Acosta AA, Given FT, Frazier AB, Cordoba RB, Luminari A. Preoperative radiation therapy in the management of squamous cell carcinoma of the vulva: Preliminary report. Am J Obstet Gynecol. 1978; 132:198–206.
2. Aitken DR, Clausen K, Klein JP et al. The extent of primary melanoma excision—A re-evaluation—How wide is wide? Ann Surg. 1983; 198:634–41.
3. Balch CM. The role of elective lymph node dissection in melanomy: Rationale, results and controversis. J Clin Oncol. 1988; 6:163.
4. Beller U, Demopoulos RI and Beckman EM. Vulvovaginal melanoma. A clinicopathologic study. J Reprod Med. 1986; 31:315–9.
5. Berman ML, Soper JT, Creasman WT, Olt GT, DiSaia PJ. Conservative surgical management of superficially invasive stage I vulvar carcinoma. Gynecol Oncol. 1989; 35:352–357.
6. Bervon E. The treatment of cancer of the vulva. Brit J Radio. 1949; 22:498.
7. Boice CR, Seraj IM, Thrasher T, King A. Microinvasive squamous carcinoma of the vulva: Present status and reassessment. Gynecol Oncol. 1984; 18:71–76.
8. Bonner JA, Perez-Tamayo C, Reid GC, Roberts JA, Morley GW. The management of vaginal melanoma. Cancer. 1988; 62:2066–2072.
9. Boronow RC, Hickman BT, Reagan MT, Smith A, Steadham RE. Combined therapy as an alternative to exenteration for locally advanced vulvovaginal cancer: II Results, complications, and dosimetric and surgical considerations. Am J Clin Oncol. 1987; 10:171–181.
10. Brand E, Fu YS, Lagasse LD, Berek JS. Vulvovaginal melanoma: Report of seven cases and literature review. Gynecol Oncol. 1984; 33:54–60.
11. Breslow A. Thickness, cross-sectional area and depth of invasion in the prognosis of cutaneous melanoma. Ann Surg. 1979; 172:902.
12. Brinton LA, Nasca PC, Mallin K, Baptiste MS, Wilbanks GD, Richart RM. Case control study of cancer of the vulva. Am J Obstet Gynecol. 1990; 15:859.
13. Buscema J, Stern JL, Woodruff JD. Early invasive carcinoma of the vulva. Am J Obstet Gynecol. 1981; 140:563–569.
14. Cavanagh D, Shepherd JH. The place of pelvic exenteration in the primary management of advanced carcinoma of the vulva. Gynecol Oncol. 1982; 13:318–322.
15. Clark WH, From L, Fernadino EA, Mihm MC. The histogenesis and biologic behaviour of primary human malignant melanoms of the skin. Cancer Res. 1969; 29:705.
16. Collins CG, Lee FYL, Lopez JJ. Invasive carcinoma of the vulva with lymph node metastases. Am J Obstet Gynecol. 1971; 109:446.
17. Chu J, Tamini HK, Figge DC. Stage I vulvar cancer: Criteria for microinvasion. Am J Obstet Gynecol. 1982; 59:716–719.
18. Chung AF, Woodruff JW, Lewis JL. Malignant melanoma of the vulva: A report of 44 cases. Obstet Gynecol. 1975; 45:638–46.
19. Daly JW, Million RR. Radical culvectomy combined with elective node irradiation for Tx N0 squamous carcinoma of the vulva. Cancer. 1974; 34:161–165.
20. Deppe G, Bruckner HW, Cohen CJ. Adriamycin treatment of advanced vulvar carcinoma. Obstet Gynecol (Supplement). 1977; 10:13.
21. Durrant KR, Mangioni C, Lacave AJ, George M, van der Burg MEL, Guthrie D, Rotmenz N, Dalesio O, Vermorken JB. Belomycin, methotrexate and CCNU in advanced inoperable squamous cell carcinoma of the vulva: a phase II study of the EORTC Gynaecological Cancer Cooperative Group (GCCG). Gynceol Oncol. 1990; 37:359–362.
22. Evans LS, Kersh CR, Constable WC, Taylor PT. Concomitant 5-fluorouracil, mitomycin-C and radiotherapy for advanced gynecologic malignancies. Int J Radiation Oncol Biol Phys. 1988; 15:901–906.
23. Fairey RN, MacKay PA, Benedet JL, Boyes DA, Turko M. Radiation treatment of carcinoma of the vulva, 1950–1980. Am J Obstet Gynecol. 1985; 151:591–7.
24. FIGO stages—1988 revision [Announcements]. Gynecol Oncol. 1989; 35:125–7.
25. Flamant F, Gerbaulet A, Nihoul-Fekete, Valteau-Couanet D, Chasagne D, Lemerle J. Long-term sequelae of conservative treatment by surgery, brachytherapy and chemotherapy for vulval and vaginal rhabdomyosarcoma in children. J Clin Oncol. 1980; 8:1847–1853.
26. Fletcher GH. Textbook of radiology. 3rd Ed. Philadelphia: Lea and Harbinger; 1988.
27. Frankendal B, Larrson LG, Westling P. Carcinoma of the vulva. Acta Radiol. 1973; 12:165–174.
28. Frischbier HJ, Thomsen K. Treatment of cancer of the vulva with high energy electrons. Am J Obstet Gynecol. 1971; 111:431–435.
29. Grimshaw RN, Ghazal Aswad S, Monaghan JM. The role of anovulvectomy in locally advanced carcinoma of the vulva. Int J Gynecol Cancer. 1991; 1:15–18.

30. Hacker NF, Berek JS, Juillard GJF, Lagasse LD. Preoperative radiation therapy for locally advanced vulvar cancer. Cancer. 1984; 54:2056–2061.

31. Hacker NF, Berek JS, Lagasse LD, Leuchter RS, Moore JG. Management of regional lymph nodes and their prognostic influence in vulvar cancer. Obstet Gynecol. 1983; 61:408–412.

32. Hacker NF, Berek JS, Lagasse LD, Nieberg RK, Leuchter RS. Individualization of treatment of stage I squamous cell vulvar carcinoma. Obstet Gynecol. 1984; 63:155–162.

33. Hacker NF, Eifel P, McGuire W, Wilkinson EJ. Vulva. In: Hoskins WJ, Perez CA and Young RC, eds. Principles and Practice of Gynecologic Oncology. Philadelphia: JB Lippincott; 1992.

34. Hacker NF, Van der Velden J. Conservative surgery for early vulvar cancer. Cancer. 1993; 71:1673–1677.

35. Hacker NF, Wain GV, Nicklin J. Resection of Bulky Positive Lymph Nodes in Cervical Cancer (abstract). Int J Gyn Cancer. 1993; 3 (Supp. 1), 2.

36. Hays DM, Shimada H, Raney RB, Tefft M, Newton W, Crist WM, Lawrence W, Ragab A, Beltangady M, Maurer HM. Clinical staging and treatment results in rhabdomyosarcoma of the female genital tract among children and adolescents. Cancer. 1988; 61:1893–1903.

37. Heaps JM, Fu YS, Montz FJ, Hacker NF, Berek JS. Surgical-pathologic variables predictive of local recurrence in squamous cell carcinoma of the vulva. Gynegol Oncol. 1990; 38:309–314.

38. Hebermalz HJ, Fischer JJ. Radiation therapy for malignant melanoma. Cancer. 1976; 38:2258–2262.

39. Henderson RH, Parsons JT, Morgan L, Million RR. Elective ilioinguinal lymph node irradiation. Int J Radiation Oncol Biol Phys. 1984; 10:811–819.

40. Hoffman JS, Kumar NB, Morley GW. Microinvasive squamous carcinoma of the vulva: Search for a definition. Obstet Gynecol. 1983; 61:615–618.

41. Homesley HD, Bundy BN, Sedlis A, Adcock L. Radiation therapy versus pelvic node resection for carcinoma of the vulva with positive groin nodes. Obstet Gynceol. 1986; 68:733–740.

42. Homesley HD, Bundy BN, Sedlis A, Yordan E, Berek JS, Jahshan A, Mortel R. Assessment of current International Federation of Gynecology and Obstetrics staging of vulvar carcinoma relative to prognostic factors for survival (A Gynecologic Oncology Group Study). Am J Obstet Gynecol. 1994; 164:997–1004.

43. Hopkins MP, Reid GC, Morley GW. The surgical management of recurrent squamous cell carcinoma of the vulva. Obstet Gynecol. 1990; 75:1001–1005.

44. Houghton CRS, Iversen T. Squamous cell carcinoma of the vagina: a clinical study of the location of the tumour. Gynecol Oncol. 1982; 13:365–372.

45. Iversen T. The value of groin palpation in epidermoid carcinoma of the vulva. Gynecol Oncol. 1981; 12:291–295.

46. Iversen T, Aas M. Lymph drainage from the vulva. Gynecol Oncol. 1983; 16:179–189.

47. Jafari K, Magalotti M. Radiation therapy in carcinoma of the vulva. Cancer. 1981; 47:686–691.

48. Kalnicki S, Zide A, Maleki N, De Wyngaert JK, Lipstein R, Dalton JF, Bloomer WD. Transmission block to simplify combined pelvic and inguinal radiation therapy. Radiology. 1987; 164:578.

49. Kalra JK, Grossman AM, Krumholz BA, Chen S, Tinker MA, Flores GT, Molho L, Cortes EP. Preoperative chemoradiotherapy for carcinoma of the vulva. Gynecol Oncol. 1981; 12:256–260.

50. Katib S, Kuten A, Steiner M, Yudelev M, Robinson E. The effectiveness of multidrug treatment of bleomycin, methotrexate and cisplatinum in advanced vaginal carcinoma. Gynecol Oncol. 1985; 21:101–102.

51. Kavanah MT, Feldman MI, Deveraux DF, Kondi ES. New surgical approach to minimize radiation associated small bowel injury in patients with pelvic malignancies requiring surgery and high-dose irradiation. Cancer. 1985; 56:1300–1304.

52. King LA, Downey GO, Savage JE, Twiggs LB, Oakley GJ, Prem KA. Resection ofthe pubic bone as an adjunct to the management of primary, recurrent or metastatic pelvic malignancies. Obstet Gynecol. 1989; 73:1022–1026.

53. Knapstein PG, Friedberg V, Sevin BU. Reconstructive surgery in gynecology. Stuttgart: Georg Thieme Verlag; 1990.

54. Kneale B, Elliot P, Fortune D. Microinvasive carcinoma of the vulva. Proceedings of the International Society for the Study of Vulvar Disease, 6th World Congress, Cambridge, England; 1981.

55. Kneale BL. Microinvasive carcinoma of the vulva: Report of the International Society for the Study of Vulvar Disease Task Force, VIIth Congress. J Reprod Med. 1984; 29:454.

56. Kucera H, Weghaupt K. The electrosurgical operation of vulvar carcinoma with postoperative irradiation of inguinal lymph nodes. Gynecol Oncol. 1988; 29:158–167.

57. Levin W, Rad FF, Goldberg G, Altaras M, Bloch B, Shelton MG. The use of concomitant chemotherapy and radiotherapy prior to surgery in advanced stage carcinoma of the vulva. Gynecol Oncol. 1986; 25:20–25.

58. Levitan Z, Gordon AN, Kaplan AL, Kaufman RH. Primary malignant melanoma of the vagina: Report of four cases and review of the literature. Gynecol Oncol. 1989; 33:85–90.

59. Lippman SM, Kavanagh JJ, Paredes-Espinoza M, Delgadillo-Madrueno F, Paredes-Casillas P, Hong WK, Holdener E, Krakoff IH. "13-cis-Retinoic Acid plus interferon alpha-2a: Highly active Systemic Therapy for Squamous Cell Carcinoma of the Cervix". J Natl Cancer Inst. 1992; 84:241–245.

60. Lippman SM, Parkinson DR, Itri LM, Weber RS, Schantz SP, Ota DM, Schusterman MA, Krakoff IH, Gutterman JU, Hong WK. "13-cis-Retinoic Acid plus Interferon alpha-2a: Effective Combination

Therapy for Advanced Squamous Cell Carcinoma of the Skin". J Natl Cancer Inst. 1992; 84:235–241.

61. Magrina JF, Webb MJ, Gaffey TA, Symmonds RE. Stage I squamous cell cancer of the vulva. Gynecol Oncol. 1979; 134:453–459.

62. Malfetano J, Piver MS, Tsukada Y. Stage III and IV Squamous cell carcinoma of the vulva. Gynecol Oncol. 1986; 23:192–198.

63. Masiel A, Buttrick P, Bitran J. Tamoxifen in the treatment of malignant melanoma. Cancer Treat Rep. 1981; 65:531.

64. Massey F. Vulvovaginal reconstruction following radical resections. Clin Obstet Gyn. 1986; 29:617–627.

65. Montana GS, Moore D, Thomas GM, Stehman FB, Lewandowski G, Bundy B. Preliminary report of concurrent chemoradiation followed by surgery for advanced vulvar carcinoma: A Gynecologic Oncology Group study. Proceedings of the International Gynecologic Cancer Society, Third Biennial Meeting, Cairns; 1991.

66. Morrow CP, DiSaia PJ. Malignant melanoma of the female genitalia: A clinical analysis. Obstet Gynecol Surv. 1976; 31:233–271.

67. Morrow CP, Rutledge FN. Melanoma of the vulva. Obstet Gynecol. 1972; 39:745–52.

68. Muss HB, Bundy BN, Christopherson WA. Mitoxantrone in the treatment of advanced vulvar and vaginal carcinoma. Am J Clin Oncol. 1989; 12:142–144.

69. Overgaard J. Radiation treatment of malignant melanoma. Int J Radiation Oncol Biol Phys. 1979; 6:41–44.

70. Pao WM, Perez CA, Kuske RR, Sommers GM, Camel HM, Galakatos AE. Radiation therapy and conservation surgery for primary and recurrent carcinoma of the vulva: Report of 40 patients and a review of the literature. Int J Radiation Oncol Biol Phys. 1988; 14:1123–1132.

71. Park JS, Jones RW, McLean MR, Currie JL, Woodruff JD, Shah KV, Kurman RJ. Possible etiologic heterogeneity of vulvar intraepithelial neoplasia. Cancer. 1991; 67:1599–1607.

72. Parker RT, Duncan I, Rampone J. Operative management of early invasive epidermoid carcinoma of the vulva. Am J Obstet Gynecol. 1975; 123:349.

73. Perez CA, Arneson AN, Galakatos A, Samanth HK. Malignant tumours of the vagina. Cancer. 1973; 31:36–44.

74. Perez CA, Camel HM, Galakatos AE, Grigsby PW, Kuske RR, Buchsbaum G, Hederman MA. Definitive irradiation in carcinoma of the vagina: Long-term evaluation of results. Int J Radiation Oncol Biol Phys. 1988; 15:1283–1290.

75. Perez CA, Gersell DJ, Hoskins WJ, McGuire WP. Vagina. In: Hoskins WJ, Perez CA, Young RC, eds. Principles and Practice of Gynecologic Oncology. Philadelphia: JB Lippincott; 1992.

76. Peters WA, Kumar NB, Morley GW, Carcinoma of the vagina: Factors influencing treatment outcome. Cancer. 1985; 55:892–897.

77. Phillips GL, Twiggs, LB, Okagaki T. Vulvar melanoma: A microstaging study. Gynecol Oncol. 1982; 14:80–8.

78. Plentl AA, Friedman EA. Lymphatic System of the Female Genitalia. Philadelphia: WB Saunders; 1971.

79. Podratz KC, Gaffey TA, Symmonds RE, Johansen KL, O'Brien PC. Melanoma of the vulva: An update. Gynecol Oncol. 1983; 16:153–168.

80. Prempree T, Amornmarn R. Radiation treatment of recurrent carcinoma of the vulva. Cancer. 1984; 54:1943–1949.

81. Puthawala A, Nisar Syed AM, Nalickk R, McNamara C, DiSaia PJ. Integrated external and interstitial radiation therapy for primary carcinoma of the vagina. Obstet Gynecol. 1983; 62:367–372.

82. Reid GC, Schmidt RW, Roberts JA, Hopkins MP, Barrett RJ, Morley GW. Primary melanoma of the vagina. Obstet Gynecol. 1989; 74:190–199.

83. Rose PG, Piver MS, Tsukada Y, Lau T. Conservative therapy for melanoma of the vulva. Am J Obstet Gynecol. 1988; 159:52–55.

84. Ross MJ, Ehrmann RL. Histologic prognosticators in Stage I squamous cell carcinoma of the vulva. Obstet Gynecol. 1987; 70:774–784.

85. Rowley KC, Gallion HH, Donaldson ES, Van Nagell JR, Higgins RV, Powell DE, Kryscio RJ, Pavlik EJ. Prognostic factors in early vulvar cancer. Gynecol Oncol. 1988; 31:43–49.

86. Rubin SC, Young J, Mikuta JJ. Squamous carcinoma of the vagina: Treatment, complications and long-term follow-up. Gynecol Oncol. 1985; 20:346–353.

87. Sedlis A, Homesley H, Bundy BN, Marshall R, Yordan E, Hacker NF, Lee JH, Whitney C. Positive groin lymph nodes in superficial squamous cell vulvar cancer—A Gynecologic Oncology Group study. Am J Obstet Gynecol. 1987; 156:1159–64.

88. Shepherd JH, McLean C, van Dam PA, Whitaker SJ, Hudson CN, Blake P, Arnott SJ. Combined chemoradiotherapy in advanced carcinoma of the vulva: Alternative to exenterative surgery. Proceedings of the International Gynecologic Cancer Society, Third Biennial Meeting, Cairns; 1991.

89. Shimuzu Y, Hasumi K, Masubuchi K. Effective chemotherapy consisting of bleomycin, vincristine, mitomycin C and cisplatin (BOMP) for a patient with inoperable vulvar cancer. Gynecol Oncol. 1990; 36:423–427.

90. Sim FH, Taylor WF, Pritchard DJ, Soule EH. Lymphadenectomy in the management of Stage I malignant melanoma: A prospective randomized study. Mayo Clin Proc. 1986; 61:697–705.

91. Simonsen E, Nordberg UB, Johnsson JE, Lamm IL, Trope C. Radiation therapy and surgery in the treatment of regional lymph nodes in squamous cell carcinoma of the vulva. Acta Radiol Oncol. 1984; 23:433–442.

92. Slayton RE, Blessing JA, Beecham J et al. Phase II trial of etoposide in the management of advanced of recurrent squamous cell carcinoma of the vulva

and carcinoma of the vagina: A Gynecologic Oncology Group study. Cancer Treat Rep. 1987; 71:869–870.

93. Stehman FB, Bundy BN, Dvoretsky PM, Creasman WT. Early stage I carcinoma of the vulva treated with ipsilateral superficial inguinal lymphadenectomy and modified radical vulvectomy: a prospective study of the Gynecologic Oncology Group. Obstet Gynecol. 1992; 79:490–7.

94. Stehman FB, Budy BN, Thomas G, Varia M, Okagaki T, Roberts J, Bell J, Heller PB. Groin Dissection versus Groin Radiation in Carcinoma of the Vulva: A Gynecologic Oncology Group Study. Int J Radiation Oncology Biol Phys. 1992; 24:289–396.

95. Stoeckel W. Zur Therapie des Vulvakarzinoms. Zentralbl Gynaecol. 1930; 54:47.

96. Struyk AP, Bouma J, van Lindert ACM, Aartsen EJ, Trimbos JB, van Lent M, Helmerhorst TJM, Schijf CPT, van der Putten HW, de Graaf J, van Wijck JA, Schilthuis MS, Heintz AP, Aalders JG. Early stage cancer of the vulva. A pilot investigation of cancer of the vulva in the Netherlands. Proceedings, International Gynecologic Cancer Society, Toronto; 1989.

97. Taussig FJ. Cancer of the vulva: An analysis of 155 cases. Am J Obstet Gynecol. 1940; 40:764.

98. Taussig FJ. Primary cancer of the vulva, vagina and female urethra: five-year results. Surg Gynecol Obstet. 1935; 60:477.

99. Tavassoli FA, Norris HJ, Smooth muscle tumors of the vulva. Gynecol Oncol. 1979; 53:213.

100. Thigpen JT, Blessing JA, Homesley HD, Berek JS, Creasman WT. Phase II trial of cisplatin in advanced or recurrent cancer of the vagina: A Gynecologic Oncology Group Study. Gynecol Oncol. 1986; 23:101–104.

101. Thigpen JT, Blessing JA, Homesley HD, Lewis GC. Phase II trials of cisplatin and piperazinedione in advanced squamous cell carcinoma of the vulva: A Gynecologic Oncology study. Gynecol Oncol. 1986; 23:358–363.

102. Thomas G, Dembo A, DePetrillo A et al. Concurrent radiation and chemotherapy in vulvar carcinoma. Gynecol Oncol. 1989; 34:263–267.

103. Tod MC. Radium implantation treatment of carcinoma of the vulva. Brit J Radiol. 1949; 22:508–512.

104. Trope C, Johnsson JE, Larsson G, Simonsen E. Bleomycin alone or combined with mitomycin C in treatment of advanced or recurrent squamous cell carcinoma of the vulva. Cancer Treat Rep. 1980; 64:639–642.

105. Van der Velden J, Kooyman CD, Van Lindert ACM, Heintz APM. A stage I-a vulvar carcinoma with an inguinal lymph node recurrence after local excision. A case report and literature review. Int J Gynecol Cancer. 1992; 2:157–159.

106. Veronesi U, Adamus J, Bandiera et al. Delayed regional lymph node dissection in Stage I melanoma of the skin of the lower extremities. Cancer. 1982; 49:2420–2430.

107. Veronesi U, Cascinelli N, Adamus J et al. Thin Stage I primary cutaneous malignant melanoma: Comparison of excision with margins of 1 or 3 cm. N Engl J Med. 1988; 318; 1159–62.

108. Way S. Carcinoma of the vulva. Am J Obstet Gynecol. 1960; 79:692.

109. Wharton JT, Gallager S, Rutledge RN. Microinvasive carcinoma of the vulva. Am J Obstet Gynecol. 1974; 118:159.

110. Wilkinson EJ, Rico MJ, Pierson KK. Microinvasive carcinoma of the vulva. Int J Gynecol Path. 1982; 1:29–39.

3 Uterine Corpus

B.-U. Sevin and R. Angioli

Introduction and Historical Review of the Development of Multimodality Treatment Concepts

Introduction

Endometrial cancer is the most common malignancy in the female genital tract. There were about 31000 new cases diagnosed in 1993 with 5700 estimated cancer-related deaths.[14] Most neoplasms of the uterine corpus are carcinomas; less than 5% are sarcomas or mixed tumors. Because of its numerical dominance, endometrial carcinoma has been the center of most investigations and therapeutic efforts.

Since 75% of all cases are diagnosed while the disease is still confined to the uterus, endometrial carcinoma has been considered a relatively benign malignancy with an actuarial 5-year survival of 67%, and of about 76% for stage 1 disease.[95] Unopposed, prolonged estrogen exposure appears to be the most common etiologic factor in the development of endometrial carcinoma. Exogenous or endogenous estrogen sources, if not opposed by progesterone, may initially lead to the development of endometrial hyperplasia and eventually to invasive carcinoma.[41] Bokhman postulated the existence of two different pathogenic types of endometrial cancers.[12] Type A is characterized by the traditional risk factors, such as obesity, diabetes mellitus, reduced fertility, ovulatory dysfunction, presence of endometrial hyperplasia, and history of exogenous or endogenous unopposed estrogen exposure. This type of neoplasm supposedly has a relatively good prognosis. In contrast, type B occurs in patients without evidence of unopposed estrogen exposure. Tumors in this group are usually poorly differentiated, metastasize early, and have a relatively poor prognosis.

The standard care in the past was a combination of surgical extirpation of the uterus and its adenxae, in combination with pre- and/or postoperative radiation.[54] The clinical FIGO-staging system served as a rough guideline for treatment planning based on more-or-less accepted clinical prognostic factors that could be identified before initiation of treatment, such as size of the uterus, histologic cell type, grade of differentiation, and disease extension beyond the uterine corpus. Surgical treatment included abdominal and vaginal hysterectomy for disease confined to the uterine corpus, and a more radical hysterectomy for more advanced disease.

Preoperative radiation was given to patients who had an enlarged uterus, unfavorable histology, and/or disease outside the uterine corpus proper. Postoperative radiation was given whenever the operative findings suggested an increased risk for treatment failure. The objective of preoperative radiation was the reduction of vaginal recurrences and improved chance of survival. The form of radiation, intracavitary or external beam, varied greatly depending mostly on the individual physician or institutional preference.

Primary adjunctive chemotherapy or hormone treatment was reserved for more extensive disease, such as intra-abdominal tumor spread, or on the small number of patients with distant metastases. Most data on chemo- and/or hormone therapy, however, were collected from patients with recurrent disease after prior surgery and radiation.

In recent years, the management of endometrial cancer has undergone profound changes. Large clinical trials have evaluated primary surgery, including surgical assessment of disease extent, and individually tailored postoperative adjunctive therapy based on individually defined surgical-pathologic findings. These efforts resulted in a change of the clinical FIGO-staging system of 1971 to a primary surgical-pathologic staging system in 1988.[26] This new system is currently under intense scrutiny, and the future will most likely see some modifications.

In contrast to uterine carcinomas, the sarcomas have received little attention. FIGO does not offer a separate staging system, and most clinicians apply the system used for endometrial carcinomas. However, it is well known that cell type more than grade is an important prognostic factor in this heterogenous group of malignancies. In contrast to carcinomas, sarcomas and mixed tumors (e.g., carcinosarcomas) have the tendency to metastasize early, not only through the lymphatic, but also through the hematogenous route. Distant metastases and recurrences are therefore not uncommon. For these reasons, combinations of surgery and radiation, as well as adjunctive systemic chemotherapy have been used in the past with uncertain therapeutic benefit.

Treatment of recurrent disease has been highly individualized, depending on the site of recurrence and prior therapy. Patients who were treated only by surgery, or with a localized recurrence outside the field of prior radiation, usually received locoregional radiation. Central recurrences in the field of radiation may, in selected cases, be explored for surgical resection, including the rare indication for pelvic exenteration. For all other cases, hormone- and/or chemotherapy have been used to provide palliation, only rarely achieving a cure.

▓ Pathology

Epithelial Tumors

Hyperplasia

Hyperplasias have been regarded precursors of endometrial carcinoma. In the past, various terminologies have been used to classify these changes and relate them to their respective risks of progressing to carcinoma. The International Society of Gynecological Pathology recommends the following classification, which seems most useful for clinical practice:

Simple (cystic without atypia) and complex (adenomatous without atypia) hyperplasias carry a low risk of progressing to frank carcinoma. The risk is one and three percent.[66] In contrast, atypical hyperplasias, simple and complex with atypia, carry a risk of progressing to cancer in 8% and 29%. Atypical hyperplasia is characterized by a combination of the respective glandular growth pattern (cystic or adenomatous) and the presence of cytologic atypia in the cells lining the glands.[41, 66] Because of the risk of progressing to invasive carcinoma, hysterectomy is the treatment of choice in cases of atypical hyperplasia,

except in young women who desire children. (see section on Diagnostic Preoperative Evaluation)

Carcinomas

Endometrial carcinoma can be present in a variety of histologic cell types and grades of differentiation, some behaving more aggressively than others (Table **1**). The grade of differentiation may be defined by the architectural growth pattern used in the FIGO grading system, expressing grade on the percent of solid growth pattern in a given specimen, or by nuclear characteristics.[67]

Of the histologic cell types, endometrioid adenocarcinomas are the most common, comprising more than 75% of all cases.[146] These tumors resemble normal endometrium. Small

Table **1**   Classification of uterine neoplasms

A) Carcinomas

Endometrioid adenocarcinoma
    papillary, secretory, ciliated cell, adeno-
    carcinoma with squamous differentiation
Mucinous carcinoma
Serous carcinoma
Clear cell carcinoma
Squamous carcinoma
Undifferentiated carcinoma
Mixed types
Miscellaneous carcinoma
Metastatic carcinoma

B) Sarcomas

Pure nonepithelial tumors
Endometrial stromal tumors:
    stromal nodule, low and high-grade stromal
    sarcoma
Smooth muscle tumors:
    leiomyoma, smooth muscle tumor of
    uncertain malignant potential, leiomyo-
    sarcoma, other smooth muscle tumors
Mixed endometrial stromal and smooth muscle
tumors:
    adenomatoid tumor, other benign and
    malignant soft tissue tumors

Mixed epithelial–nonepithelial tumors
Benign tumors:
    adenofibroma, adenomyoma
Malignant tumors:
    adenosarcoma (homologous, heterologous),
    carcinofibroma, carcinosarcoma
    (homologous, heterologous)

areas of differentiation (metaplasia) into squamous, papillary, secretory, and ciliated cells, however, can be observed; some of these are thought to be a response to unopposed estrogen exposure.[46] These tumors with minor variations in differentiation need to be clearly separated from tumors in which different histologic cell types make up the major cellular component (>50%) of the tumor specimen.[41, 66, 146] Tumors with significant, benign, squamous metaplasia (also called adenoacanthoma) are quite common and considered relatively benign. According to the International Society of Gynecological Pathology, the following malignant cell types should be identified as separate entities: mucinous, serous, clear cell, squamous, and undifferentiated carcinomas. Except for the mucinous carcinoma, all of these neoplasms are thought to have a worse prognosis than endometrioid carcinomas. Mixed cell types contain more than one cell type, each comprising more than 30% of the tumor. Metastatic disease from extrauterine sites (most commonly the breast, colon, and stomach) have been observed on rare occasions. Another interesting pathologic entity is the occurrence of synchronous endometrial and ovarian cancer with identical morphology. The primary site is usually assigned on the basis of morphology and the most advanced tumor stage at each site.

Mesenchymal Tumors

Sarcomas are a histologically diverse group of neoplasms that comprise less then 5% of all uterine neoplasms. Symptoms and clinical presentation of these tumors are similar to those seen in endometrial carcinoma. Symptoms of uterine sarcomas, in addition to abnormal uterine bleeding, are pelvic pain and an enlarged uterus (frequently with a friable tumor protruding through the cervical os). However, the correct diagnosis is frequently not made preoperatively, but only on the hysterectomy specimen. Since there is no separate staging system for uterine sarcomas, they are generally staged by the FIGO system used for endometrial carcinoma (see pages 34, 35). Major prognostic parameters are surgical stage, depth of invasion, and histologic grade. In contrast to carcinomas, these tumors have a tendency to spread not only by lymphatic, but also hematogenous route. The recent classification of the International Society

of Gynecological Pathology differentiates between pure nonepithelial and mixed epithelial–nonepithelial uterine sarcomas (Table **1**).

While the majority of these neoplasms are quite aggressive, with early distant metastatic spread and poor survival, the well-differentiated leiomyosarcomas, endometrial stromal sarcomas, and adenosarcomas usually show only locoregional growth and have a relatively good prognosis. Histologic grading of sarcomas, however, has been controversial. It is generally accepted that a combination of cellular and nuclear features, as well as number of mitosis is required to make the correct diagnosis. Unusual histologic presentations, however, are quite common.

Pure Nonepithelial Tumors

The most common malignant tumors in this category are the leiomyosarcomas (LMS) and endometrial stromal sarcomas (ESS). Compared with LMS, ESS seem to have a better prognosis, with a 5-year survival of 67% and 39%, respectively.[87] Well-differentiated tumors (G1–2) have a better prognosis with a 5-year survival of 83%, compared to 33% for grade 3–4 tumors.

Mixed Epithelial–Nonepithelial Tumors

This group of neoplasms is characterized by the presence of a mixture of stromal and epithelial components. The nomenclature of each is determined by the benign or malignant nature of each component. The most common type is the carcinosarcoma (CS), which is synonymous with malignant mixed mesodermal tumor (MMT) and malignant mixed müllerian tumor. In these tumors, both components are malignant. The epithelial component is usually an adenocarcinoma with different degrees of differentiation, similar to those seen in pure carcinomas. For descriptive purposes, the same terminology used for pure carcinomas in regard to histologic type and grade of differentiation is applied to these mixed tumors. The stromal components may be of homologous differentiation, typical for pure sarcomas originating from the uterus (e.g., leiomyosarcoma, derived from smooth muscle), or of heterologous differentiation, typical for sarcomas originating from extrauterine sites (e.g., rhabdomyosarcoma, derived from striated muscle).

The prognosis for patients with CS is generally worse than for LMS and ESS, mainly because of the more advanced disease state at the time of diagnosis. An overall 5-year survival of 21% was reported in 610 patients, with most tumor-related deaths occurring within 18 months of diagnosis.[9] Myometrial invasion seems to be an important predictor of treatment failure in stage I–II disease, but even patients without myometrial invasion had recurrent disease in 25% of the cases.

Primary Disease

Staging and Surgical Procedures

Overview

Staging of endometrial cancer has undergone profound changes in recent years. In 1971, FIGO accepted a clinical system to define prognostic parameters that relied on diagnostic procedures that could be done prior to treatment planning (Table 2).[32] In 1988, FIGO changed to a surgical-pathological system, which is applied to all patients undergoing primary surgery (Table 3).[26] However, almost all current published data use the clinical staging system of 1971 as stage reference.

Since the majority of cases (>75%) are diagnosed in stage I, when the cancer is confined to the uterine corpus, other accepted prognostic indicators, such as grade of differentiation and uterine size, are only applied to stage I but not to more advanced disease. Most authors agreed that histologic grade is an important indicator for prognosis, with 5-year survival differences in stage I for grade 1, 2 and 3 being 81%, 74% and 50%, respectively.[54] Uterine size differentiating between stage IA and IB, with 5-year survival rates of 85% and 67%,[54] may only be of significance if cancer growth is the cause for uterine enlargement and not a benign condition, such as uterine fibroids.

Stage II is defined by involvement of the endocervical canal and/or cervix with cancer, as assessed by endocervical curettage and/or cervical biopsy ("carcinoma corpori i colli"). Only 10–15% of patients with endometrial carcinoma have stage II disease, but their prognosis is, compared to stage I, considerably worse (57% vs. 76%.[83] The assessment of endocervical tumor

Table **2** Clinical staging for endometrial carcinoma (FIGO; 1971)

Stage 0	Atypical hyperplasia or carcinoma in situ Histological findings suspicious of malignancy
Stage I	Carcinoma is confined to the corpus
IA	The length of the uterine cavity is 8 cm or less
IB	The length of the uterine cavity is more than 8 cm

Stage I cases should be subgrouped with regard to the histological type of the adenocarcinoma as follows:

G1—highly differentiated adenomatous carcinoma
G2—moderately differentiated adenomatous carcinoma with partly solid areas
G3—predominantly solid or entirely undifferentiated carcinoma

Stage II	The carcinoma has involved the corpus and the cervix, but has not extended outside the uterus
Stage III	The carcinoma has extended outside the uterus, but has not extended outside the true pelvis
Stage IV	The carcinoma has extended outside the true pelvis or has obviously involved the mucosa of the bladder or rectum. A bullous edema as such does not permit a case to be allotted to stage IV disease
IVA	Spread of growth to adjacent organs
IVB	Spread of growth to distant organs

involvement, in cases without ectocervical tumor growth, is limited by the inaccuracy of the endocervical curettage, which yields false negative and positive results in over 30% of cases. Stage III disease is defined by clinically assessable disease outside the uterus, including pelvic structures and the vagina, but not outside the true pelvis, and stage IV disease includes all other cases of distant metastasis. These two entities constitute only 8% and 4% of all endometrial cancers, but they have a very poor 5-year survival of 30% and 11%, respectively.[95]

Studies using surgery as the initial step to diagnose disease extent and treat primary endometrial cancer demonstrated that in addition to

Table **3**   Surgical staging system for endometrial carcinoma (FIGO, 1988)

Stage IA   G123 Tumor limited to endometrium
Stage IB   G123 Invasion to < 1/2 myometrium
Stage IC   G123 Invasion to > 1/2 myometrium

Stage IIA   G123 Endocervical glandular involvement only
Stage IIB   G123 Cervical stroma invasion

Stage IIIA   G123 Tumor invades serosa and/or adnexa and/or positive peritoneal cytology
Stage IIIB   G123 Metastases to pelvic and/or para-aortic lymph nodes

Stage IVA   G123 Tumor invasion of bladder and/or
Stage IVB   bowel mucosa distant metastases including intra-abdominal and/or inguinal lymph nodes

Histopathology: Degree of differentiation
G1   5% or less of a nonsquamous or nonmorular solid growth pattern
G2   5–50% of a nonsquamous or nonmorular solid growth pattern
G3   More than 50% of a nonsquamous or nonmorular solid growth pattern

Notes on pathological grading:
1) Notable nuclear atypia, inappropriate for the architectural grade, raises the grade of a grade 1 or 2 tumor by one
2) In serous adenocarcinomas, clear cell adenocarcinomas, and squamous cell carcinomas, nuclear grading takes precedence
3) Adenocarcinoma with squamous differentiation are graded according to the nuclear grade of the glandular component

histologic grade, the depth of myometrial invasion and surgically proven disease beyond the uterine corpus, such as endocervix, adnexae, and lymph nodes (Figures **1** and **2**, page X), were powerful prognostic parameters for survival.

In 1970, Lewis and Stallworthy published an excellent study on 129 patients treated by radical hysterectomy, pelvic lymphadenectomy, and individualized perioperative radiation, pointing the way to our current approach to endometrial carcinoma.[71] If disease was confined to the uterine corpus, the rate of pelvic lymph node metastases was 11.2%, but was 36.2% in cases with deep myometrial invasion and 26.3% with poorly differentiated tumors. The uncorrected 5-year survival rates were 74% overall and 36.4% for patients with pelvic lymph node metastases.

Only 56.5% of the patients died from recurrent endometrial cancer. The authors emphasize the fact "that of the seven patients with positive nodes who died, only one had a pelvic recurrence. It would seem from these findings that surgical excision of the lymphatic nodes plus postoperative radiation has had a favorable influence on prognosis."

In 1974, the Gynecologic Oncology Group (GOG) initiated a prospective study on surgical staging of FIGO Stage I endometrial carcinoma.[16, 28] Two-hundred and twenty-two patients underwent primary surgery, including peritoneal washing, extrafascial total abdominal hysterectomy, bilateral salpingo-oophorectomy, and pelvic node dissection. In 156 selected patients, a para-aortic node dissection was also performed. Similar to the data reported by Lewis and Stallworthy, pelvic node metastases were found in 10.4% (26% for grade 3 tumors). In addition, an unexpectedly high incidence of metastases to the para-aortic nodes (7.7–10.8%), adnexae (7.6%), and positive peritoneal cytology (11.7%) was observed. These data led to a larger prospective study by the GOG on stage I and II (occult) endometrial carcinoma between 1977 and 1983 (GOG #33), into which 1180 women were entered.[25, 82] The first publication reports the surgical pathologic spread patterns in 621 evaluable patients with clinical stage I disease.[25] Pelvic and para-aortic lymph node metastases were found in 9% and 6%, respectively, positive peritoneal cytology in 12%, and other extrauterine metastases in 6%. Significant risk factors for nodal metastasis are summarized in Table **4**.

It became obvious that there is a strong interdependence of risk factors; such as clinical stage, histologic grade, depth of myometrial invasion, extrauterine disease, and lymph node metastasis. Of particular importance were grade and depth of myometrial invasion (Table **5**). Since only clinical stage and histologic grade are easily determined without surgical exploration, it is of particular interest to the clinician, faced with the management decision in a newly diagnosed patient, to anticipate the need for node dissection in this elderly, frequently obese patient population, which carries considerable risks of perioperative complications. A breakdown of these data in regard to node metastasis and clinical (FIGO 1971) stage I and II disease allows the clinician to plan surgical management to a certain extent based on FIGO stage and grade (Table **6**). Assess-

Table **4**   Risk factors and frequency of lymph node metastasis (LNM) in percent (GOG #33)

Risk factor	N	Pelvic LNM	Aortic LNM
Stage			
IA	346	7%	3%
IB	275	13%	8%
Histology			
Adenocarcinoma	180	9%	5%
Adenoacanthoma	41	10%	0%
Adenosquamous	99	12%	9%
Others	22	9%	18%
Grade			
1	180	3%	2%
2	288	9%	5%
3	153	18%	11%
Myometrial invasion			
Endometrial only	87	1%	1%
Superficial	279	5%	3%
Middle	116	6%	1%
Deep	139	25%	17%
Peritoneal cytology			
Negative	537	7%	4%
Positive	75	25%	19%
Site of tumor location			
Fundus	524	8%	4%
Isthmus-Cervix	97	16%	14%
Adnexal involvement			
Positive	34	32%	20%
negative	587	8%	5%
Other extrauterine metastasis			
Positive	35	51%	23%
Negative	586	7%	4%
Capillary-like space involvement			
Positive	93	27%	19%
Negative	528	7%	9%

Table **5**   Grade (G) and depth of invasion (DI) versus pelvic node metastasis (GOG #33)

DI	N	G1	G2	G3
Endometrium only	86	0%	3%	0%
Inner 1/3	281	3%	5%	9%
Middle 1/3	115	0%	9%	4%
Deep 1/3	139	11%	19%	34%

Table **6**   FIGO stage versus lymph node metastasis (LNM) (GOG #33)

Stage	N	Pelvic LNM	Aortic LNM
IA G1	101	2%	0%
G2	169	8%	4%
G3	76	11%	7%
IB G1	79	4%	4%
G2	119	10%	7%
G3	77	26%	16%

currence, the patients may be spared adjunctive radiation, which in itself carries significant risk for complications in this elderly patient population (see following section).

The GOG studies also demonstrated that in the majority of patients with stage I and II occult endometrial carcinoma that had grade 1–2 tumors (77.7%), disease was limited to the uterine fundus (77.4%), and 75% had < 2/3 myometrial invasion.[82] In this study of 895 patients, 58.4% had none of the identified risk factors for recurrence (node metastasis, gross disease outside the uterus, positive cytology or adnexae, capillary space involvement, or isthmus/cervix invasion). Patients without these risk factors may therefore be spared postoperative therapy altogether, avoiding associated complications and cost. In 1988, FIGO changed to a surgical–pathologic staging system (Tables **3–5**), which should be applied to all patients treated primarily by surgery. However, patients who will not undergo primary surgery, or only TAH-BSO without surgical staging, should be staged with the clinical staging system of 1971.

Diagnostic Preoperative Evaluation

Most endometrial neoplasms are diagnosed in patients presenting with the most common

ment of myometrial invasion during surgery further defines the risk of pelvic and/or aortic node metastasis. Intraoperatively, the clinician can thus evaluate the risk–benefit ratio between performing a lymphadenectomy or not and the surgical risks for each individual patient. This issue is of importance, since the lymph node dissection is primarily a diagnostic procedure and only of potential therapeutic benefit if the removed nodes contain tumor. However, if the nodes are negative and the pathologic evaluation of the uterus itself suggests a low risk for re-

symptom, that of irregular vaginal, especially postmenopausal, bleeding. Since most endometrial carcinomas are diagnosed in menopause (75%), postmenopausal bleeding should be seen as a symptom that requires the clinician to either diagnose or rule out the presence of cancer. With increasing use of postmenopausal estrogen replacement therapy, the need for close surveillance of these patients is imperative. Although the likelihood of diagnosing endometrial cancer in women with postmenopausal bleeding is less than 20%, tissue must be obtained from the endometrial cavity for histological evaluation. This can be done with a relatively simple office procedure, using a variety of techniques, such as endometrial cytology, the Vabra aspirator, the Pipelle, or other endometrial biopsy tools.[52, 57] If these methods fail to make the diagnosis of endometrial cancer, a fractional dilatation and curettage needs to be done to make the diagnosis or rule out cancer (Fig. **1**). In premenopausal women, persistent menometrorrhagia requires histological assessment of endometrial tissue, preferentially by fractional curettage. Since not all patients are candidates for surgical staging according to FIGO (1988), it is advisable to perform the diagnostic procedures (Table **7A**) required for clinical staging (FIGO 1971).

Other diagnostic procedures may be done in the hope of better defining the depth of myometrial invasion, and/or extrauterine disease

Table **7**   Staging of endometrial carcinoma

A) *Procedures for clinical staging (FIGO, 1971)*

General physical examination*

Pelvic examination* (inspection and palpation)

Endocervical curettage

Measure uterine length (</= 8 cm, > 8 cm)

Intravenous pyelogram

Chest X-ray

Cystoscopy* and sigmoidoscopy*

B) *Procedures for surgical staging (FIGO, 1988)*

Midline incision

Peritoneal lavage

Inspection and palpation of pelvic and abdominal organs, biopsy of tumor suspicious sites

Extrafascial hysterectomy

Bilateral salpingo-oophorectomy

Bilateral pelvic and aortic lymph node dissection

* Areas suspicious for tumor need to be biopsied to obtain morphologic confirmation of cancer

spread with the aid of abdominal or vaginal ultrasonography (US),[93] Computerized Tomography (CT), or Nuclear Magnetic Resonance (NMR). The latter two studies are costly and not necessary for patients who will undergo surgical staging.

Intraoperative Procedures

In clinical stage I and II disease, primary staging laparotomy and TAH-BSO should be standard care for all surgically suited patients (Table **7B**). Since a large number of patients are considered to have low risk for extrauterine disease spread, node metastases, and recurrence, this extensive surgical staging procedure appears too radical to many clinicians, especially in this patient population who are frequently elderly, obese, and afflicted with multiple medical problems. In patients with a moderate or high risk for perioperative complications, a more individualized surgical approach, based on risk factors that can be defined pre- and intraoperatively, appears more appropriate in the overall treatment scheme of multimodal therapy of stage I and II disease (Fig. **2**). In patients with biopsy-proven involvement of the ectocervix, a modified radical hysterectomy may be selected as in primary cervix cancer.

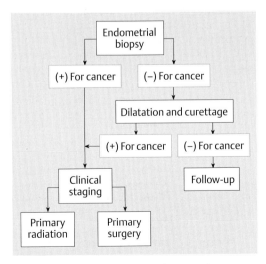

Fig. **1**   Endometrial carcinoma diagnosis (symptoms suggestive of endometrial neoplasm)

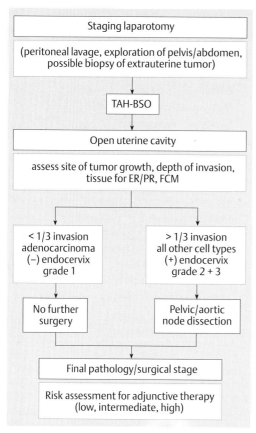

Fig. 2 Endometrial carcinoma: Primary surgery (operable patients: stages I and II occ.)

node metastases were suspicious because of nodal enlargement.[82] Removing only palpable nodes appears insufficient to assure the absence of node metastases. Only a complete, bilateral pelvic and aortic lymphadenectomy, removing more than 30–40 nodes, can do this. The therapeutic value of a lymphadenectomy is still uncertain. Considering the potential morbidity, the risk of this procedure should be offset by the risk of node metastasis. The indication for an aortic lymph node dissection is of particular importance for this discussion. In the GOG trial, only 25% of the patients had one or more of the high risk factors, such as grossly positive pelvic nodes, gross adnexal metastasis, outer one-third myometrial invasion, or suspicious aortic nodes, but 98% of cases with aortic node metastases were found in these patients.[82] Selecting patients for aortic node dissection based on these risk factors intraoperatively may be more prudent. The surgeon may elect *not* to perform an aortic LND in the patient with a low risk for node metastases, especially if the surgical risk is significant. On the other hand, the surgeon may elect to *only* perform an aortic LND in a patient who will receive pelvic radiation based on already established pre- or intraoperatively defined risk factors, such as deep myometrial or cervical invasion. Similarly, in the presence of histologically confirmed metastasis, a selected removal of palpably enlarged lymph nodes may render a more extensive lymphadenectomy unnecessary, unless the clinician believes in the therapeutic value of lymphadenectomy for microscopic disease. Resecting *enlarged* lymph nodes probably does have therapeutic benefits in the form of "tumor debulking," as suggested by Lewis.[71] It is obvious that the issue of LND requires careful evaluation of all of these factors, and the decision should be made in the context of multimodality treatment, individualized for the overall benefit to the patient (Fig. 3).

Patients with increased risk for abdominal surgery such as obesity, cardiovascular disease, and/or diabetes mellitus, may still be candidates for vaginal hysterectomy, specially in stage I (G1–2) disease. Postoperative radiation can be added for surgical risk factors defined on the uterine specimen.[11]

Assessment of the location of tumor growth (fundus vs. isthmus) or cervical involvement and depth of myometrial invasion should be done either by gross inspection or by frozen section analysis. At this point, tumor tissue should be submitted for special studies, such as estrogen and progesterone receptors, flow cytometry (FCM), or other laboratory studies.

One of the main questions to be answered intraoperatively, after hysterectomy, is the need for and the extent of a lymph node dissection (LND). Optimally, a pelvic and para-aortic LND is performed in all patients as required by FIGO (1988). This LND is primarily a diagnostic procedure. The diagnostic accuracy of detecting node metastasis increases with the number of nodes removed. Selected node "sampling" will certainly reduce the yield of node positivity. In the GOG study, only 46% of histologically proven aortic

In clinical stage III and IV disease, primary surgery and tumor debulking (Fig. 2), followed by individualized adjunctive radiation and/or chemotherapy may be selected. Alternative

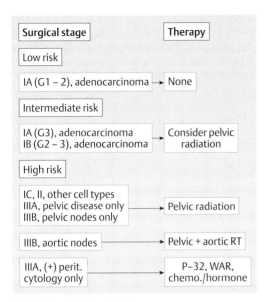

Fig. **3** Endometrial carcinoma: Postoperative adjunctive therapy

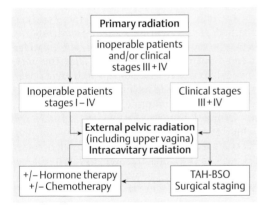

Fig. **4** Endometrial carcinoma

options are primary radiation, followed by adjunctive hormone and/or chemotherapy, or abdominal (vaginal) hysterectomy (Fig. **4**).

Treatment of endometrial sarcomas should be surgical, as described for carcinomas, including careful surgical staging.[6] For clinical stage I disease, TAH-BSO, and in more advanced disease, maximal tumor debulking is the treatment of choice. Prognosis differs depending on cell type and surgically defined disease extent.

Postoperative Adjunctive Therapy

An important aspect of these recent clinical–pathologic studies,[25, 82] besides precisely assessing disease extent, is the planning of adjunctive therapy: Which patient would or would not benefit from postoperative therapy, and what would constitute optimal treatment in the high-risk patient? Previously, the standard care was a combination of pre- and/or postoperative radiation in combination with an extrafascial hysterectomy.

The first prospective study on postoperative therapy after primary surgery and surgical staging was done by the Gynecologic Oncology Group (GOG # 34).[81] Only surgically staged patients (GOG study # 33), with pathologically defined risk factors for recurrence, such as > 50% myometrial invasion, cervical involvement, lymph node metastasis, or adnexal metastases were eligible. Of the 224 patients entered, 181 were evaluable. All patients without aortic node metastases received 5000 rads of pelvic radiation. Patients with aortic node metastases received additional 4500 rads of aortic radiation. After radiation, patients were also randomized to receive doxorubicin chemotherapy or no further therapy. Results from this study indicate that postoperative radiation, with or without chemotherapy, is fairly well tolerated in this surgically staged patient population: serious complications included small bowel obstructions in 6.9% and treatment related deaths in 2.8%. Overall, 5-year survival was good (63.5%), even in patients with pelvic node metastases (68%), but only 26% with aortic node metastases. The effect of doxorubicin could not be determined because the number of evaluable patients was insufficient. This and other studies support the current concept of postoperative adjunctive therapy as outlined in Figure **3**.

Patients who had primary TAH-BSO without node dissection and were found to have increased risk factors for metastasis/recurrence (e.g., deep myometrial invasion) should receive postoperative RT. In the presence of 0–1, 2, and 3–4 of the following surgically defined risk factors (cervical involvement, grade 3, > 1/3 myometrial invasion, vascular invasion, and positive peritoneal cytology) 5-year survival rates of 97%, 66%, and 17%, respectively, were observed in patients managed with individualized postoperative radiation.[55]

It has been emphasized that a large number of patients were not considered high risk for recurrence; 48.1% received no adjunctive therapy.[82] Surgical staging is not only important for identifying the patients who may benefit from adjunctive treatment, but for identifying patients, who according to our current understanding, do *not* require adjunctive treatment after appropriate surgery. Since adjunctive radiation in this elderly patient population is associated with considerable risk, it is important to avoid unnecessary radiation with its associated costs and complications.

A benefit of adjunctive therapy for patients with uterine sarcoma has not been clearly established. In the past, postoperative radiation and/or chemotherapy were applied, but without clear benefit to patient survival. Recurrence rates are high, even in disease that appears confined to the uterus. Differences may exist between the different cell types ESS, LMS, and CS. Except for LMS, no difference in overall recurrence rates was observed in sarcomas treated with or without postoperative radiation.[74] The site of first recurrence has been studied to determine the benefit of postoperative pelvic radiation in preventing pelvic recurrences. No clear benefit was observed in carcinosarcomas. In LMS, the pelvic, as well as the overall recurrence rates were reduced by pelvic radiation. These data seem to support the value of radiation. However, the number of patients in the study was small, radiation was given according to physician's preference, and the 3-year survival was only 31%.[74] Most patients died with widespread disease. The discouraging results with radiation led to clinical trials with adjuvant systemic therapy. Current data and management recommendations will be discussed in the sections on radiation and systemic therapy.

▨ Radiation Therapy

A short history of radiation therapy for endometrial cancer will be presented, followed by a descriptive presentation of external, intracavitary, and intraperitoneal radiation. These modes of radiotherapy are also used for other gynecologic neoplasms. The general discussion in this chapter, therefore, also applies (with some modifications) to radiation given for cancer of the vulva, cervix, and ovary. On pages 45–49, specific treatment recommendations for endometrial carcinomas and sarcomas are discussed. On pages 49, 50, the management of radiation-related complications is discussed, which again applies also to other gynecologic malignancies.

History of Radiation Therapy

In the past, the treatment of choice for endometrial cancer was surgery. In the early 1900s, the use of radiation for cervical cancer patients was already well known, but only very few authors reported experience of radiotherapy for endometrial cancer. When Howard Kelly reported his experience in 327 uterine cancer patients treated with radium in 1916, he pointed out that the excellent results obtained with surgery prevented the investigation of other treatment methods for endometrial cancer. Despite this consideration, he reported in the same article about five patients with endometrial carcinoma, treated with intrauterine radium at the time of curettage.[60] In some of these patients, he observed no evidence of disease at the time of the hysterectomy a few weeks later.

In 1935, Heyman introduced the Stockholm method of intrauterine radiation and reported a 5-year survival rate of 60% in stage I patients treated with radiation alone.[47] With this technique, radioactive tubes or capsules were inserted into the uterus to maximize the radiation dose delivered to the tumor.

External beam radiation was initially delivered by orthovoltage X-ray machines, until the ^{60}Cobalt teletherapy unit, using the high energy ^{60}C isotope as radioactive source, was developed in 1951. It became the most commonly used unit in clinical practice. In the 1960s, linear accelerators, using high frequency electronic waves to accelerate electrons, were developed for medical use and are now the most commonly used systems in radiation oncology.

In 1936, Arneson published a literature review of different treatment modalities for endometrial carcinoma.[8] He found 5-year survival rates of 53% in 473 operable patients treated with irradiation alone, 57% in 927 patients treated with surgery alone, and 60% in 91 patients treated with combination irradiation followed by surgery. This report focused the attention on the value of intracavitary and external preoperative radiotherapy. Primary external pelvic radiotherapy was considered more advantageous because it was supposed to decrease the risk of lymphatic and transtubal tumor spread, reduce tumor volume inside the uterine cavity, and facilitate insertion of intrauterine radium applicators.

In the 1940s, the importance of lymph node metastasis in endometrial cancer patients became known[46a] and radiation after surgery for patients with positive lymph nodes was recommended. Starting in the late 1950s, two schools of thought developed in regard to the management of patients with endometrial cancer. The oldest of these suggested the use of radium and/or external radiation therapy *prior* to surgery, while the other one advocated primary surgery *followed* by radiotherapy *only* for patients with an increased risk for recurrence. The main arguments for combining RT with surgery were reduction of vaginal recurrence and improvement for survival. Since radiation therapy alone showed lower survival data then surgery alone or combination therapy, it was usually reserved for patients not suitable for surgery.[54]

External Beam Radiation

External beam irradiation, also known as teletherapy, is frequently used to treat endometrial cancer, usually in combination with surgery, brachytherapy, or both. Radiation energy output of teletherapy units, ^{60}Cobalt, and linear accelerators, is commonly measured in megavoltage (MeV), ranging from 4 to 25 MeV. The actual dose delivered to the tumor depends on a variety of factors: the quality and energy of the source, the distance and media between the radiation source and the tumor, and the size of the radiation field. The absorbed dose describes the energy of radiation delivered, and is expressed either as "Rads" (rad = 0.01 Joule/kg) or "Gray" (1 Gy = 1 J/kg; 1 cGy = 0.001 J/kg). Verification of the appropriate size and location of the radiation field is usually done with computerized tomography (CT). Calculation of radiation delivered to the tumor and surrounding structures is computerized, providing the clinician with isodose distribution diagrams, which represent points of equal doses projected onto the various planes of the radiated tissue volume.

The field of pelvic radiation should include the primary tumor, pelvic lymph nodes, and the vaginal cuff. Standard approaches include either a two-field or a four-field technique. The two-field technique uses parallel opposing anterior and posterior fields. The upper border extends from the level of the pelvic brim between L4 and L5 to the upper half of the vagina (Figs. **1** and **2**, see page X). The lateral border of the field is placed 1–2 cm from the pelvic brim, but spares the hip joint. The fields are treated daily with 180–200 cGy per treatment fraction; treatment schedules vary between institutions. The average suggested weekly dose is 900–1000 cGy, up to a total of 4500–5500 cGy. In case of macroscopic lymph node metastasis, a higher dose is delivered, in small fields, to the tumor bearing area.

Some institutions prefer the four-field technique, which minimizes damage to skin and subcutaneous tissue. This is particularly useful in obese patients, for whom the distance from skin to tumor is large. Radiation falloff increases with distance of the tumor from the radiation source. To deliver a fixed dose of radiation to the tumor in an obese patient requires an increase in the dose. This increases the dose delivered to the skin of that area. The four-field technique allows the same dose to be delivered to the tumor without increasing the skin dose. While the two fields previously described are placed in the same position, two additional fields are located laterally. The anterior border of the lateral field is placed 1 cm anterior to the pubic symphysis to cover external iliac lymph nodes and the posterior border between S2 and S3 (or at S1) to irradiate presacral lymph nodes (Figs. **1** and **2**, see page X). If intracavitary radiation is also given, the central portion of the radiation field may need shielding to prevent overexposure to parts of the bladder and rectum.

Patients with para-aortic node involvement should be treated with a cranial extension of the pelvic fields. The aortic fields are usually 8 cm wide and extend upward from the top of the pelvic fields for a mean of 18 cm, including the lymphatics of the renal vessels. Lower aortic fields with a mean height of 9 cm may also be used in selected cases of common ileac node involvement. The average total dose of para-aortic node irradiation is about 4500 cGy, but an additional boost of 350–500 cGy may be added with small fields to areas of lymph node metastasis.

Whole abdominal radiotherapy (WAR) has been applied to the treatment of peritoneal metastasis, which is obviously an unfavorable prognostic factor for patients with endometrial carcinoma. Three different techniques have been described to irradiate the whole abdomen: the open field, the moving strip,[38] and the so-called "Stanford technique." Open-field abdominal external beam radiotherapy radiates the entire abdomen and pelvis in one field that extends from at least 1 cm above the diaphragm to the inferior margin of the obturator foramen, covering at least the upper two-thirds of the vagina, and laterally 2 cm beyond the peritoneal reflections.[101] The average total dose delivered to the abdomen is 2000–2400 cGy with a daily fraction of 100–120 cGy. The open-field WAR allows a homogeneous distribution of radiation to the abdomen. Pelvic radiation extending from the bottom of the obturator foramen to the 4th–5th lumbar vertebra and 1 cm lateral to the bony pelvis is usually added, delivering an average of 2000–2500 cGy to the pelvis. Areas of residual tumor growth or lymph node metastasis may be individually boosted.

The moving-strip technique of WAR was developed in England during the 1940s, and first applied in the United States at the M. D. Anderson Hospital by Delclos.[27] It's aim was to minimize radiation damage and improve the systemic tolerance compared to the classic whole abdominal field technique. With this technique, the abdomen is radiated in small segments, starting at the lower pelvis, and slowly moving the field of radiation cranially, until the entire abdomen is radiated. The surface of the body to be irradiated is divided into 2.5 cm strips. Four lead collimators of 2.5 × 24, 5.0 × 24, 7.5 × 24, and 10 × 24 cm are used to obtain four field sizes. Each single strip is irradiated on one day from the front, and on the next day from the back, with an increase in width of 2.5 cm, until four strips have been irradiated. Then the 10 cm collimator is moved upward by 2.5 cm every day, irradiating front and back, until the last strip is reached. Finally, field sizes are reduced by 2.5 cm per application, until the last area is fully irradiated. With the moving-strip technique, a total dose of 2600–2800 cGy is delivered to the abdomen.[38] The whole treatment is given in 30 to 40 days, with a daily dose of 350 cGy to any specific area. To avoid RT damage to kidneys and liver, the kidneys are shielded from the back with two one-half value layers (HVL) of lead and the liver from the front and back with one HVL of lead, which

reduces the radiation dose by 50%. Additional pelvic irradiation of up to 2000 cGy may be delivered before or after moving-strip irradiation. The total dose of radiation delivered to the tumor can be the same with both methods, but the open-field technique is given in a shorter time period, and therefore is more effective from a biological point of view. Irradiating only a small volume of the abdomen at any one time results in better patient tolerance.

Another modification is the Stanford technique, which combines open-field WAR with additional radiation to areas that are typical sites of tumor metastasis, such as the diaphragm, pelvic and para-aortic lymph nodes, and vaginal cuff.[78] Radiation is delivered in four phases. First, the entire peritoneal cavity is irradiated with fields that extend from 1 cm above the diaphragm down to the upper two-thirds of the vagina, and laterally 2 cm beyond the peritoneal reflections. During this first phase, a total of 3000 cGy (150 cGy × 20) are delivered to the upper abdomen, para-aortic lymph nodes, pelvis, and vagina. The liver is shielded to receive only 2250 cGy and the kidneys 2000 cGy. In the second phase, an additional 1200 cGy (150 cGy × 8) are delivered to the central half of the diaphragm, the para-aortic nodes, the pelvis, and upper two-thirds of the vagina. During the third phase, an additional 900 cGy (180 cGy × 5) are delivered to the pelvis and vagina, and 720 cGy to the vagina in the fourth phase.

Total radiation: 3000 cGy (*Liver:* 2250 cGy; *Kidney:* 2000 cGy), *Diaphragm and para-aortic region:* 4200 cGy, *Pelvis:* 5100 cGy, *Vagina (upper 2/3):* 5820 cGy.

Intracavitary Radiation

Intracavitary radiation, also called brachytherapy, delivers high doses of radiation to a limited tissue volume. The rationale behind intrauterine radiation is to maximize the radiation dose delivered to the tumor and minimize radiation to adjacent organs. Vaginal irradiation is mainly directed to the vaginal cuff and upper third to the vagina to prevent vaginal recurrence. A variety of applicators were designed to insert radioactive sources into the uterine cavity and cervix (Heyman capsules, uterine tandem) and the vagina (vaginal cylinders or ovoids). The placement of radioactive "hot" [226]Radium ([226]Ra) sources into the uterine cavity was the first method of radiation treatment for endometrial carcinoma. Later, afterloading devices were developed to protect the medical personnel from unnecessary radiation exposure and to improve the dose distribution from these radioactive sources. In recent years, high-dose radiation has been applied to treat endometrial carcinoma, using applicators designed for cervix cancer.

The dose of intrauterine radiation can be measured by multiplying the number of milligrams radium (or equivalents) by the time of exposure in hours (mg-Hr). Alternatively, radiation dose can be expressed in gamma radiation equivalents at specified anatomic points, relative to the radiation source (e.g., cGy/hour to point A). Today, computerized calculations of isodose distribution curves provide a fairly accurate measure in centigrade/hour for all commercially available brachytherapy devices. This permits the calculation of total radiation (intracavitary and external) delivered to any point within the three-dimensional field of radiation. The International Commission on Radiation Units and Measurements (ICRU) recommended the concept of "reference volume" to report intracavitary therapy.[51] Reference volume describes the three-dimensional volume at which the total absorbed radiation dose (intracavitary and external) has a fixed value. In an individual patient treated with a standard application of low dose intracavitary radiation and external beam radiation, the isodose curve of 6000 cGy would define the reference volume as recommended by the ICRU. In this chapter, we will use mg-hrs of radium (or their equivalent) to describe doses used for intracavitary radiation and gamma radiation equivalents in cGy for doses delivered to the vaginal surface.

Intrauterine Applicators

Heyman capsules are small metallic or plastic cylinders of varying diameter, each containing 5–10 mg radium. The size of capsules are chosen to allow an insertion of 10 to 15 capsules depending on the size of the uterine cavity. Since then, intrauterine afterloading devices have been developed (Simon capsules) which are 2–3 cm long and 6–10 mm in diameter. After computerized calculation of dose requirements, small ^{137}Cesium (^{137}Cs) sources, with an equivalent of

14–19 mg radium, are inserted into the empty shells in a shielded environment. The disadvantage of these afterloading tubes is the increased size and stiffness, reducing the probability of achieving optimal placement with the uterine cavity.

The major benefit from Heyman packings can be expected when the uterine cavity is enlarged and/or distorted by tumor. Capsules are used to stretch the cavity to place the highest possible number of capsules in closest proximity to the tumor. Stretching the uterine cavity reduces the thickness of neoplastic tissue that needs to be irradiated. However, serious complications, such as uterine perforation, can occur. When perforation occurs, external radiotherapy is given instead of intracavitary. The use of small capsules is advocated to better cover the tumor and to reduce the risk of uterine rupture. Placing Heyman capsules requires skill and experience. When the uterine cavity is small, uterine tandems should be used. Usual doses range from 2000 to 6000 mg-hrs. Most of the authors recommend two applications of 2500–3000 mg-hrs of intrauterine radium equivalent, given 2 to 3 weeks apart. When a hysterectomy is not contemplated, a third application is indicated.

When the uterine cavity is small and no gross irregularities are observed within the cavity, Heyman packings offer little or no advantages over the tandem used for cervical carcinoma. The number of radiation sources is similar with either technique. The tandem is loaded with three sources of 20–15–10 mg radium. Uterine tandems offer the advantage of radiating the lower part of the uterus and endocervix, and they prevent excessive anteflexion or retroflexion of the uterus, avoiding excessive radiation to the bladder or rectosigmoid.

Vaginal Applicators

Vaginal brachytherapy, which has been considered an important part of preoperative or postoperative radiotherapy in preventing vaginal vault recurrence, is performed with ovoids. The ovoids are placed lateral on each side into the vaginal fornix or with centrally placed small cylinders. Intrauterine and vaginal applicators are usually placed simultaneously. If the vagina is narrow, vaginal radiation may be done only once between intrauterine applications. In either case, it is important to distend the vagina to the maximum capacity. This is achieved by choosing the most appropriate applicators and individual spacers. In patients with tumors in the lower vagina, vaginal brachytherapy can be extended by placing radioactive sources into the lower segments of a vaginal cylinder. The total surface dose of vaginal brachytherapy should be approximately 7000–8000 cGy, given in divided doses at the time of intrauterine therapy, or 7000 cGy in case of a single application, delivered between the two intrauterine treatments.

Afterloading Systems

To irradiate the uterine cavity, lower uterine segment, endocervix, and vagina more adequately and to minimize personnel exposure to radiation, the old "hot" brachytherapy techniques have been improved with the development of a variety of afterloading systems. These systems allow the placement of unloaded applicator shells in the operating room and perform computerized dose calculations before the insertion of the "hot" radiation sources in a shielded room. During the last 20 years, the classic "hot" radium or cesium applicators have been replaced with low and medium-dose (radium or cesium) or high-dose (cobalt or iridium) afterloading techniques.

Low-Dose Brachytherapy

The rigid afterloading uterine tandem described by Fletcher for cervical cancer offers the advantage of reducing the uterine flexion almost automatically.[33] This tandem can be used in combination with the Heyman capsules and vaginal colpostats to irradiate the endocervix and paracervical area. Standard loading of the tandem uses 5-5-15 to 10-10-15 mg radium or cesium. Afterloading radium therapy can also be delivered to the vaginal vault with a colpostat or with afterloading vaginal cylinders. The size of colpostats is chosen to stretch the vaginal fornix and minimize the radiation dose delivered to the mucosa of bladder and rectum. The basic loading is 15, 20, and 25 mg radium into colpostats of 2, 2.5, and 3 cm diameters, respectively. It is possible to use colpostats of different size for each side, if one of the fornixes is obliterated. The size of the colpostats can also be changed when there is evidence of vaginal vault shrinkage during therapy.

High-Dose Brachytherapy

Recently, high-dose remote afterloading methods have been developed to deliver cobalt or iridium into the uterine cavity and vagina. The high-dose afterloading techniques allow individualization of radiation dose delivered to the uterus and vagina by adjusting the transit time of high-intensity radiation sources through the applicator shell. Radiation is delivered by moving a long train, of up to nine small ^{60}Co sources, together with a short train of two ^{60}Co sources through small tubes placed into the uterus and upper vagina. The uterine tube is placed centrally and up into the uterine fundus, creating a bulb-shaped isodose curve, which corresponds to the shape of the uterus. This bulb-shaped curve may be increased in width by prolonging the treatment time with the short train. With this technique, a safe daily fraction dose of 5–8 Gy for 5–6 fractions in one week is recommended.[115, 116] Tumor control with this new method, used as preoperative or postoperative radiotherapy, appears comparable with low-dose radiation. However, further studies are necessary to define the advantages of this method in comparison with the previously described techniques. Benefits include lack of RT-exposure to personnel and short duration of treatment, making this a safe outpatient procedure. Side effects (i.e., vaginal fibrosis and shortening) with increased incidence of dyspareunia have been described.

Intraperitoneal Radiation

The role of intraperitoneal radiation (ip RT) in the management of endometrial cancer patients is still unclear. Radioactive phosphorus (P-32), a pure beta-ray emitter, is currently used. The effect of radiation is limited to the superficial 2 mm of the tissue surface. The technique utilized for intraperitoneal P-32 is the same as that used for ovarian carcinoma. The available data suggest that it is a safe treatment when used alone; however, severe complications may occur when combined with pelvic radiation.[117] The main indication for ip P-32 is malignant peritoneal cytology, which will be discussed in detail below. The recommended treatment is a one-time instillation of 15–20 mCi P-32 radiocolloid, in 500 to 1000 mL normal saline, into the peritoneal cavity. To ensure optimal distribution of the radioactive material, a diagnostic abdominal scintigram is recommended before therapy, and the patient must be turned from side to side, and head to toe, after instillation of the radiocolloid solution.

Specific Treatment Recommendations

Radiotherapy is frequently combined with surgery for the treatment of endometrial cancer. It can be given pre- and/or postoperatively, depending on the therapeutic philosophy applied, or alone, if the patient is unable to undergo surgery.

The aim of preoperative irradiation is to shrink the tumor, reduce the risk of tumor spread during surgery, and prevent tumor recurrences. Arguments for preoperative radiation include the theoretical concept that the invasive tumor front is the most sensitive to irradiation, since it is well oxygenated and not necrotic. Occult fingers of the invasive cancer that are often the cause for recurrence may be treated by irradiation, while the central mass can be safely removed by surgery. In addition, the cytotoxic effects of radiation on tumor cells and the sealing of lymphatic and microvascular channels are considered important in preventing the spread and implantation of viable tumor cells in surgical wounds or distant sites at the time of operation. Preoperative irradiation is also considered advantageous, since blood supply is disrupted by surgery, possibly creating hypoxic areas that make the tumor less sensitive to irradiation. Arguments against preoperative radiation focus on the fact that a large number of patients with early disease are treated unnecessarily.

One of the most common indications for postoperative radiotherapy is the treatment of known or suspected local residual tumor after surgical resection of visible or microscopic disease. A major advantage of using postoperative RT is the possibility of selecting patients with a high risk for recurrences, based on accurate histopathological assessment of tumor extent and metastatic spread through surgical staging, thus avoiding radiating in patients with a low risk for recurrences. In addition, by individually tailoring the field and type of radiation to the location of disease spread for each patient, undertreatment is avoided.

Patients with major medical problems, which may prevent surgery, can be treated with external and/or intracavitary radiation only, however, the probability for cure is significantly reduced compared to a combination of radiation and surgery. Persistent intrauterine disease after radiation is the most common reason for treatment failure. This is possibly related to tumor volume and hypoxia.

This section will discuss radiation therapy recommendations, stage by stage, starting with pre- and postoperative RT, followed by RT without surgery.

Stage I

The optimal treatment method for stage I endometrial carcinoma has not been precisely defined. While the surgical approach of choice is total abdominal hysterectomy with bilateral salpingo-oophorectomy (TAH-BSO), the practice of combining surgery with irradiation still remains controversial. Most of the data collected in the past years have shown that indiscriminately combining surgery with radiation in stage I is not beneficial when compared with surgery alone. These data were reviewed by Jones in 1975.[54] In recent years, much attention has been focused on the importance of tumor grade and myometrial invasion of the lesions in regard to prognosis. This was not considered in Jones's paper. It has been clearly demonstrated that these factors correlate with incidence of lymph node metastasis, recurrence, and 5-year survival, as previously discussed in this chapter.

Many authors reported a decrease of local recurrence and longer 5-year survival rates combining surgery with radiation. Even authors who showed no difference in survival in patients treated with surgery alone compared to surgery and radiation, found a significantly lower incidence of local recurrence in patients treated with the combination.[1] A recent GOG study, which evaluated 895 patients with clinical stage I or occult stage II endometrial carcinoma, showed 7.4% vaginal and 16.8% pelvic recurrence among patients who received postoperative pelvic radiation and an incidence of 18.2% vaginal and 31.8% pelvic recurrence in patients treated with surgery alone.[82] Even if these data do not take other prognostic factors into consideration, it is interesting to note that the authors reported no recurrences in patients treated with vaginal implants, while vaginal recurrences were found in 7.4% of patients treated with external RT. When adjuvant therapy was delivered to patients with grade 2 lesions and more than one-third myometrial invasion, or with grade 3 lesions, the incidence of local/regional recurrence was 32.4%, while it was 48.4% in patients treated without adjuvant RT. Pelvic radiation did not reduce the incidence of recurrences in patients with grade 2 lesions and less than one-third of myometrial invasion. The potential benefits of RT may be offset by RT-related early and late complications (see below). In addition, patients who develop a pelvic recurrence after surgery will have a good chance of being cured with radiation (see below). No data are available comparing overall survival after postoperative radiation with delayed radiation for recurrent disease.

In our opinion, the primary modality of treatment for stage I is surgery. Due to the positive results obtained with this approach and the potential risk of complications from radiation, patients with low risk for vaginal or pelvic recurrence (surgical stages IA G1 – 2) should *not* be treated with adjuvant RT (Fig. **3**). Patients with intermediate risk (stages IA G3, IB G2 – 3) *may be* treated with adjuvant radiation, based on the patient's preference. The definition of intermediate risk, however, is not clear at this point. The GOG is currently conducting a prospective randomized study, comparing pelvic radiation (5040 cGY) with no postoperative therapy in intermediate-risk patients after surgical staging (GOG #99). Patients with surgical stages IB, IC, IIA – B, and all cell types and grades, except papillary, serous, and clear cell carcinoma are eligible.

Patients with a surgically defined high risk for treatment failure should be treated with individually tailored adjunctive therapy (Fig. **3**).

Lymph Node Metastasis

Patients with outer third myometrial invasion, metastases to pelvic lymph nodes, and/or other extrauterine sites constitute 98% of the cases with positive aortic nodes.[25] External radiation to the pelvic (4500 – 5000 cGY) and aortic (4500 cGy) region is recommended for these patients. Patients treated with postoperative pelvic- and aortic radiation had 5-year disease-free survival of 36%[82] and 5-year overall survival of 47%.[101]

Intraperitoneal Tumor Spread

Very little information is available regarding treatment results of this rare finding of histologically proven tumor in the peritonel cavity. Pelvic radiation, WAR, or systemic chemotherapy have been recommended. Pelvic radiation (5000 cGy) is indicated for disease limited to the pelvis and may be combined with chemo- and/or hormone therapy (see below). Primary chemotherapy or WAR is recommended for extrapelvic disease, depending on size and location of tumor growth. The use of WAR for disease of more than 1 cm appears unlikely to succeed.

Malignant Peritoneal Cytology

The role of peritoneal cytology as an independent prognostic factor has not been clearly determined.[45] In Heath's studys the prognosis of endometrial cancer with malignant cells in the peritoneal washing was worse then without malignant cells. In 1981, Creasman et al. reported a significant correlation of positive peritoneal washing with high-grade lesions, deep myometrial invasion, and pelvic or para-aortic lymph node involvement in patients with stage I endometrial cancer. In cases with negative peritoneal washing, the conventional prognostic factors predicted patient's outcome, however, good prognostic factors tended to be neutralized by positive washing.[23] Positive peritoneal washings have been found in about 11% of cases in stage I.[80] They are associated with other risk factors, such as grade (G1: 8.3% versus G3: 15.9%) and depth of invasion (deep: 7.6% versus superficial: 1.2%).[82] Patients with greater than one-third myometrial invasion have a 3-year disease-free survival of 30% and 87%, with and without positive peritoneal cytology, respectively. If malignant cytology was the *only* evidence of extrauterine disease in otherwise low-risk patients, no difference in survival was observed,[45, 55, 80] which is contrary to the observations made by Creasman et al.[23]

Intraperitoneal (ip) chromic phosphate P-32 was felt to be the appropriate therapy for patients with positive peritoneal cytology. Although ip RT appears to improve disease-free survival in clinical stage I patients with positive peritoneal cytology (68% vs. 27% 3-year disease-free survival), the disease-free survival for patients with less then one-third of myometrial invasion or grade 1 tumors is independent from peritoneal cytology.[45] Soper et al. reported a predicted disease-free survival beyond 24 months of 89% and 94% in patients with positive peritoneal washing with clinical and surgical stage I, respectively, treated with intraperitoneal P-32.[117] They observed no intra-abdominal recurrence in stage II and III patients treated with intraperitoneal P-32, even though the disease-free survival was still poor in this group. When intraperitoneal P-32 was used alone, intestinal morbidity requiring surgical intervention was not observed,[5, 117] but a combination of P-32 with external pelvic radiotherapy resulted in a 29% incidence of bowel complications, requiring surgical intervention.[117] It appears therefore prudent to treat patients with positive cytology and disease limited to the uterus with ip P-32, possibly in combination with hormone and/or chemotherapy, but not external radiation. Patients with other extrauterine diseases should receive external radiation, possibly WAR, and/or chemo/hormone therapy.

Myometrial Invasion

In the GOG study, 390 patients had myometrial invasion as the only risk factor (stages IB and IC). Of these, 49% received postoperative radiation (132 external, 58 vaginal cuff) in a nonrandomized fashion.[82] It is obvious that treatment selection was based on individual risk factors and physician preference: Patients with inner versus outer-third myometrial invasion received radiation in 44% versus 96%, respectively.[82] Nine of sixty patients (15%) with > one-third myometrial invasion and grade 2 or 3 lesions recurred after external radiation, in contrast to three of ten (30%) who received no adjunctive therapy, and none of five who received vaginal cuff radiation only. The benefit of external, compared with vaginal cuff radiation, is still uncertain in patients with stage I disease. Piver reported no recurrence in patients with stage IB (grade 1–2) treated with vaginal cuff radiation, but 10% in patients with stage IB (grade 3) or IC disease treated with external radiation.[97] Again, these were not comparable risk populations. Future studies are needed to answer these questions. Until then, we recommend external beam radiation, including the upper vagina, for patients with stage IB grade 3 and all stage IC diseases. Intracavitary radiation to the vaginal cuff can also be considered.

Lymph–Vascular Space Invasion

Lymph–vascular space invasion is a significant risk factor for tumor spread and recurrence; however, its prognostic importance when present as the sole risk factor is not known.[34] Most clinicians recommend adjunctive external radiation for these patients.

Tumor Grade

Tumor grade and depth of invasion are the most important prognostic indicators in stage I disease. With our current knowledge, the treatment recommendations in Figure **3** appear to be most appropriate.

Cell Type

Certain cell types are known to be associated with high risk for recurrence, which is generally due to early metastatic spread. Papillary serous and clear cell adenocarcinomas warrant aggressive adjunctive therapy, even if the disease appears to be confined to the uterus.[2, 3, 69] Because of their tendency for distant spread, chemotherapy is recommended with or without radiation.

Cervix Involvement

Involvement of the cervix constitutes clinical stage II disease if diagnosed preoperatively and will be discussed below. Occult disease, found in the surgical specimen without obvious ectocervical involvement, is subdivided into surgical stages IIA and IIB, with glandular and stromal invasion, respectively (Table **3**). Endocervical involvement is associated with increased risk for lymph node metastasis, other high-risk factors, and treatment failure, and most patients reported have been treated with a combination of surgery and radiation. However, no information is available in regard to the prognostic significance in patients with surgical stage II, without extrauterine disease. Postoperative external, with or without intracavitary radiation, is recommended. If so treated, patients with stage IIA have a significant better prognosis compared with stage IIB disease, with most recurrence occurring at extrapelvic sites.[30]

Radiation without Surgery

Radiotherapy alone for stage I provides a 5-year disease free survival of only 52%.[108] These results do not compare well with surgery alone or surgery in combination with RT. Therefore, it is suggested that only cases with specific contra-indication for surgery should be treated with RT alone. It has been shown that combined external and intracavitary radiotherapy is superior to intracavity therapy alone in all stages, except for stage IA grade 1 disease, where intracavitary irradiation alone is acceptable for inoperable patients.[125] However, a recent report suggests that intracavitary radiation is adequate therapy for all inoperable patients with clinical stage IA or IB disease, irrespective of grade.[70] Giving a mean of 5500 mg-hrs with three Heyman packings, they report no differences in corrected 5-year survival between stages IA (76%) and IB (72%), but profound differences between grade 1 (77%), grade 2 (68%) and grade 3 (53%) tumors. Most of the recurrences reappeared in the uterus (12.9%) and the vagina (5.3%). The mean age of these 171 patients was 71 years, and their uncorrected survival for stages IA and IB was 46% and 30%, respectively. This report emphasizes the importance of reduced life expectancy in this patient population with advanced age and poor health, which rendered these patients inoperable to begin with. These aspects should be taken into serious considera-tion when planning treatment.

Stage II

In 1969, Boronow suggested that patients with clinical stage II should be treated with radiation followed by surgery.[15] Preoperative +/– post-operative radiation was the most accepted therapy for patients with stage II endometrial carcinoma at the majority of institutions. How-ever, the management of these patients has been the subject of controversy in recent years. In 1982, Onsrud reported that only 56% of patients classified preoperatively as stage II were actually confirmed histopathologically to have endo-cervical tumor involvement.[91] Authors who prefer postoperative to preoperative RT adjuvant treatment stress the importance of overstaging due to false positive endocervical curettage. Most reported studies have shown better results com-bining surgery with radiation than with surgery

or radiation alone.[7, 37, 40, 73] More aggressive treatment in these patients (in comparison with stage I patients), is justified because of 5-year survival rates of 59% vs. 74%, and an incidence of pelvic node metastasis of 37% vs. 10% in patients with cervical involvement, compared with patients without cervical involvement. Larson et al. recently reported no pelvic recurrences in 69 patients treated with combined therapy.[68] Other authors reported incidence of pelvic recurrence between 0% and 19% after combination therapy.[17, 61, 91, 102, 106, 120] Considering the very low incidence of cervical involvement and the good results achieved with preoperative radiotherapy, Trimble and Jones III treated patients with stage II endo-metrial carcinoma (without gross cervical in-volvement) with intrauterine tandem and vaginal ovoids, delivering 3000 rads at point A, followed by surgery after 24–48 hours. The 5-year survival rate was 76%.[142] They reported no increase of incidence of recurrence in these patients compared with those patients treated more aggressively with external pelvic and intra-cavitary radiation followed by surgery. Greven et al. have shown that postoperative radiation can achieve the same results as preoperative RT.[39] They reported a 5-year survival rate of 86.8% in a small group of patients with clinical stage II endometrial carcinoma treated with postopera-tive pelvic RT, with or without intravaginal RT, which is comparable to results obtained with preoperative RT.

In conclusion, there are three choices for treatment of clinical stage II endometrial cancer. The first method consists of radical hysterectomy and pelvic lymphadenectomy with adjunctive radiotherapy, if lymph nodes are positive. This aggressive treatment causes an incrased inci-dence of complication (bowel and bladder damage and edema of the legs) and therefore should be limited to clinical stage II with gross cervical involvement. The second choice, which was utilized the most in the past, is external pelvic radiation (4000–5000 cGY) followed by TAH-BSO. The third possibility, the treatment we prefer, is TAH-BSO with careful surgical staging, followed by individually tailored irradiation. Performing the surgery prior to radiation treat-ment allows the physician to differentiate clinical stage II from surgical stage II. We recommend postoperative radiotherapy in surgically con-firmed stage II (Fig. **3**). Radiation therapy without surgery should, as in stage I, be reserved only for inoperable patients.

Stage III and IV

The incidence of advanced stages of endometrial cancer is very low, with 8.1% of all cases being stage III and 3.9% stage IV.[95] The scarcity of this clinical entity makes experience in management limited; therefore, optimal treatment has not been defined. The primary treatment for advanced endometrial carcinoma has been radiotherapy followed by surgery. At the Division of Gynecologic Oncology of the University of Miami School of Medicine, we observed a 5-year survival in 17% of clinical stage III patients treated with surgery alone, 25% in patients treated with radiation alone, and 38% in the group treated with surgery in combination with radiation.[98] These results are in accordance with the literature, showing that radiation plays an important role in the management of clinical stage III disease. Five-year survival can be improved with surgery when the tumor is resectable. The role of radiotherapy in stage IV is palliative, directed to local control of symptomatic tumors. Radiation treatment is usually started with external beam irradiation, and if the tumor responds, intracavitary RT may offer an additional advantage. For this stage, treatment needs to be individualized. Hysterectomy should be part of the overall treatment plan whenever possible because of the high rate of persistent disease in the uterine cavity and the risk of uterine bleeding.

We believe that the therapeutic outcome of patients with stage III and IV endometrial carcinoma may be improved with the use of effective systemic therapy, such as hormone and chemotherapy (see below).

Radiation for Mesenchymal Tumors

Radiation therapy for uterine sarcomas has been used in a similar fashion as for endometrial carcinomas. The data on the benefit of either primary or postoperative pelvic radiation, however, are poor due to a lack of prospective studies.[6] Most patients in reported series are treated by physician discretion, frequently in combination with chemotherapy. Recurrence rates are high, even in disease that appears confined to the uterus. Most recurrences occur in the abdominal cavity and

the lung. Only less than 25% occur in the pelvis. A review of the literature by Hannigan et al. of Stage I–II CS suggests an overall reduction of pelvic recurrences from 34% to 16% with pelvic radiation.[44] In a prospective GOG study on stage I–II uterine sarcoma, pelvic radiation reduced pelvic recurrence only in heterologous CS (29% vs. 16%) and LMS (17% vs. 0%), but the overall recurrence rates were 65% vs. 61% for CS and 70% vs. 77% for LMS, respectively.[74] Adjuvant chemotherapy did not seem to influence treatment results. Most patients died with widespread disease. It must be assumed that the observed differences in treatment outcome are more likely a reflection of differences in patient disease extent than the result of treatment. Spanos et al. reported no intra-abdominal recurrence after whole abdominal radiation in five patients with pathologic evidence of disease in the upper abdomen, suggesting that WAR may be of benefit in selected cases.[119]

Management of Complications

Side effects of radiation, including serious complications, are related to the dose and the field of radiation, as well as the age and medical condition of the patient. Increasing age, obesity, chronic illness, such as diabetes mellitus or arteriosclerosis, and previous abdominal surgery increase the risk for radiation complications. Most data in the gynecological literature on radiation complications are based on patients radiated for cervical carcinoma using standard external and low-dose intracavitary radiation. These may not apply to the generally older patients with endometrial cancer. High-dose radiation is another variable that is not well tested in this patient population. Complications of radiation treatment may develop during or after treatment. Acute complications that occur during treatment are usually less severe and are medically treatable. Only rarely is it necessary to interrupt treatment. Posttreatment complications generally occur within 2 years after irradiation, sometimes requiring surgical intervention.

Radiation complications in stage I patients treated with external radiotherapy are lower if only vaginal irradiation is delivered, compared with vaginal and pelvic radiation. In a series of 605 patients treated with vaginal or vaginal plus pelvic external irradiation, complications were observed in 7.4% and 15.6%, respectively.[50]

Serious complications after external postoperative radiotherapy were observed in 4–6.5% of the cases.[76, 141] In the GOG study on stage I and occult stage II (previously mentioned), complications were observed in 4.2% of the cases treated with postoperative intracavitary only and in 37.8% of patients treated with external radiation. Most of these complications were mild; however, 13% had moderate complications requiring treatment interruption, and four had severe complications requiring surgery.[82]

In a reported series of 401 patients treated with preoperative intracavitary high-dose afterloading radiation, the incidence of early intestinal radiation reactions was 15.7%, while incidence of early bladder reactions was 2.2%. Late intestinal reactions were observed in 15.0% and late bladder reaction in 4.7% of the cases.[115] The same Swedish group reported complications requiring surgery in 6.6% of the cases.[114] In a series of 404 patients treated with postoperative vaginal irradiation with high-dose afterloading technique, the incidence of early radiation reactions was 30.9% and late reactions 15.8%. Serious complications were observed in 6.9%.[116] These data suggest that high-dose intracavitary radiation is associated with more early and late complications than with low-dose radiation.

The acute problems during treatment involve the small and large intestine and the bladder. During pelvic irradiation, diarrhea and abdominal cramps are frequent. A low-residue bland diet and symptomatic medical treatment are usually sufficient to alleviate the symptoms. If symptoms persist and are severe, radiation treatment should be temporarily ceased. When abdominal radiotherapy is delivered, anorexia, nausea, vomiting, and abdominal cramps are common. If low-residue diet and symptomatic therapy (antiemetic) do not eliminate severe symptoms, therapy should be temporarily suspended. Pelvic radiotherapy is also accompanied by bladder irritation. Urinary frequency, urgency, pain, and dysuria may be alleviated by antispastic treatment. Bacterial cystitis requires antibiotic therapy.

Posttreatment complications may involve the vaginal vault, the large and small bowel, and the bladder. Vaginal vault necrosis should be treated immediately to avoid severe complications, such as vesicovaginal, rectovaginal, and more rarely, enterovaginal fistulae. Vaginal douches with hydrogen peroxide or sodium hypochlorite solutions are often beneficial for relieving symptoms. The most common large-bowel complication is proctosigmoiditis. It usually responds well to steroid enemas, sedatives, and antidiarrheal medication. Persistent bleeding or uncontrollable severe rectal pain and tenesmus may, on rare occasion, require surgery. Surgery is required in the case of rectovaginal fistula or rectosigmoid obstruction. When surgery is required, the treatment of choice is usually diverting colostomy. Intra-abdominal large-bowel perforation after radiation is usually fatal and must be prevented. Early surgical intervention is advised.

Small-bowel complications usually present as bowel obstruction. The primary treatment of choice is conservative management with nasogastric suction and intravenous fluids, possibly hyperalimentation. If this fails, surgical exploration with lysis of adhesions, bypass at the level of obstruction, or bowel resection may be necessary. The concurrent presence of fever and ileus may herald a threatening bowel perforation. Under these circumstances, exploratory surgery must be performed as soon as possible to avoid more serious complications, such as peritonitis, which again carries a high mortality risk. Alternatively, the combination of fever and paralytic ileus may be the result of a pelvic or abdominal abscess. Ultrasonography or computerized tomography should be done. If an abscess is found, this may be drained percutaneously or transvaginally, under antibiotic coverage, avoiding surgery.

Bladder complications from radiation may be severe and difficult to manage. The most common severe bladder complication is hemorrhagic cystitis with bleeding. The initial treatment for hemorrhagic cystitis is elimination of bladder irritants from the diet, urine acidification, and bladder sedatives. If bacteria are present, urine culture and specific antibiotic therapy are indicated. Bladder irrigation with cold saline solution or diluted silver nitrate may control bleeding. When the bleeding does not cease and constant bladder irrigation is not beneficial, urinary diversion may be necessary. Radiation related vesicovaginal fistulas require surgical intervention, frequently urinary diversion. The absence of tumor should be demonstrated before selecting the surgical procedure.

Systemic Therapy

Endometrial Carcinomas

Endometrial cancer is characterized by early symptoms, therefore, most of the cases are diagnosed at early stages. The most effective treatments for these stages, as previously discussed in this chapter, are surgery with or without radiation. Therefore, only a limited number of patients are candidates for primary systemic therapy. Patients with advanced disease at the time of diagnosis, represent only 10–15% of the patients with endometrial cancer. However, most data on systemic therapy have been obtained in patients with recurrent disease. Most of the clinical trials are performed on a small number of patients. The heterogenous patient population in different studies makes it difficult to compare reports from different institutions. In early studies, no attempts were made to separate patients with advanced primary disease from those with recurrent disease or those receiving treatment as first-line regimen from those who had already been treated with chemotherapy. For practical purposes, we will discuss systemic therapy using hormones, single agent chemotherapy, combination chemotherapy, and hormone chemotherapy combinations, in sequence.

Hormone Therapy

Most of the endometrial cancers present as adenocarcinoma, which is considered a hormone sensitive tumor. The ethiopathology of endo-

metrial cancer has clearly shown that estrogens promote tumor cell growth,[31] while progestins and antiestrogens are useful drugs for the treatment of this disease.[127] The most significant historical study on hormone treatment of endometrial cancer with progestational agents was reported by Kelley in 1961.[59] Since then, numerous investigators have used progestins for treatment of advanced and recurrent disease. The most commonly used hormones are hydroxyprogesterone, megestrol, and medroxyprogesterone.

Most of the studies on advanced and recurrent cancer are of limited statistical value because of the small number of patients encountered. Hormone receptor status of the tumor plays an important role in defining response probability to progestin therapy, but has not always been analyzed. Table **8** shows the response rates of patients with endometrial cancer to hormone treatment in relation to progesterone receptor status. The overall response to progestin therapy is 32%. Hormone receptor positive tumors have response rates of 69% to progestins compared to 9% in receptor negative tumors (Table **8**). Since receptor expression is directly related to the grade of differentiation, a better response to progestins is also observed in well rather than in poorly differentiated tumors. However, progestin therapy does not appear dose related. One GOG study (GOG #81) showed the response to 200 mg/d medroxyprogesterone acetate to be slightly better than to 1000 mg/d in terms of progression-free interval at 2 months, with no further benefits later.[128] In summary,

Table **8** Hormone receptor status and response to progestin therapy	Investigation	Number of responses (%)			
		Regardless of receptor status	Receptor positive	Receptor negative	Ref.
	Martin '79	14/19 (74)	13/14 (93)	1/5 (20)	77
	McCarthy '79	4/13 (31)	4/5 (80)	0/8 (0)	79
	Bernaard '80	5/11 (46)	5/6 (83)	0/5 (0)	10
	Creasman '80	4/13 (31)	3/5 (60)	1/8 (12)	24
	Kauppila '82	4/19 (21)	2/3 (67)	2/16 (13)	58
	Pollow '83	9/22 (41)	9/9 (100)	0/13 (0)	100
	Quinn '85	3/20 (15)	3/7 (43)	0/13 (0)	104
	Thigpen '85	7/35 (20)	4/10 (40)	3/25 (12)	130
	Ehrlich '88	10/38 (26)	6/12 (50)	4/26 (15)	29
	Total	60/190 (32)	49/71 (69)	11/119 (9)	

progestins are indeed effective treatment in patients with endometrial cancer and should be considered first-line therapy in patients with progesterone receptor positive and well-differentiated tumors.

Tamoxifen, a partial estrogen agonist (considered by some authors an antiestrogen), has been used in several trials to treat patients with endometrial cancer. Although Bonte reported a response rate of 53%,[13] the average reported response rate is 18%.[103, 111, 124] The high response rate reported by Bonte is most likely related to the selection of patients. Most of them were previously responsive to progestin therapy and had well or moderately well-differentiated tumors.[13]

Besides medroxyprogesterone and tamoxifen, other hormone treatments have been used, such as hydroxyprogesterone caproate and megestrol acetate, with average response rates of 29% and 20%, respectively.[59, 64, 96, 99, 105] Gonadotropin-releasing hormone analogs have also been used to treat endometrial cancer.[35]

Recently, several investigators have used hormone combinations,[62, 126] but a clear advantage over conventional progestin therapy has not yet been demonstrated. Long-term use of progestins has been shown to reduce the progesterone receptor levels in tumor tissue. Based on in vivo laboratory evidence indicating that tamoxifen increases progesterone receptor levels in tumor tissue, the current GOG trial #119 evaluates the effects of tamoxifen 40 mg/d and intermittent Provera 200 mg/d, given every other week.

Single Agent Chemotherapy

The consideration of the high incidence of treatment failures in patients with advanced endometrial cancer, particularly when hormone receptor negative, has led to the investigation of several cytotoxic drugs during the last 20 years. At least 21 single agents have been used in clinical trials.[94] Doxorubicin, cisplatin, carboplatin, and 5-fluorouracil have been shown to be the most active drugs (Table **9**). Doxorubicin is presently considered the most active single agent, with response rates varying between 19% and 37%. The response to chemotherapy in patients with endometrial cancer decreases in those who received prior treatment. In the case of cisplatin, for example, the response rate in patients who

had previous chemotherapy is 4% compared to 20% in patients not previously treated with chemotherapy. The GOG is currently evaluating the effec of ifosfamide in combination with the uroprotector mesna and high-dose Paclitaxel with G-CSF.

Combination Chemotherapy

In recent years, the number of combination chemotherapy trials for patients with advanced and recurrent endometrial cancer has increased. Early studies have shown promising results. The three most effective single agents in gynecologic malignancies; doxorubicin, cisplatin, and cyclophosphamide have been used in combination (PAC) for endometrial carcinoma, showing in one of the largest prospective studies a response rate of 47%, but with only a 4.8 months median response duration (Table **9**). This study was not compared with single agent treatment.[18] The interpretation of reported treatment results is often difficult because most clinical trials include only a small number of patients and/or are done without a control group to compare single agent vs. combination treatment effects. One large phase III randomized trial on combination vs. single agent treatment (GOG # 48), evaluated the effect of doxorubicin 60 mg/m² vs. doxorubicin 60 mg/m² plus cyclophosphamide 500 mg/m² q 3 weeks × 8 courses in 202 patients with advanced primary or recurrent disease, who had failed to respond to hormone therapy. Although the drug combination showed a slightly higher response rate compared to doxorubicin alone (32% vs. 22%), survival in the two groups was not significantly different (7.6 vs. 6.8 months).[129]

Another randomized phase III GOG study (GOG # 107) compared the effect of doxorubicin 60 mg/m² vs. doxorubicin 60 mg/m² plus cisplatin 50 mg/m² every 3 weeks in patients with measurable disease.[139] Preliminary results of this study showed that the combination treatment is more effective in terms of response rate with a total of 45% responses (CR + PR) vs. 27% response in the single agent group. Progression-free interval and survival are still under analysis.[139]

Combination Hormone Chemotherapy

Chemotherapy has also been used in combination with hormone treatment. A randomized phase III GOG study evaluated the effect of megestrol acetate plus cyclophosphamide, doxo-rubicin, and 5-fluorouracil (M-CAF) vs. megestrol acetate plus melphalan and 5-fluorouracil (M-MF) in 155 patients.[21] In this study, the survival rates were similar in the two groups, 10.1 months for M-CAF vs. 10.6 months in M-MF. The response rate was 36% in the M-CAF group vs. 38% in the M-MF group. These results were not superior to doxorubicin therapy used as single agent. Table **9** summarizes two large randomized trials on combination chemotherapy plus hormones. Both studies showed that prior hormonal treatment did not influence the response and that the addition of hormones to combination chemotherapy does not seem to enhance response rates.[21, 49]

In conclusion, even though systemic therapy for advanced and recurrent adenocarcinoma of the endometrium is not highly effective, it is the only approach that offers some hope of clinical remission. Hormone therapy should always be considered first and is the treatment of choice in patients with hormone receptor positive and grade 1 or 2 tumors. High-risk patients, patients with hormone receptor negative tumor, or those who have failed hormone treatment are treated either with doxorubicin alone, or in combination with cisplatin. In consideration of the poor results obtained in terms of both remission of disease and disease-free survival, patients with advanced and recurrent adenocarcinoma of the endometrium should be entered in clinical trials whenever possible.

A current GOG study (GOG # 122) is evaluating the effect of WAR vs. cisplatin 50 mg/m^2 and doxorubicin 60 mg/m^2 in patients with advanced (stage III–IV) endometrial carcinoma with less than or up to 2 cm residual disease after surgery. Patients with measurable disease are eligible for GOG protocol # 139, which evaluates the effect of doxorubicin 60 mg/m^2, plus cisplatin 50 mg/m^2 given in the standard fashion vs. the circadian-timed sequence, which consists in delivering the doxorubicin at 6 o'clock AM and cisplatin at 6 o'clock PM.

Uterine Sarcomas

Uterine sarcomas are a heterogeneous group of rare diseases, that constitute less than 5% of all uterine neoplasm. Most of the treatment studies are nonrandomized and are performed on a small number of patients. This makes it difficult to analzye data and draw clear conclusions. The International Society of Gynecological Pathology has recently grouped these tumors into two main histopathological categories; carcinosarcomas (CS) and leiomyosarcoma (LMS), in an attempt to collect a higher number of patients with neoplasms with similar behavior and to better analyze the results. Although well-differentiated leiomyosarcomas, endometrial stromal sarcomas, and adenosarcomas have a relatively good prognosis, the overall recurrence rate for uterine sarcomas is above 50% including early stages. The high recurrence rate and the fre-

Table **9** Systemic treatment for endometrial carcinoma

Author	Drug(s)	No. of pts.	Prior chemo.	Response (%)	Ref.
Carbone PP '74	F	34	?	21	19
Horton J '78	A	21	no	19	48
Thigpen JT '79 (GOG)	A	43	no	37	138
Long HJ '88	Cp	26	no	27	72
Thigpen JT '84 (GOG)	P	25	yes	4	135
Thigpen JT '89 (GOG)	P	49	no	20	131
Trope C '84	PA	20	no	60	143
Thigpen '85 (GOG)	CA/A	202	no	32/22	129
Burke TW '91	PAC	102	no	47	18
Thigpen '93 (GOG)	PA/A	223	no	45/27	139
Horton J '82	m-CA/m-CAF	114	no	27/16	49
Cohen C '84 (GOG)	m-CAF/m-MF	155	no	36/38	21

A = doxorubicin; C = cyclophosphamide; Cp = carboplatin; F = 5FU; M = melphalan;
m = megestrol Acetate; P = cisplatin.

quency of distant metastasis make these tumors candidates for systemic therapy. Most of the data reported so far in the literature refer to the category of pure nonepithelial tumors as leiomyosarcomas (LMS) and for the category of the mixed epithelial–nonepithelial tumors to mixed mesodermal sarcomas (MMT) or carcinosarcomas (CS).

Hormone Therapy

Hormone receptor status was also evaluated in uterine sarcomas. Although Soper et al. have found the highest receptor level in MMT,[118] most studies have shown that ESS has the highest estrogen receptor and progesterone receptor content.[104,123,145] However, hormone therapy has not been studied extensively in uterine sarcomas. Except for ESS, reponse to hormone therapy in sarcomas has been poor, and does not seem to correlate with hormone receptor status.[145]

Early Disease

Although recurrence rates in early stages are considerably high in uterine sarcomas, as previously discussed, there is little experience with adjuvant systemic therapy for these conditions. The most representative study is a randomized GOG trial that evaluated the effect of doxorubicin vs. no further therapy in patients (with stage I and II sarcoma, with no residual disease after surgery.[89] This study showed no statistically significant difference in the two arms in regard to overall disease-free interval, recurrence rate or survival. However, patients who received adjuvant chemotherapy, had lower recurrence rates (41 % vs. 53 %) and longer median survival (74 vs. 55 months) then patients without further therapy. Recurrence rate in patients with leiomyosarcoma was 44 % (11/25 patients) in the chemotherapy arm, vs. 61 % (14/23 patients) in the no-further-therapy arm, and in patients with mixed mesodermal sarcoma 39 % (17/44 patients) vs. 51 % (25/49 patients), respectively. Other trials[107] have shown that adjuvant chemotherapy does not reduce the incidence of recurrences in patients with limited disease. However, they all suffer from the low number of patients included in these trials.

Advanced Disease

Several trials have shown that chemotherapy is effective in primary, advanced, and recurrent uterine sarcoma. Most of the clinical trials do not differentiate between these two groups of patients, and they will be discussed together in this chapter. There seems to be a difference in chemotherapy response between carcinosarcomas and pure sarcomas.

Single-Agent Chemotherapy

Ifosfamide and cisplatin are the most active single agents used to treat carcinosarcomas (Table **10**). Ifosfamide, given with the uroprotector mesna, is considered the most active single agent. Cisplatin has similar activity when used as

Table **10** Systemic therapy for uterine sarcomas: single agents

Author	Drug	Schedule	No. of pats.	Prior chemo.	Response (%)	Ref.
a) carcinosarcomas						
Omura GA '83 (GOG)	Doxo	60 mg/m^2 q3w	41	no	10	90
Thigpen JT '86 (GOG)	DDP	50 mg/m^2 q3w	28	yes	18	136
Sutton GP '89 (GOG)	Ifos./mesna	1.5 gm/m^2/d q4w	28	yes	32	122
Thigpen JT '91 (GOG)	DDP	50 mg/m^2 q3w	63	no	19	133
b) leiomyosarcomas						
Omura GA '83 (GOG)	Doxo	60 mg/m^2 q3w	28	no	25	90
Thigpen JT '86 (GOG)	DDP	50 mg/m^2 q3w	19	yes	5	137
Sutton GP '90 (GOG)	Ifos./mesna	1.5 gm/m^2/d q4w	28	no	14	121
Thigpen JT '91 (GOG)	DDP	50 mg/m^2 q3w	33	no	3	133

Table **11** Systemic treatment for uterine sarcomas: combination therapy

Author	Treatment	No of pts.	Response (%)	Ref.
a) carcinosarcomas				
Hanningan EV '83	Vinc + Act-D + CYT	35	26	43
Omura GA '83 (GOG)	Doxo + DTIC	31	23	90
Muss HB '85 (GOG)	Doxo +/– CTX	20	25	85
Baker TR '91	DDP + Doxo + DTCI	6	33	9
Sutton GP '93 (GOG)	Doxo + Ifosf./mesna	27	37	122
b) leiomyosarcomas				
Omura GA '83 (GOG)	Doxo + DTIC	20	30	90
Muss HB '85 (GOG)	Doxo +/– CTX	23	13	85

first and second-line chemotherapy. Doxorubicin, etoposide, mitoxantrone, and piperazinedione have little or no activity in these tumors, with response rates varying from 0% to 10%.[36, 84, 90, 113, 134]

The most effective single agent chemotherapy in leiomyosarcomas is doxorubicin (Table **10**). One arm of a phase III clinical study evaluating the effect of doxorubicin as single agent at 60 mg/m^2 every 3 weeks, compared to a combination of doxorubicin and DTIC (Table **11**), resulted in a total of seven (25%) responses among 28 patients with advanced or recurrent leiomyosarcoma.[90] Other single agents such as ifosfamide, cisplatin, etoposide, mitoxantrone, and piperazinedione have shown minimal activity with response rate between 0% and 14%.[84, 112, 121, 133, 134, 136] In leiomyosarcomas, the effect of cisplatin shows poor results when given as first or second-line chemotherapy.[137]

Combination Chemotherapy

Combination chemotherapy for the treatment of uterine sarcomas has been evaluated with phase III randomized trials to compare standard treatment with new regimens. Leiomyosarcomas respond better to doxorubicin, while the most active agents for carcinosarcomas are ifosfamide and cisplatin. Therefore, prospective clinical studies should differentiate between these histological types of sarcoma. The two GOG phase III studies conducted on combination chemotherapy failled to show a significant difference between doxorubicin vs. multiple agents regimen (Table **11**). The first of such studies evaluated the effect of doxorubicin vs. doxorubicin plus dimethyl triazininoimidazole

carboxamide (DTIC) in advanced and recurrent uterine sarcomas.[90] Although this study showed that mixed mesodermal sarcomas are slightly more sensitive to combination treatment than to single agent, with a response rate of 23% vs. 10%, this discrepency was not significantly different. The two arms had similar effects on leiomyosarcomas (25% vs. 30%). The second GOG study (GOG #42) evaluated the effect of doxorubicin vs. doxorubicin plus cyclophosphamide in advanced and recurrent uterine sarcomas.[85] This study failed to show a difference in response rates between the two regimens. Cell type did not influence response rate, progression-free interval, or survival.

The preliminary results of the GOG study # 87 F, which evaluated the effect of ifosfamide 5.0 g/m^2/24 hrs plus MESNA 6.0 g/m^2/36 hrs plus doxorubicin 50 mg/m^2 q 3 wks in patients with LMS, showed an overall respone rate of 37%, but the toxicity of this regimen was severe.[122] Table **11** summarizes several studies on combination chemotherapy for carcinosarcomas, but the lack of randomization and the limited number of patients make the interpretation of such studies difficult. Currently, GOG protocol # 108 is studying ifosfamide and MESNA with or without cisplatin in advanced and recurrent carcinosarcoma.

Follow-up Management

The objectives of patient management after completed treatment for endometrial cancer are early detection of recurrent disease, management of treatment related complications (see pages 49, 50), and prevention of other events that may reduce length and/or quality of life, including general medical and psychological support of these elderly patients. Estrogen replacement therapy is one important issue in this context and will be discussed below.

Detection of Tumor Recurrence

Overall, about 33% of all patients treated for endometrial cancer will die within 5 years from recurrent cancer and intercurrent diseases.[95] Risk factors for disease recurrence were discussed in detail in the section on staging and surgical procedures. Most recurrences are diagnosed within 2 years after diagnosis, and less then 10% after 5 years. The time of recurrence is inversely related to the stage of disease.[1] Half of the recurrences occur in the pelvis and vagina. The other half occur either as distant or as combined pelvic and distant recurrences. The site of first recurrence depends to a certain extent on the histology of the tumor, disease extent, and whether the patient was treated with or without pelvic radiation. Preferred sites of recurrence are the vagina, pelvis, abdomen, lung, liver, and bone. Symptoms of recurrent endometrial cancer include vaginal bleeding (30%), pelvic pain (15%), and a variety of other complaints; however, more then 33% of patients are asymptomatic. Efforts to detect recurrent disease should focus on the first 2 years, and be more intense in patients with increased risk factors. Recommended follow-up procedures in the asymptomatic patient are summarized in Table **12**. Repeated, careful, general physical and pelvic exam and PAP smear from the upper and lower vagina are most important. Chest X-ray and IVP have traditionally been used to detect pulmonary and pelvic recurrences. However, detection of pelvic and/or abdominal disease is difficult and may warrant repeated CT-scans of pelvis and abdomen with contrast studies of the upper GI and urinary tract. Close monitoring of blood chemistry, including liver function studies and tumor markers, such as Ca 125, may help identify patients who harbor subclinical disease.[86] Ca 125 may be elevated in patients with endometrial carcinoma in up to 60% of the cases, and therefore may be a useful marker for the diagnosis and treatment of recurrent disease. Patients treated only with radiotherapy may undergo endometrial biopsy or curettage 3 and 12 months after completion of therapy to detect persistent intrauterine disease.

Hormone Replacement Therapy

During the last 10 years, hormone replacement therapy (HRT) has been recommended in menopausal women. Numerous controlled clinical trials have shown that HRT prevents postmenopausal osteoporosis to a certain extent. Estrogens also lower low-density lipoproteins (LDL) and raise the level of high-density lipoproteins (HDL), which leads to a reduction of cardiovascular disease and related deaths in patients who take estrogens after menopause. HRT is also commonly used to relieve other menopausal symptoms, such as atrophy and dryness of vagina and skin, as well as vasomotor symptoms such as hot flushes.

Since endometrial cancer is a well-known hormone-sensitive tumor, HRT in patients with endometrial cancer has been controversial for the last several years. Unfortunately, we don't have sufficient data to offer a clear recommendation. The patient must be informed concerning risks and benefits of HRT to enable her to make a decision.

Table **12**   Endometrial carcinoma: Follow-up procedures after therapy

	1–2 years	3–5 years	> 5 years
Exam + PAP	q. 3 months	q. 6 months	q. 12 months
Chest X-ray	q. 6 months	q. 12 months	PRN*
IVP or CT-scan	q. 12 months	PRN*	PRN*
Tumor marker	q. 3 months	q. 6 months	q. 12 months
Blood chemistry	q. 3 months	q. 6 months	q. 12 months

* When indicated.

The ACOG Committee Opinion,[4] of August 1993 states that HRT can be safely used in patients with a history of endometrial cancer that are presently free of disease, but the patient need to be informed of the possible risk of early recurrence. The prognostic factors of endometrial cancer, discussed early in this chapter, are an integral part of patient counseling. HRT may enhance tumor growth in any patients with endometrial cancer. HRT may be considered even in high risk patients, especially if the patient considers the benefits of the amelioration of postmenopausal symptoms more important than the risk of tumor growth stimulation. Since estrogens may enhance growth of hormone dependent tumors, they should be given in combination with progestins to patients at risk for endometrial cancer.

Recurrent Disease

Because there is a high cure rate for patients with endometrial carcinoma, this neoplasm has been considered a "benign malignancy." Therefore, treatment modalities for recurrent disease have tended to evolve slowly. Nevertheless, the overall recurrence rate is about 33%.[95] The treatment for recurrent endometrial cancer must be individualized, based on the site and size of recurrence. Previous therapy plays an important role in the choice of treatment. Surgery, radiotherapy, hormone-, and/or chemotherapy may be used alone, or in combination, depending on the characteristics of the lesion. In this section, we will discuss treatment options that generally apply to both carcinomas and sarcomas. For systemic therapy modalities, we refer to the section on systemic therapy, which covers both advanced primary and recurrent disease.

▦ Diagnostic and Surgical Procedures

For practical reasons, we seperate different sites of recurrence, pelvic (uterus, vagina, pelvis) from distant (abdomen, lung, liver, etc.), as well as patients previously treated with or without radiation. Since combined pelvic and distant metastases are common, a complete metastatic workup to define the precise disease extent should precede any treatment selection.

Persistent disease inside the uterine cavity in patients treated with pelvic radiation alone, is either symptomatic (vaginal bleeding) or diagnosed by PAP smear and/or endometrial biopsy. Some of these patients, who were at the time of primary therapy not thought to be candidates for abdominal hysterectomy, could well be candidates for vaginal hysterectomy as a potential curative procedure. Preoperatively, metastatic disease beyond the uterus needs to be ruled out with pelvic–abdominal CT-scan and chest X-ray.

Most *vaginal recurrences* are symptomatic (vaginal bleeding) or detected by exfoliate cytology and/or palpation. A biopsy should be taken to confirm the diagnosis. Patients who previously did not receive radiation are candidates for potentially curative radiation. Patients who had only vaginal vault radiation may be candidates for additional external pelvic and intercavitary radiation. Patients with superficial vaginal recurrence may be treated with wide surgical excision, including a partial or total vaginectomy. However, the risk of an incomplete tumor resection is considerable. Selected patients with a central pelvic recurrence may be candidates for pelvic exenteration, as described for cancer of the cervix. The absence of pelvic side-wall involvement and extrapelvic disease needs to be confirmed with a thorough metastatic workup. Patient selection in regard to operability is imperative for this ultraradical surgical therapy. However, since it offers the possibility for cure, it should be considered even in this elderly patient population.

Pelvic recurrences, not involving the vaginal mucosa are usually diagnosed by pelvic examination or routine X-rays (CT-scan, IVP). Pelvic pain, ureteral obstruction, leg edema, rectal bleeding, and small-bowel obstruction may all indicate the presence of pelvic recurrence. However, radiation-related complications may present similar symptoms. A careful metastatic workup is necessary to define the presence and the extent of the disease. Transvaginal or abdominal fine needle aspiration cytology, which can be done with ultrasound or CT guidance, may provide morphologic confirmation of recurrent disease, avoiding exploratory surgery.[109] Patients not previously treated with radiation are candidates for curative therapy with radiation. Patients with bulky disease, which may be too large to be cured with radiation alone, may benefit from surgical debulking prior to radiation. If disease appears unresectable or the patient is not suited for surgery, a combination of radiation and chemohormone therapy may provide optimal palliation, however the likelyhood for cure is small. Patients already treated with radiation may benefit from systemic therapy for palliation. Cytoreductive surgery, as described for ovarian carcinoma; does not seem to improve the overall poor prognosis.

Distant metastases to the upper abdomen, liver, and lung are only amenable to palliative sytemic therapy as discussed in the section on Systemic Therapy, whereby histology and receptor status of the tumor provide the basic guidelines for drug selection. Locoregional radiation may be considered in selected cases for alleviation of pain.

▓ Radiation Therapy

Aggressive radiation therapy is the treatment of choice in previously unradiated patients with vaginal and/or pelvic recurrence. In resectable lesions, radiotherapy may be combined with surgery. Some investigators have observed higher cure rates in apical vaginal lesions compared with distal vaginal lesions.[1] Radiotherapy in patients with locoregional recurrence may be applied as intracavitary or interstitial implants when the lesion is small. Large vaginal vault lesions are best treated with the whole pelvis, followed by intracavitary radiation. Radiation dosimetry should be individualized depending on the size and location of the recurrent tumor. If surgical tumor debulking is considered, radiation therapy may be given as intraoperative, interstitial and/or postoperative radiation. A variety of hot and afterloading interstitial radiation sources are currently available. Careful treatment planning before surgery should be done jointly with the radiation oncologist to optimally prepare for such a highly individualized treatment plan.

▓ Systemic Therapy

The reader is referred to pages 51–55, in which hormone and chemotherapy for advanced primary and recurrent uterine carcinomas and sarcomas are discussed.

Research

▓ Clinical Studies

Validity of new FIGO staging system: Several recent studies support the understanding that surgical is superior to clinical staging.[75] The added procedures required for surgical staging seem to only minimally increase perioperative morbidity.[92] Equivalencies of risk factors, however, need to be further defined. Stage III A, which equates adnexal tumor involvement with positive peritoneal cytology, is one example. Another issue is the assignment of surgical stage based on uterine pathology itself, without performing a diagnostic pelvic and aortic node dissection.[147]

Radicality of surgery: A host of issues must be further studied, addressing the issue of optimal surgery in this generally elderly patient population. "Too much" as well as a "too little" surgical intervention raises questions regarding the need for pelvic and PAND node dissection and vaginal cuff resection in the low-risk patient, the number of nodes removed, the radicality of the parametrial resection in stage II disease, and also the value of tumor debulking in patients with abdominal metastases. On the conservative side, the adequacy of vaginal and laparoscopic assited surgical staging (LASS) with vaginal hysterectomy (LAVH) needs to be studied further.[20]

Adjunctive postoperative therapy for intermediate-risk carcinoma with external pelvic and/or vaginal radiation is currently under investigation. Future data will possibly assist the clinician in the management of these patients. Optimal postoperative therapy of advanced (stage III–IV) carcinoma and sarcoma has not yet been defined and requires further study.

Tumor markers: Ca125 has been reported to be elevated in 78% of patients with advanced and recurrent endometrial carcinoma, but negative in almost 100% of stage I–II disease.[86] The value of monitoring Ca125 values during therapy of metastatic disease must be investigated.

▓ Prognostic Factors

A variety of factors have been studied on tumor tissues that relate to metastatic potential and prognosis. In addition to nuclear estrogen and progesterone receptors,[56] epidermal growth factor receptors,[144] proliferation markers,[149] and a variety of oncogens[42, 140] have been identified as being related to the degree of malignant alteration, disease progression, and survival. DNA aneuploidy and rate of cell proliferation, studied either by flow cytometry, morphometry, or immunohistochemisty, all support the current understanding that aneuploid tumors and those with a high fraction of proliferating cells have histologically undifferentiated tumors, advanced disease in regards to depth of invasion, metastatic spread, and poor prognosis. This has been shown for endometrial carcinomas and sarcomas.[55, 147, 148] Interrelation between these different markers is usually quite good, but at this point it is difficult to say whether one factor is more significant than the others. Multivariate analyses, comparing these factors simultaneously, need to be done to answer these questions.

Laboratory Studies

Prediction of chemotherapy response by in vitro testing may help drug selection in patients with advanced primary and recurrent uterine neoplasms, such as in ovarian and breast cancer.[63, 110] Radiation sensitivity and the effect of treatment combinations (chemohormone, chemoradiation, etc.) can be tested and may aid individualization of combination therapy for these patients. Preliminary data, for instance, suggest that combination hormone chemotherapy is only advantageous in receptor-positive tumors that have only partial sensitivity to chemotherapy, while the cytostatic effect of progesterone does not increase overall cell kill in highly sensitive tumors.[88] Whether genetherapy with oligonucleotides[53] can be translated into clinical practice still needs to be shown. However, it is this kind of preclinical resarch on cell lines and fresh tumor tissue that may lead to novel treatment modalities in the future.

References

1. Aalders JG, Abeler V, Kolstad P. Recurrent adenocarcinoma of the endometrium: a clinical and histopathological study of 379 patients. Gynecol Oncol. 1984; 17:85–103.
2. Abeler VM, Kjorstad KE. Serous papillary carcinoma of the endometrium: a histopathological study of 22 cases. Gynecol Oncol. 1990; 39:266–271.
3. Abeler VM, Kjorstad KE. Clear cell carcinoma of the endometrium: a histopathological and clinial study of 97 cases. Gynecol Oncol. 1991; 40:207–217.
4. ACOG Committee Opinion. Estrogen replacement therapy and endometrial cancer. ACOG committee on Gynecologic practice; 1993; August 126.
5. Alderman SJ, Dillon TF, Krummerman MS. Postoperative use of radioactive phosphorus in Stage I ovarian carcinoma. Obstet Gynecol. 1977; 49:659–662.
6. Alì S, Wells M. Mixed mullerian tumors of the uterine corpus: a review. Int J Gynecol Cancer. 1993; 3:1–11.
7. Andersen ES. Stage II endometrial carcinoma: prognostic factors and the results of treatment. Gynecol Oncol. 1990; 38:220–223.
8. Arneson A. Clinical results and histologic changes following the radiation treatment of cancer of the corpus uteri. Am J Roentgenol. 1936; 36:461–476.
9. Baker TR, Piver S, Calgar H, Piedmonte M. Prospective trial of cisplatin, adriamycin, and dacarbazine in metastatic mixed mesodermal sarcomas of the uterus and ovary. Am J Oncol. 1991; 14:246–250.
10. Bernaard TJ, Friberg LG, Koenders AJM, Kullander S. Do estrogen and progesterone receptors (ER and PR) in metastasizing endometrial cancer predict the response to gestagen therapy? Acta Obstet Gynecol Scand. 1980; 59:155–159.
11. Bloss JD, Berman ML, Bloss LP, Buller RE. Use of vaginal hysterectomy for the management of stage I endometrial cancer in the medically compromised patient. Gynecol Oncol. 1991; 40:74–77.
12. Bokhman IV. Two pathogenetic types of endometrial carcinoma. Gynecol Oncol. 1983; 15:10–17.
13. Bonte J, Ide P, Billet G, Wynants P. Tamoxifen as a possible chemotherapeutic agent in endometrial adenocarcinoma. Gynecol Oncol. 1981; 11:140–161.
14. Boring CC, Squires TS, Tong T. Cancer Statistics, 1993. CA – A cancer journal for clinicians; 1993; 43:7–26.
15. Boronow RC. Carcinoma of the corpus: treatment at M.D. Anderson Hospital. In cancer of the uterus and ovary. Chicago: Year Book Medical Publishers; 1969; 35–61.
16. Boronow RC, Morrow CP, Creasman WT, DiSaia PJ, Silverberg SG, Miller A, Blessing JA. Surgical staging in endometrial cancer: clinical-pathologic findings of a prospective study. Obstet Gynecol. 1984; 63:825–832.
17. Bruckman JF, Goodtman RL, Muthy A, Marck A. Combined irradiation and surgery in the treatment of Stage II carcinoma of the endometrium. Cancer. 1978; 42:1146–1151.
18. Burke TW, Stringer CA, Morris M, Freedman RS, Gershenson DM, Kavanagh JJ, Edwards CL. Prospective treatment of advanced or recurrent endometrial carcinoma with cisplatin, doxorubicin, and cyclophosphamide. Gynecol Oncol. 1991; 40:264–267.
19. Carbone PP, Carter SK. Endometrial cancer: approach to development of effective chemotherapy. Gynecol Oncol. 1974; 2:348.

20. Childers JM, Brzechffa PR, Hatch KD, Surwit EA. Laparoscopically assisted surgical staging (LASS) in endometrial cancer. Gynecol Oncol. 1993; 51:33–38.
21. Cohen C, Bruckner H, Deppe G, Blessing JA, Homesley H, Lee JH, Watring W. Multidrug treatment of advanced and recurrent endometrial carcinoma: a Gynecologic Oncology Group study. Obstet Gynecol. 1984; 63:719–726.
22. Committee on gynecologic practice. Estrogen replacement therapy and endometrial cancer. ACOG committe opinion; August, 1993; 126.
23. Creasman WT, DiSaia PJ, Blessing J, Wilkinson RH, Johnston W, Weed J. Prognostic significance of peritoneal cytology in patients with endometrial cancer and preliminary data concerning therapy with intraperitoneal radiopharmaceuticals. Am J Obstet Gynecol. 1981; 141:921–929.
24. Creasman WT, Mccarthy KS Jr, Barton TK, McCarthy KS Jr. Clinical correlates of estrogen and progesterone-biding proteins in human endometrial adenocarcinoma. Obstet Gynecol. 1980; 55:363–370.
25. Creasman WT, Morrow CP, Bundy BN, Homesley HD, Graham JE, Heller PB. Surgical pathologic spread patterns of endometrial cancer. Cancer. 1987; 60:2035–2041.
26. Creasman WT. Announcement: FIGO stages-1988 revisions. Gynecol Oncol. 1989; 35:125–127.
27. Declos L, Braun EJ, Herrera JR, Sampiere VA, Roosenbeek EV. Whole abdominal irradiation by cobalt-60 moving-strip technic. Radiology. 1963; 81:632–641.
28. DiSaia P, Creasman W, Boronow R, Blessing J. Risk factors and recurrent patterns in stage I endometrial cancer. Am J Obstet Gynecol. 1985; 151:1009–1015.
29. Ehrlich CE, Young PCM, Stehman GP, Sutton GP, Alford WM. Steroid receptors and clinical outcome in patients with adenocarcinoma of the endometrium. Am J Obstet Gynecol. 1988; 158:796–807.
30. Fanning J, Alvarez PM, Tsukada Y, Piver MS. Prognostic significance of extent of cervical involvement by endometrial cancer. Gynecol Oncol. 1991; 40:46–47.
31. FDA. Food and Drug Administration. Estrogen and endometrial cancer. FDA Drug Bull. 1976; 6:18–20.
32. FIGO. Classification and staging of malignant tumors in the female pelvis. Int J Gynecol Obstet. 1971; 9:172.
33. Fletcher GH, Rutledge FN, Declos L. Adenocarcinoma of the uterus. In: Textbook of radiotherapy, Fletcher GH 3rd Ed. Lea and Febiger; 1980: 789–808.
34. Gal D, Recio FO, Zamurovic D, Tancer L. Lymphvascular space involvement-A prognostic indicator in endometrial adenocarcinoma. Gynecol Oncol. 1991; 42:142–145.
35. Gallagher CJ, Olive TRD, Gram Dh et al. Gonadotropin releasing hormone analogue treatment for recurrent progestagen resistent endometrial cancer. Proc Am Soc Clin Oncol. 1992; 11:223.
36. Gershenson DM, Kavanagh JJ, Copeland LJ. Cisplatin therapy for disseminated mixed mesodermal sarcoma of the uterus. J Clin Oncol. 1987; 5:618–24.
37. Greenberg SB, Glassburn JR, Antoniades J, Brady LW. Management of carcinoma of the uterus Stage II. Cancer Clin Trials. 1980; 4:183–186.
38. Greer BE, Hamburger AD. Treatment of intraperitoneal metastatic adenocarcinoma of the endometrium by the whole-abdomen moving-strip technique and pelvic boost irradiation. Gynecol Oncol. 1983; 16:365–373.
39. Greven K, Olds W. Radiotherapy in the management of endometrial carcinoma with cervical involvement. Cancer. 1987; 60:1737–1740.
40. Grisby PW, Perez CA, Camel HM, Kao MS, Galaktos AE. Stage II carcinoma of the endometrium: results of therapy and prognostic factors. Int J Radiat Oncol Biol Phys. 1985; 11:1915–1923.
41. Gusberg SB. Diagnosis and principles of treatment of cancer of the endometrium. In: Gusberg SB, Shingleton HM, Deepe G, eds. Female genital cancer, New York: Churchill; 1988:337–360.
42. Hachisuga T, Fuhuda K, Uchijoma M, Matusuo N, Iwasaka T, Suginiomi. Immunochemical study of P-53 expression in endometrial carcinoma: correlation with markers of proliferation cells and clinicopathologic features. Int. J Gynecol Cancer. 1993; 3:363–368.
43. Hannigan E, Curtin JP, Silverberg SG, Thigpen JT, Spanos WJ. Corpus: mesenchymal tumors. Ed Hoskins. 1992; 29:695–714.
44. Hanningan EV, Freedman RS, Elder KW, Rutledge FN. Treatment of advanced uterin sarcoma with vincristine, actinomycin D and cyclophosphamide. Gynecol Oncol. 1983; 15:224–229.
45. Heath R, Rosenman J, Varia M, Walton L. Peritoneal fluid cytology in endometrial cancer: its significance and the role of chromic phosphate (32P) therapy. Int J Radiat Oncol Biol Phys. 1988; 15:815–822.
46. Hendrikson MR, Kempson RL. Endometrial hyperplasia, metaplasia and carcinoma. In: Fox H ed., Haines and Taylor: obstetrical and gynecological pathology 1987; Edinburg: Churchill-Livingstone:354–405.
46a. Henrikson E. The lymphatic spread of carcinoma of the cervix and of the body of the uterus: a study of 420 necropsies. Am J Obstet Gynecol. 1949; 58:924–942.
47. Heyman J. The so-called Stockholm Method and the results of treatment of uterine cancer at the Radiumhemmet. Acta Radiol. 1935; 16:129.
48. Horton J, Begg CB, Arseneault J, Bruckner H, Creech R, Hahn RG. Comparison of adriamycin with cyclophosphamide in patients with advanced endometrial cancer. Cancer Treat Rep. 1978; 62:159–161.
49. Horton J, Elson P, Gordon P, Hahn R, Creech R. Combination chemotherapy for advanced endometrial cancer. Cancer. 1982; 49:2441–2445.

51. ICRU. International commission on radiation units and measurements. Dose and volume specification for reporting intracavitary therapy in gynecology. Bethesda, MD, international commission on radiation units. 1985; Report 38:1–16.

52. Iversen OE, Segadal E. The value of endometrial cytology. A comparative study of the Gravlee jet-washer, Isaac cell sampler, and endoscann versus curettage in 600 patients. Obstet Gynecol. 1985; 40:14–21.

53. Janicek M, Nguyen H, Sevin B-U, Unal A, Scott W, Averette HE. Combination gene therapy targeting MYC and P53 in endometrial cancer cell lines. Proceedings of ASCO 1994; 13:122.

54. Jones HW. Treatment of adenocarcinoma of the endometrium: review. Obstet Gynecol Survey. 1975; 30:147–169.

55. Kadar N, Malfetano JH, Homesley HD. Determinants of survival of surgically staged patients with endometrial carcinoma histologically confined to the uterus: implications for therapy. Obstet Gynecol. 1992; 80:655–659.

56. Kadar N, Malfetano JH, Homesley HD. Steroid receptor concentration in endometrial carcinoma: effect of survival in surgically staged patients. Gynecol Oncol. 1993; 50:281–286.

57. Kaunitz AM, Mosciello A, Ostrowski M, Rovira EZ. Comparison of endometrial biopsy with the endometrial pipette and vabra aspirator. J Rep Med. 1988; 33:427–431.

58. Kauppila A, Kujansuu E, Vihko R. Cytosol estrogen and progestin receptors in endometrial carcinoma of patients treated with surgery, radiotherapy and progestin. Cancer. 1982; 50:2157–2162.

59. Kelley RM, Baker WH. Progestational agents in the treatment of carcinoma of the endometrium. Engl J Med. 1961; 264:216–222.

60. Kelly H. Radium therapy in cancer of the uterus. Trans Am Gynecol Soc. 1916; 41:532.

61. Kinsella TJ, Bloomer WD, Lavin PT, Knapp RC. Stage II endometrial carcinoma 10-year follow-up of combined radiation and surgical treatment. Gynecol Oncol. 1980; 10:290–297.

62. Kline RC, Freedman RS, Jones LA, Atkinson EN. Treatment of recurrent or metastatic poorly differentiated adenocarcinoma of the endometrium with tamoxifen and medroxyprogesterone acetate. Cancer Treat Rep. 1987; 71:327–328.

63. Köchli OR, Sevin BU, Haller U. Chemosensitivity testing in gynecologic malignancies and breast cancer. Basel Switzerland: Karger AG; 1994.

64. Kohorn EI. Gestagens and endometrial carcinoma. Gynecol Oncol. 1976; 4:398–411.

65. Kucera H, Vaura N, Weghaupt K. Benefit of external irradiation in pathologic stage I endometrial carcinoma: a prospective clinical trial of 605 patients who received postoperative vaginal irradiation and additional pelvic irradiation in the presence of unfavorable prognostic factors. Gynecol Oncol. 1990; 38:99–104.

66. Kurman RJ, Kaminisky PF, Norris HJ. The behavior of endometrial hyperplasia. A long-term study of "untreated" hyperplasia in 170 patients. Cancer. 1985; 56:403–412.

67. Kurman RJ, Norris HJ. Endometrial carcinoma. In: Kurman RJ, ed. Blaustein's pathology of the female genital tract 3rd ed. New York: Springer; 1987: 338–372.

68. Larson DM, Copeland LJ, Gallager HS, Kong JP, Wharton JT, Stringer CA. Stage II endometrial carcinoma: results and complications of a combined radiotherapeutic-surgical approach. Cancer. 1988; 61:1528–1534.

69. Lee KR, Belinson JL. Papillary serous adenocarcinoma of the endometrium: a clinicopathologic study of 19 cases. Gynecol Oncol. 1992; 46:51–54.

70. Lehoczky O, Bosze P, Ungar L, Tottossy B. Stage I endometrial carcinoma: treatment of non-operable patients with intracavitary radiation therapy alone. Gynecol Oncol. 1991; 43:211–216.

71. Lewis BV, Stallworthy JA, Cowell R. Adenocarcinoma of the body of the uterus. J Obstet Gynecol Br Commonw. 1970; 77:343–348.

72. Long HJ, Pfeife DM, Wieand HS, Hrook JE, Edmonson JH, Buchner JC. Phase II evaluation of carboplatin in advanced endometrial carcinoma. JNCI. 1988; 80:276–278.

73. Madoc-Jones H. Adenocarcinoma of the endometrium. Stage II. Problems in definition and management. Int J Radiat Oncol Biol Phys. 1980; 6:887–890.

74. Major FJ, Blessing JA, Silverberg SG, Morrow CP, Creasman WT, Carrie JL, Jordan CP, Brady MF. Prognostic factors in early-stage uterine sarcoma. Cancer. 1993; 71:1202–1209.

75. Mangioni C, DePalo G, Marcebini F, Del Vecchio M. Surgical pathologic staging in apparent stage I endometrial carcinoma. Int J Gynecol Cancer. 1993; 3:373–384.

76. Marchetti DL, Caglar H, Driscoll DL, Hereshchyshyn MM. Pelvic radiation in stage I endometrial adenocarcinoma with high-risk attributes. Gynecol Oncol. 1990; 37:51–54.

77. Martin PM, Rolland PH, Gammerre M, Serment H, Toga M. Estradiol and progesterone receptors in normal and neoplastic endometrium: Correlation between receptors, histopathological examination, and clinical responses under progestin therapy. Int J Cancer. 1979; 23:321–329.

78. Martinez A, Podraz K, Schray M, Malkasian G. Result of whole abdominopelvic irradiation with nodal boost for patients with endometrial cancer at high risk of failure in the peritoneal cavity. Hematology Oncology Clinics of N Am. 1988; 2, (3):431–446.

79. McCarthy KS Jr, Barton TK, Fetter BF, Creasman WT, McCarthy KS Sr. Correlation of estrogen and progesteron receptors with histologial differentiation in endometrial adenocarcinoma. Am J Pathol. 1979; 96:171–182.

80. Milosevic MF, Dembo AJ, Thomas GM. The clinical significance of malignant peritoneal cytology in stage I endometrial carcinoma. Int J Gynecol Cancer. 1992; 2:225–235.

81. Morrow CP, Bundy B, Homesley H, Creasman WT, Hornback NB, Kurman R, Thigpen JT. Doxorubicin as an adjuvant following surgery and radiation therapy in patients with high risk endometrial carcinoma, Stage I and occult Stage II: a Gynecologic Oncology Group study. Gynecol Oncol. 1990; 36:166–171.

82. Morrow CP, Bundy BN, Kurman RJ, Creasman WT, Heller P, Homesley HD, Graham JE. Relationship between surgical-pathologial risk factors and outcome in clinical Stage I and II carcinoma of the endometrium: a Gynecological Oncology Group study. Gynecol Oncol. 1991; 40:55–65.

83. Morrow CP, DiSaia PJ, Townsend DE. Current management of endometrial carcinoma. Obstet Gynecol. 1973; 42:399–406.

84. Muss HB, Bundy BN, Adcock L, Belcham J. Mitoxantrone in the treatment of advanced uterine sarcoma. A phase II trial of the Gynecologic Oncology Group. Am J Clin Oncol. 1990; 13:32–34.

85. Muss HB, Bundy BN, DiSaia PJ, Homesley HD, Fowler WC, Creasman W, Yordan E. Treatment of recurrent or advanced uterine sarcoma: a randomized trial of doxorubicin versus doxorubicin and cylophosphamide: a phase III trial of the Gynecologic Oncology Group. Cancer. 1985; 55:1648–1653.

86. Neloff JM. Ca 125 and tumor markers in gynecologic cancer. Chemotherapy of gynecologic cancer. 2nd ed. Gunter Deppe, ed. New York: J Wiley-Liss and Sons, Inc.; 1990.

87. Nordal RN, Kjorstad KE, Stenwing AE, Trope CG. Leiomyosarcoma (LMS) and endometrial stromal sarcoma (ESS) of the uterus. A survey of patients treated in Norwegian Radium Hospital 1976–1985. Int J Gynecol Cancer. 1993; 3:110–115.

88. Nguyen HN, Sevin BU, Averette HE, Perras JP, Ramos R, Penalver M, Donato D. The effect of provera on chemotherapy in uterine cancer cell lines. Gynecol Oncol. 1991; 42:165–177.

89. Omura GA, Blessing JA, Major F. A randomized clinical trial of adjuvant adriamycin in uterine sarcomas: a Gynecologic Oncology Group study. J Clin Oncol. 1985; 3:1240–1245.

90. Omura GA, Major FJ, Blessing JA. A randomized study of adriamycin with and without dimethyl triazinoimidazole carboxamide in advanced uterine sarcomas. Cancer. 1983; 52:626–632.

91. Onsrud M, Aalders J, Abeler V, Taylor P. Endometrial carcinoma with cervical involvement (Stage II): Prognostic factors and value of combined radiological-surgical treatment. Gynecol Oncol. 1982; 13:76–86.

92. Orr JW, Hallaway RW, Orr PF, Holimon JL. Surgical staging of uterine cancer: an analysis of perioperative morbidity. Gynecol Oncol. 1991; 42:209–216.

93. Osmers R, Volksen M, Shauer A. Vaginosonography of early detection of endometrial carcinoma? Lancet. 1990; 335:1569–1571.

94. Park RC, Grisby PW, Muss HB, Norris HJ. Corpus: Epithelial Tumors. JP Lippincott Company, ed. In: Gynecologic Oncology. Hoskins WJ, Perez CA, Young RC. 1992:663–693.

95. Petterson F. Annual report of the results of the treatment in gynecological cancer. Int J Gynecol Obstet. 1991; 36 (suppl):132–237.

96. Piver MS, Barlow JJ, Lurain JR, Blumenson LE. Medroxyprogesterone acetate (Depo-Provera) vs. hyroxyprogesterone caproate (Delalutin) in women with metastatic endometrial adenocarcinoma. Cancer. 1980; 45:268–272.

97. Piver MS, Hempling RE. A prospective trial of postoperative vaginal radium/cesium for grade 1–2 less than 50% myometrial invasion and pelvic radiation therapy for grade 3 or deep myometrial invasion in surgical stage I endometrial adenocarcinoma. Cancer. 1990; 66:1133–42.

98. Pliskow S, Penalver M, Averette HE. Stage III and stage IV endometrial carcinoma: a review of 41 cases. Gynecol Oncol. 1990; 38:210–215.

99. Podraz KC, O'Brien PC, Malkasian GD Jr, Decker DG, Jefferies JA, Edmonson JH. Effects of progestational agents in treatment of endometrial carcinoma. Obstet Gynecol. 1985; 66:106–110.

100. Pollow K, Manz B, Grill JH. Estrogen and progesteron receptors in endometrial cancer. In: Jasoni VM, ed. Steroids and Endometrial Cancer. New York: New York Raven Press; 1983:33–60.

101. Potish RA, Twiggs LB, Adcock LL, Prem LL. Role of whole abdomonal radiation therapy in the management of endometrial cancer; prognostic importance of factors indicating peritoneal metastases. Gynecol Oncol. 1985; 21:80–86.

102. Prempree T, Patanaphan V, Salazar OM. Influence of treatment and tumor grade on prognosis of Stage II carcinoma of the endometrium. Acta Radiol Oncol. 1982; 21:225–229.

103. Quinn MA, Campbell JJ. Tamoxifen therapy in advanced/recurrent endometrial carcinoma. Gynecol Oncol. 1989; 32:1–3.

104. Quinn MA, Cauchi M, Fortune D. Endometrial carcinoma: steroid receptors and response to medroxyprogesterone acetate. Gynecol Oncol. 21; 1985:314–319.

105. Reifenstein EC Jr. The treatment of advanced endometrial cancer with hydroxyprogesterone caproate [review]. Gynecol Oncol. 1974; 2:377–414.

106. Roberts DWT. Carcinoma of body of the uterus at Chelsea Hospital for Women 1943–1954. J Obstet Gynaecol Br Commonw. 1961; 68:132–138.

107. Rose PG, Boutselis JG, Sachs L. Adjuvant therapy for stage I uterine sarcoma. Am J Obstet Gynecol 1987; 156:660–663.

108. Rustowski J, Kupsc W. Factors influencing the results of radiotherapy in cases of inoperable endometrial cancer. Gynecol Oncol. 1982; 14:185–193.

109. Sevin BU, Nadji M, Greening SE, Ng APB, Nordqvist SRB, Girtanner RE, Averette HE. Fine needle aspiration cytology in gynecologic oncology – Early detection of occult persistent or recurrent cancer after radiation therapy. Gynecol Oncol. 1980; 9:351–360.

110. Sevin BU, Perras JP, Averette HE, Donato DM, Penalver MA. Chemosensitivity testing in ovarian cancer. Cancer. 1993; 71 : 1422–1437.

111. Slavik M, Petty WM, Blesing JA, Creasman WT, Homesley HD. Phase II clinical study of tamoxifen in advanced endometrial adenocarcinoma: A Gynecologic Oncology Group study. Cancer Treat Rep. 1984; 68 : 809–811.

112. Slayton RE, Blessing J, Angel C, Berman M. Phase II trial of etoposide in the management of advanced or recurrent leiomyosarcoma of the uterus: a Gynecologic Oncology Group study. Cancer Treat Rep. 1987B; 71 : 1303–1304.

113. Slayton RE, Blessing JA, DiSaia PJ, Christopher WA. Phase II trial of etoposide in the management of advanced or recurrent mixed mesodermal sarcomas of the uterus: a Gynecologic Oncology Group study. Cancer Treat Rep. 1987A; 71 : 661–662.

114. Sobre B, Frankendal B, Risberg B. Intracavitary irradiation of endometrial carcinoma stage I by a high dose-rate afterloading technique. Gynecol Oncol. 1989; 33 : 135–145.

115. Sobre B, Kjellgren Stenson S. Prognosis of endometrial carcinoma stage in two Swedish regions. Acta Oncologica. 1990A; 29 (1) : 29–37.

116. Sobre BG, Smeds AC. Postoperative vaginal irradiation with high dose rate afterloading technique in endometrial carcinoma stage I. Int J Radiat Oncol Biol Phys. 1990B; 18 : 305–314.

117. Soper JT, Creasman T, Clarke-Pearson D, Sullivan DC, Vergadoro F, Johnston WW. Intraperitoneal chromic phosphate P32 suspension therapy of malignant peritoneal cytology in endometrial carcinoma. Am J Obstet Gynecol. 1985; 153 : 191–196.

118. Soper JT, McCarthy KS, Hinshaw W. Cytoplasmatic estrogen and progesterone receptor content of uterine sarcomas. Am J Obstet Gynecol. 1984; 150 : 342–348.

119. Spanos WJ, Peters LJ, Oswald MJ. Pattern of recurrence in malignant mixed mullerian tumor of the uterus. Cancer. 1986; 57 : 311.

120. Surwitt EA, Fowler WC, Rogoff EE, Jelovser F, Parker RT, Creasman WT. Stage II carcinoma of the endometrium. Int J Radiat Oncol Biol Phys. 1979; 5 : 323–326.

121. Sutton G, Blessing JA, McGuire W, Photopoulos G, DiSaia P. Phase II trial of ifosfamide and mesna in leiomyosarcomas of the uterus. Gynecol Oncol. 1990; 36 : 295–299.

122. Sutton GP, Blessing JA, Rosenshein N et al. Phase II trial of ifosfamide and mesna in mixed mesodermal tumors of the uterus (a Gynecologic Oncology Group study). Am J Obstet Gynecol. 1989; 161 : 309–314.

123. Sutton GP, Stehman FB, Michael H, Young PCM, Ehrlich CE. Estrogen and progesterone reptors in uterine sarcomas. Obstet Gynecol. 1986; 68 : 709–714.

124. Swenerton KD. Treatment of advanced endometrial adenocarcinoma with tamoxifen. Cancer Treat Rep. 1980; 64 : 805–811.

125. Taghian A, Pernot M, Hoffstetter S, Luporsi E, Bey P. Radiation therapy alone for medically inoperable patients with adenocarcinoma of the endometrium. Int J Radiat Oncol Biol Phys. 1988; 15 : 1135–1140.

126. Tatman JL, Freedman RS, Scott W, Atkinson EN. Treatment of advanced endometrial adenocarcinoma with cyclic sequential ethinyl estradiol and medroxyprogesterone acetate. Eur J Cancer Clin Oncol. 1989; 25 : 1619–1621.

127. Thigpen JT. Chemotherapy for advanced or recurrent gynecologic cancer. Cancer. 1987; 20 : 2104–2116.

128. Thigpen JT. Chemotherapy of cancers of the female genital tract. In: Perry M., ed. The Chemotherapy Source Book. Baltimore, MD: Williams & Wilkins; 1992: 58 : 1039–1067

129. Thigpen JT, Blessing J, DiSaia P. A randomized comparison of adriamycin with or without cyclophosphamide in the treatment of advanced or recurrent endometrial carcinoma (abstr). Proc Am Soc Clin Oncol. 1985A; 4 : 115.

130. Thigpen JT, Blessing J, DiSaia P, Ehrlich C. Treatment of advanced or recurrent endometrial carcinoma with medroxyprogesteroe acetate (MPA): a Gynecologic Oncology Group study (abstr). Gynecol Oncol. 1985B; 20 : 250.

131. Thigpen JT, Blessing J, Homesley H, Creasman W, Sutton G. Phase II trial of cisplatin as first-line chemotherapy in patients with advanced or recurrent endometrial carcinoma: a Gynecologic Oncology Group study. Gynecol Oncol. 1989; 33 : 68–70.

132. Thigpen JT, Blessing JA et al. Doxorubicin +/- cisplatin in advanced or recurrent endometrial carcinoma: a gynecologic oncology group study. Proc Am Soc Clin Oncol. 1993; 12 : 261.

133. Thigpen JT, Blessing J, Beechman J, Homesley H, Yordan E. Phase II trial of cisplatin as first-line chemotherapy in patients with advanced or recurrent uterine sarcomas: a Gynecologic Oncology Group study. J Clin Oncol. 1991; 9 : 1962–1966.

134. Thigpen JT, Blessing JA, Homesley HD, Hacker N, Curry SL. Phase II trial of piperazinedione in patients with advanced or recurrent uterine sarcoma. Am J Clin Oncol. 1985; 8 : 350–352.

135. Thigpen JT, Blessing JA, Lagasse LD, DiSaia PJ, Homesley HD. Phase II trial of cisplatin as second-line chemotherapy in patients with advanced or recurrent endometrial carcinoma. Am J Clin Oncol. 1984; 7 : 253–256.

136. Thigpen JT, Blessing JA, Orr JW Jr, DiSaia PJ. Phase II trial of cisplatin in the treatment of patients with advanced or recurrent mixed mesodermal sarcomas of the uterus: a Gynecologic Oncology Group study. Cancer Treat Rep. 1986A; 70 : 271–274.

137. Thigpen JT, Blessing JA, Wilbanks GD. Cisplatin as second-line chemotherapy in the treatment of advanced or recurrent leiomyosarcoma of the uterus. Am J Cin Oncol. 1986B; 9 : 18–20.

138. Thigpen JT, Buchsbaum HJ, Mangan C, Blessing JA. Phase II trial of adriamycin in the treatment of advanced and recurrent endometrial carcinoma: a Gynecologic Oncology Group study. Cancer Treat Rep. 1979; 63:21–27.

139. Thigpen JT, Blessing J, Homesley H, Malfetano J, DiSaia P, Yordan E. Phase III trial of doxorubicin +/– cisplatin in advanced or recurrent endometrial carcinoma: a Gynecologic Oncology Group (GOG) Study. Proceedings of ASCO. 1993; 12(830):261.

140. Tidy JA, Wrede D. Tumor suppressor genes: new pathways in gynecologic cancer. Int J Gynecol cancer. 1992; 2:1–8.

141. Torrisi JR, Barnes WA, Popescu G, Whitfield G, Barter J, Lewandowski G, Delgado G. Postoperative adjuvant external-beam radiotherapy in surgical stage I endometrial carcinoma. Cancer. 1989; 64:1414–1417.

142. Trimble EL, Jones III HW. Management of Stage II endometrial adenocarcinoma. Obstet Gynecol. 1988; 71:323–326.

143. Trope C, Johnson JE, Simonsen E, Christiansen H, Carallin-Stahl E, Horvat G. Treatment of recurrent endometrial adenocarcinoma with a combination of doxorubicin and cisplatin. Am J Obstet Gynecol. 1984; 139:379–381.

144. Van Dam P, Lowe DG, Watson JU, James M, Chard T, Hudson CN, Shepherd JH. Multiparameter flow-cytometric quantitation of epidermal growth factor receptor and c-erb B-2 oncoprotein in normal and neoplastic tissues of the female genital tract. Gynecol Oncol. 1991; 42:256–264.

145. Wade K, Quinn MA, Hammond I, Williams K, Cauchi M. Uterine sarcoma: steroid receptors and response to hormonal therapy. Gynecol Oncol. 1990; 39:364–367.

146. Wilson TO, Podratz KC, Gaffey THA, Malkasian GD, O'Brian PC, Naessens JM. Evaluation of unfavorable histologic subtypes in endometrial carcinoma. Am J Obstet Gynecol. 1990; 162:418–426.

147. Wolfson AH, Sightler SE, Markoe AM, Schwade JG, Averette HE, Ganjei P, Hilsenbeck SG, The prognostic significance of surgical staging for carcinoma of the endometrium. Gynecol Oncol. 1992; 45:142–146.

148. Wolfson AH, Wolfson DJ, Sittler SY, Breton L, Markoe AM, Schwade JG, Houdek PV, Averette HE, Sevin B-U, Penalver M, Duncan RC, Ganjei P. A multivariate analysis of clinicopathologic factors for predicting outcome in uterine sarcomas. Gynecol Oncol. 1994; 52:56–62.

149. Yabushita H, Masuda T, Sawaguchi K, Noguchi M, Nahinishi M. Growth Potential of endometrial cancer assessed by a Ki-G7 Ag/DNA dual-color flow-cytometry asay. Gynecol Oncol. 1992; 44:263–267.

4 Gestational Trophoblastic Disease

O. R. Köchli and B.-U. Sevin

Introduction

Gestational trophoblastic neoplasia (GTN), also called gestational trophoblastic diseases (GTD), includes a spectrum of interrelated tumors:

- Hydatidiform mole,
- Invasive mole,
- Choriocarcinoma,
- Placental site trophoblastic tumor.

Although this chapter follows the outline of the book, beginning with surgical procedures, we would like to emphasize that chemotherapy is most important in treatment, especially in the case of malignant GTN.

Choriocarcinoma can occur after a hydatidiform mole, a nonmolar abortion, or a term birth, while only a hydatidiform mole can lead to an invasive mole. Persistent GTN most commonly arises from a hydatidiform mole, although it theoretically may follow any type of pregnancy: spontaneous or therapeutic abortion, term, or ectopic pregnancy (Fig. 1). Over the last 30 years, gestational trophoblastic disease has developed from one of the most fatal malignancies in women to one of the potentially most curable, due to the development of effective chemotherapy. Li et al.[49] (1956) reported the first complete and sustained remission in three patients with metastatic choriocarcinoma by using methotrexate. In 1961, Hertz et al.[41] reported 5-year cure rates and experiences with chemotherapy in patients with metastatic choriocarcinoma and related trophoblastic tumors. Since then, much has been learned about the therapy for GTN, and due to the improvements in chemotherapy, GTN is currently known to be the most curable gynecological malignancy. Through the aggressive use of multimodality therapy, such as single and combination chemotherapy regimens, surgery, and radiotherapy, the results have significantly improved. These improvements have been obtained not only because GTN were found to be very sensitive to different chemotherapeutic agents, but also because a very sensitive marker (human chorionic gonadotropins (hCG), produced by the tumor) had made the diagnosis and assessment of the treatment response very easy. In addition, through large clinical trials, prognostic risk factors have been identified and put into a scoring system to individualize treatment.

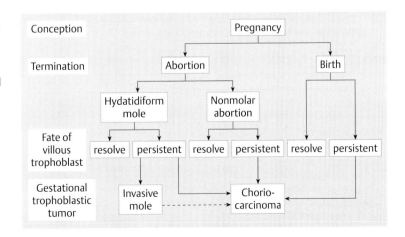

Fig. 1 Antecendent pregnancy and gestational trophoblastic tumors (modified and reprinted with permission from Lawler SD, 1987). Placental site tumors arise from trophoblast of placental bed

Primary Disease

▣ Staging and Surgical Procedures

An overview of the management of gestational trophoblastic neoplasms is given in Figure **2**.

Typical symptoms of GTN lead the clinician to the possible diagnosis of gestational trophoblastic neoplasm (see Tables **1** and **2**). Once the diagnosis has been made, it is important to determine whether the patient has a malignant disease or a hydatidiform mole. To decide upon the optimal therapy for malignant GTN, a complete evaluation of the patient is necessary. The classic workup for malignant GTN is shown in Table **3**. After diagnosing malignant metastatic or nonmetastatic disease, a staging system should be applied to define the appropriate treatment. Over the years, various classification systems have been developed to assess th risk of treatment failure, but none has been universally applied. Because treatment protocols are based on diverse classifications, it is difficult to make interinstitutional comparisons. As shown in Figure **2**, patients are categorized based on anatomical extent of disease and likelihood of response to various chemotherapeutic protocols.

Staging

There are currently three prognostic staging–scoring systems available[25]: The FIGO staging

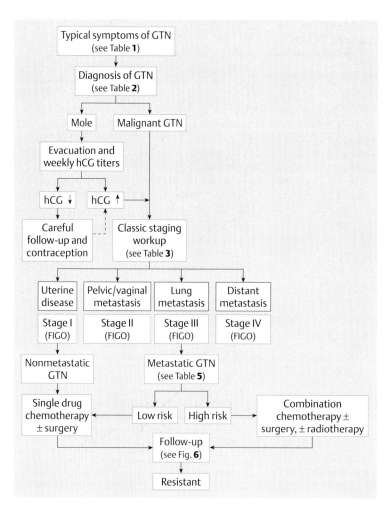

Fig. **2**   Management of GTN

Table **1** Symptoms of GTN

Complete hydatidiform mole[a]	Malignant GTN[b]
– uterine bleeding in the first half of pregnancy – spontanous passage of typical molar tissue – excessive uterine size – lower abdominal pain – elevated beta-hCG (higher than normal pregnancy values) – toxemia early in pregnancy (< 24 weeks) – hyperemesis gravidarum – hyperthyroidism – absent fetal heart beat – chest pain, dyspnea, tachypnea, and tachycardia, respiratory distress due to trophoblastic embolization (2 %, Berkowitz 1989) – prominent ovarian theca lutein cysts	– irregular vaginal bleeding – persistently elevated serum hCG levels – theca lutein cysts – uterine subinvolution – excessive uterine asymmetric enlargement – abdominal pain (uterine perforation) – pain, hemoptysis, or melena because of perforation by a metastatic lesion – evidence of increased intracranial pressure from intracerebral hemorrhage: headache, seizures, hemiplegia – pulmonary symptoms, such as dyspnea, cough, chest pain – right upper-quadrant pain with extensive liver metastases – hematuria from renal involvement

[a] Patients with partial moles most often present with signs and symptoms of a missed abortion or an incomplete abortion. The diagnosis is made after pathological review of the curettage (Szulman 1982).
[b] Invasive mole and choriocarcinoma (FIGO I–IV).
The relative incidence of common metastatic sites are: lungs 80 %, vagina 30 %, pelvis 20 %, brain 10 %, liver 10 %, bowel, kidney, spleen < 5 %, other < 5 %, undetermined with persistent hCG titer after hysterectomy < 5 % (Berkowitz 1981).

Table **2** Diagnosis

Hydatidiform mole	Malignant GTN
– symptoms (see Table **1**) – ultrasound (abdominal or vaginal) – serum beta-hCG (higher than normal pregnancy values) – chest X-ray – amniocentesis – tissue diagnosis	– symptoms for malignant GTN (see Table **1**) – ultrasound – persistently elevated or rising hCG level after any pregnancy – radiological studies of various organs – tissue diagnosis: curettage, biopsy of metastatic lesions, hysterectomy specimen or placenta[a]

[a] Biopsy of lesions is rarely performed because of the risk of uncontrollable bleeding that can occur.

Table **3** Classic metastatic work-up

– chest X-ray film if normal: CT scan of the lungs (Mutch 1986)
– ultrasound, CT scan, or MRI of abdomen and pelvis
– computed tomographic scan of the head (CT scan or MRI)
– intravenous pyelogram, if indicated
– measurement of cerebral spinal fluid hCG titer, if any metastatic disease has been diagnosed and the brain scan is negative
(The plasma/CSF hCG ratio tends to be < 60 : 1 when cerebral metastases are present (Bagshawe 1976)).
– selective angiography is rarely indicated

All patients with persistent GTN should undergo careful metastatic work-up before starting treatment. A complete history and physical examination; measurement of serum beta-hCG titer; hepatic, thyroid, and renal function tests; and a complete count of peripheral white blood cells and platelets are indicated. The metastatic work-up should include the examinations shown in this table.

Table **4a**   Old staging of gestational trophoblastic neoplasia (FIGO)

Stage I	Confined to uterine corpus
Stage II	Metastases to pelvis and vagina
Stage III	Metastases to lung
Stage IV	Distant metastases

Table **4b**   New staging of gestational trophoblastic neoplasia (FIGO)

Stage I	Disease confined to uterus
Stage I	Disease confined to uterus
Stage I A	Disease confined to uterus with no risk factors
Stage I B	Disease confined to uterus with one risk factor
Stage I C	Disease confined to uterus with two risk factors
Stage II	Gestational trophoblastic tumor extending outside uterus but limited to genital structures (adnexa, vagina, broad ligament)
Stage II A	Gestational trophoblastic tumor involving genital structures without risk factors
Stage II B	Gestational trophoblastic tumor extending outside uterus but limited to genital structues with one risk factor
Stage II C	Gestational trophoblastic tumor extending outside uterus but limited to genital structures with two risk factors
Stage III	Gestational trophoblastic tumor extending to lungs with or without known genital tract involvement
Stage III A	Gestational trophoblastic tumor extending to lungs with or without known genital tract involvement and with no risk factors
Stage III B	Gestational trophoblastic tumor extending to lungs with or without known genital tract involvement and with one risk factor
Stage III C	Gestational trophoblastic tumor extending to lungs with or without known genital tract involvement and with two risk factors
Stage IV	All other metastatic sites
Stage IV A	All other metastatic sites without risk factors
Stage IV B	All other metastatic sites with one risk factor
Stage IV C	All other metastatic sites with two risk factors

Risk factors affecting staging include the following: (1) human chorionic gonadotropin > 100000 mIU/ml and (2) duration of disease > 6 months from termination of antecedent pregnancy. The following factors should be considered and noted in reporting: (1) Prior chemotherapy has been given for known gestational trophoblastic tumor; (2) placental site tumors should be reported separately; (3) histologic verification of disease is not required.

system, the NIH prognosis classification, and the WHO scoring system. It has been proposed that the WHO scoring system is best suited to identify the high-risk patient.[56a] An inquiry among 180 members of the Society of Gynecologic Oncologists in the United States showed that in 1990, over 70% used the NIH classification; only 15% used the WHO scoring system. The original FIGO system (1982) was used by 3% only.

FIGO Clinical Staging

An anatomical staging system of GTN was adopted at the meeting of the International Society for the Study of Trophoblastic Neoplasms in Hong Kong in 1979. The International Federation of Gynecology and Obstetrics (FIGO) adopted this staging system in 1982 (see Table **4a**). At its meeting in Singapore, the Oncology Committee of the FIGO revised the staging for GTN. Classic anatomic staging is combined with prognostic factors and is now recommended by FIGO (see Table **4b**).

National Institute of Health (NIH) Classification of Gestational Trophoblastic Neoplasia: Clinical Classification of Prognostic Groups

The clinical classification used by most investigators and major U.S. Trophoblastic Disease

Table **5**   Prognostic group clinical classification: NIH classification of gestational trophoblastic neoplasia

I. Nonmetastatic GTN

II. Metastatic GTN
   A. Low-risk group
      1. short duration (last pregnancy < 4 months)
      2. low pretreatment hCG titer (< 100000 IU/24 h urine or < 40000 mIU/ml serum)
      3. no metastases in brain or liver
      4. no prior chemotherapy
      5. antecedent pregnant event is not a term delivery (mole, ectopic pregnancy, spontaneous abortion)
   B. High-risk group
      1. long duration (last pregnancy > 4 months)
      2. high pretreatment hCG titer (> 100000 IU/ 24 h urine or > 40 000 mIU/ml serum)
      3. brain or liver metastases
      4. significant, unsuccessful prior chemotherapy
      5. term pregnancy

Centers, e.g., Southeastern Trophoblastic Disease Center, separates patients with metastatic disease into "good" and "poor" prognostic categories.[38] Three prognostic groups of patients were formed (see Table **5**).

WHO Prognostic Scoring System

A more comprehensive scoring system has been devised by Bagshawe,[2] in which a variety of factors affecting prognosis are assigned numerically weighted scores. The additive totals are then used to divide patients into three groups: low, medium, and high-risk groups.[2, 4] This classification, which is difficult to apply universally, allows identification of some patients as "low risk," who would in other staging systems be categorized as "high-risk patients." However, patients with nonmetastatic neoplasia, who are known to have a very good prognosis, may be classified, at least theoretically, into a higher risk group. For these reasons, it is important to point out which scoring or staging system has been used to identify "high-risk patients." In 1983, the World Health Organization (WHO) adopted a modified prognostic scoring system proposed by Bagshawe based on: the patient's age, parity, type of antecedent pregnancy, time interval between the antecedent pregnancy and the trophoblastic tumor event, hCG level, paternal and maternal blood type, number and site of metastases, largest tumor mass, and previous chemotherapy.[84] Modifications of this system have been used by many investigators. Wong et al.[82] delete the ABO blood types and do not allow the uterus to be included in the assessment of the largest tumor. This scoring system seems to be more useful and readily acceptable to many experts in the field of GTN. The scoring system published by the World Health Organization is shown in Table **6**. The total score for a patient is obtained by adding the individual scores for each prognostic factor.

Table **6**   WHO prognostic scoring system

Risk factor	0	1	2	4
Age	$\leq$ 39	> 39		
Antecedent pregnancy	Hydatidiform mole	Nonmolar abortion	Term	–
Interval between pregnancy event and treatment (in months)[a]	< 4	– 6	7 – 12	> 12
hCG (IU/L)[b]	< 10^3	– 10^4	– 10^5	> 10^5
ABO blood groups Female × male		$0 \times A$	B	
No. of metastases	–	1 – 4	– 8	> 8
Site of metastases	–	spleen, kidney	gastrointestinal tract, liver	brain
Largest tumor mass, including uterine (cm)		3 – 5	> 5	
Prior chemotherapy (drugs)			single drug	two or more

[a] Interval is the time (months) between the end of an antecedent pregnancy and the start of chemotherapy.
[b] Immediate pretherapy plasma hCG-level

Risk groups:
$\leq$ 4 low-risk group
5 – 7 middle-risk group
$\leq$ 8 high-risk group

In more recent publications, a subset of patients within the traditional "high-risk group" (Table **5**), who account for most deaths from GTN, were called "ultrahigh-risk patients." Identification of these "ultrahigh-risk patients" within the traditional "high-risk" category can be accomplished in a number of different ways. Patients who have prognostic scores ≥ 8 when using the WHO-System (Table **6**), are placed into this group. Patients with three or more traditional "high-risk" factors (Table **5**) are also accepted in this group with the poorest prognosis.[76] It is important to define the selection criteria for this subset of patients.

Surgical Procedures

Hydatidiform Mole

After a molar pregnancy is diagnosed and associated medical complications (such as pre-eclampsia, anemia, etc.) are treated, a decision must be made concerning the most appropriate treatment.

The method most often used is suction curettage followed by sharp curettage. In some patients, a hysterectomy may be considered, particularly if bleeding is heavy. It should be noted that a hydatidiform mole is seldom diagnosed in the first trimester of pregnancy, when emptying the uterus by conventional curettage would be easy and safe.

Suction curettage, followed by sharp curettage, is the preferred method of evacuation. After the dilatation of the cervix, the evacuation is performed carefully to avoid perforation. During and after the evacuation, oxytocin is infused i.v. for several hours to stimulate uterine contractions. A gentle sharp curettage follows. The specimens obtained from suction and sharp curettage should be submitted separately to pathology.

Hysterectomy. Termination of a molar pregnancy by means of primary hysterectomy is the preferred method in the management of patients who wish sterilization and are in good medical condition. The ovaries may be preserved at the time of surgery even if theca lutein cysts are present.

Nonmetastatic Disease

For patients who request sterilization and have nonmetastatic GTN, hysterectomy followed by single agent adjuvant chemotherapy is the treatment of choice. In placental-site trophoblastic tumor, a D & C is often curative and essential to establish the diagnosis. If the disease persists, hysterectomy is absolutely necessary and the only curative treatment because it is usually resistent to chemotherapy. However, there are very limited reports on this rare event. In cases where complete surgical resection can be performed, a good prognosis can usually be expected.[23, 27, 55] The behavior of placental site trophoblastic tumor remains difficult to predict.[26] Long-term follow-up, including monitoring of serum beta-hCG, is recommended. However, it should be noted that low beta-hCG at first presentation is typical for placental site trophoblastic tumors.[5] Previous studies have shown a very poor prognosis in those patients who present with extrauterine metastatic disease. Resistance to chemotherapy is thought to correlate with the predominant cell type, which resembles the intermediate trophoblast. Although it is documented that some patients with persistent placental site trophoblastic tumor may benefit from combination chemotherapy, with the EMA-CO protocol, surgery continues to offer the best chance of long-term survival.[23]

Metastatic Disease

In the management of metastatic disease, chemotherapy is the first-line treatment modality of choice. Surgery should be avoided as much as possible, but sometimes it is necessary for curing the patient or to control complications. Vaginal, pulmonary, hepatic, and cerebral metastases may require surgical intervention. Hysterectomy may be necessary to control uterine hemorrhage or sepsis and to reduce the tumor burden. Hysterectomy may also be required to eradicate persistent disease in the uterus if all evidence of metastatic disease has disappeared and the beta-hCG titer remains elevated after several courses of chemotherapy. When vaginal metastases bleed substantially, packing may be necessary. Bleeding may also be controlled with intra-arterial embolization, avoiding surgery. Thoracotomy may be performed when a patient has a persistent pulmonary metastasis despite intensive combination chemotherapy.[28] Hepatic resection may be necessary when acute bleeding cannot be stopped or when a metastatic focus is resistant to chemotherapy. Although radiation therapy and combinatin chemotherapy are the first therapy modalities for cerebral metastasis, craniotomy may be required to control bleeding or to provide acute intracranial decompression.[40]

Chemotherapy

Hydatidiform Mole

Prophylactic adjunctive single-drug chemotherapy (methotrexate, actinomycin D) after evacuation of a hydatidiform mole is controversial. It should be considered when follow-up is not available or is unreliable, especially in patients with "high-risk" hydatidiform mole (see Table **7**).

After a molar evacuation, persistent uterine disease occurs in 15% of patients (3.4% in "low-risk" patients and 31% in "high-risk" patients) and metastases in 4% of patients (0.6% in "low-risk" patients and 8.8% in "high-risk" patients).[29] These results published by Goldstein et al.[29] were obtained in 858 patients with hydatidiform moles managed by evacuation without prophylactic chemotherapy. Patients with any one of the signs (1) beta-hCG level > 100 000 mIU/ml, (2) excessive uterine enlargement, (3) theca lutein cysts > 6 cm in diameter, were classified as "high-risk" patients. In this study, 4% of the "low-risk," and almost 40% of the "high-risk" patients had persistent GTN.

Malignant GTN

Careful clinical staging has led to more appropriate individualization of therapy, providing re-

Table **7** "High-risk" hydatidiform mole (Curry 1975, Morrow 1977)

- hCG-titer > 100 000 mIU/ml
- theca-lutein cysts > 6 cm
- excessive uterine enlargement
- maternal age > 40 yrs.
- toxemia
- coagulopathy
- hyperthyroidism
- trophoblastic embolization
- prior choriocarcinoma tumor

duced toxicity for patients with low-risk disease, while identifying high-risk patients for whom a more toxic multiagent chemotherapy will be required (see pages 66). Since 1956, the primary treatment for malignant GTN has been chemotherapy. A variety of agents have been utilized, including methotrexate (with or without folinic acid), actinomycin D, 5-fluorouracil, vincristine, and others (more recently, also cis-platinum and etoposide).

Nonmetastatic and Metastatic "Low-Risk" GTN

As shown in Figure **3**, the treatment with chemotherapy is very similar for patients with nonmetastatic trophoblastic tumors and for patients with metastatic trophoblastic tumors in the "low-risk" group.[15a, 62, 82] A rise in titer of beta-hCG is defined as numerical doubling of the value over 2 weeks. A plateau value is defined as a titer which neither declines nor doubles over a 3-week period of evaluation. Single-agent chemotherapy with either actinomycin D or methotrexate has achieved excellent and comparable results in both nonmetastatic and "low-risk" metastatic GTN.[10, 15a, 49, 62, 65, 69, 71, 74, 83] For patients with nonmetastatic GTN, methotrexate 0.4 mg/kg i.m. or i.v. daily for 5 days per treatment course has traditionally been the treatment of choice.[37] Today, there are several protocols available, containing either methotrexate (with or without folinic acid) or actinomycin-D as single agent (see appendix). Actinomycin-D can be given in a 5-day regimen or as a bolus. For women with nonmetastatic disease, a unique regimen using weekly intramuscular methotrexate was evaluated,[44] and can be recommended for patients with postmolar nonmetastatic GTN. There is insufficient evidence of efficacy to recommend its use in treatment of women with nonmetastatic GTN arising after nonmolar gestations. Most single-agent chemotherapy courses are repeated every 12–14 days. An optimal regimen should maximize response rate while minimizing morbidity. Therefore, the selection of chemotherapy should be influenced by the associated systemic toxicity. Actinomycin D is the appropriate therapeutic agent for patients with compromised liver and renal functions. Patients who fail to respond to one single agent are switched to the other single agent. Patients who develop resistance to two

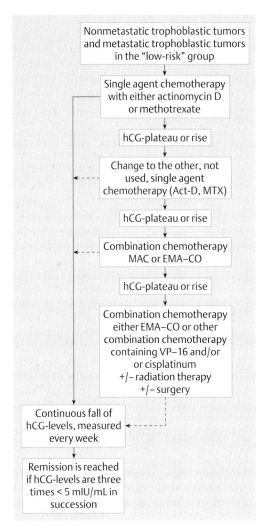

Fig. 3   Management of nonmetastatic and metastatic GTN at "low risk"

single-agent chemotherapy regimens are then treated with combination chemotherapy used for "high-risk" disease.

In recent years, efforts have been made to develop new chemotherapeutic protocols that maximize response rates and minimize morbidity, hospitalization, and costs, without compromising the outcome of the patient. In the search for more efficient, less expensive, and yet safe treatment for managing patients with nonmetastatic and low-risk metastatic GTN, single-dose protocols for actinomycin-D and methotrexate have

been devised.[44, 63, 69] In a GOG study, 94% of 31 patients with nonmetastatic GTN achieved remission with actinomycin-D alone (1.25 mg/m^2 i.v.; every 14 days) after a median of four courses. They considered this regimen now treatment of choice.[63]

Berkowitz et al.[10] do not recommend chemotherapy at predetermined fixed time intervals, but rather based on the repeated beta-hCG regression curve. Only one course of chemotherapy induced remission in 121 (82.3%) patients with nonmetastatic GTN treated with the 8-day MTX-FA regimen (see appendix). The mean number of chemotherapy courses necessary to achieve remission was 1.5 in patients with the 8-day MTX-FA regimen without fixed time intervals, but 3.5 in patients with nonmetastatic GTN who were treated with the same regimen at fixed intervals.[70] When chemotherapy is given on the basis of the beta-hCG regression curve, a high remission rate may be achieved, while limiting chemotherapy exposure and risk of tumor relapse.[10] With this method, a second course of chemotherapy is administered only under the following conditions: (1) if the beta-hCG titer plateaus for more than 3 consecutive weeks or begins to rise again; (2) if the beta-hCG titer does not decline by one log within 18 days after completion of the first treatment; (3) if old metastases enlarge or recur; (4) if new lesions develop.[10, 11, 15] If a second course is necessary, the same dosage of MTX is given, when the first response was adequate (fall in the beta-hCG level by one log after a course of chemotherapy). If the response was inadequate, the MTX-dosage is increased, if the response to two consecutive courses of MTX-FA is inadequate, actinomycin-D is given. In the appendix, several chemotherapy protocols are shown containing methotrexate and actinomycin-D. The results are comparable in terms of remission rates and side effects.[7, 10, 15a, 44, 63, 65, 69, 70, 82]

Approximately 85% of patients with nonmetastatic GTN are cured by initial chemotherapy. The remaining patients may achieve permanent remission with additional chemotherapy. Surgery may play a role in the cure of those patients. Fewer than 5% of patients require hysterectomy for cure.

Forty to fifty percent of patients with "low-risk" metastatic GTN develop resistance to the first chemotherapeutic agent.[15a, 32, 36] With these cases, it is necessary to change to a second agent as early as possible (e.g., actinomycin-D). Approximately 10–15% of patients treated for low-risk metastatic GTN with two sequential single agents (methotrexate and actinomycin-D) require combination chemotherapy with or without other modalities, such as surgery. Several studies, however, have shown virtually 100% cure rates in patients with "low-risk" metastatic disease.[8, 18, 31, 32, 36, 40, 45, 51, 64]

Metastatic "High-Risk" GTN

In Figure **4**, the management of metastatic GTN with "high-risk" is shown. Analysis of a recent Gynecologic Oncology Group (GOG) randomized trial and the experience at the New England Trophoblastic Disease Center, strongly suggests that the chemotherapy of choice in a patient with a prognostic score ≤ 7 is the traditional MAC chemotherapy. However, this therapy is inadequate for patients with prognostic scores of ≥ 8 ("ultrahigh-risk patients"). Superior results in these patients have been achieved with alternative regimens that contain VP-16.[3, 76, 83] The MAC-protocol (see appendix) has achieved satisfactory remission rates (63–80%), with acceptable levels of toxicity.[12, 53] The EMA-CO regimen (see appendix), first formulated by Bagshawe, incorporates VP-16, which has been reported to be a highly effective antitumor agent in GTN.[3, 60] The EMA-CO regimen is a modification of the CHAMOCA regimen (= modified Bagshawe protocol, that includes CTX, hydroxyurea, actinomycin-D, MTX-FA, vincristine, and adriamycin). In a randomized clinical trial, comparing MAC and CHAMOCA for the treatment of "high-risk" patients, the GOG found that the cure rate was higher in those patients who were treated with the MAC regimen, compared to those patients treated with the CHAMOCA protocol.[20] Life-threatening toxicity occurred in 45% of the patients receiving CHAMOCA, compared to 9% of the patients on the MAC regimen. Although this study was criticized because patients in the CHAMOCA group had the highest prognostic scores, it still demonstrated that MAC is as effective as CHAMOCA in treating "high-risk" patients and is certainly less toxic.

Because the EMA-CO regimen has been shown to be highly effective (with a remission rate of 83% in patients with "high-risk" GTN) and has proven to be less toxic than the CHAMOCA regimen, it is the regimen of choice for

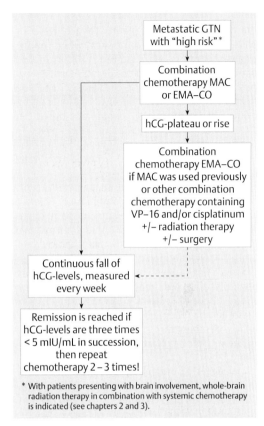

Fig. **4**   Management of metastatic GTN at "high risk"

"high-risk" patients at present, with prognostic scores ≥ 8. For such patients (Table **6**; in some publications "ultrahigh-risk patients"), the MAC chemotherapy seems to be inadequate. Superior results in these patients have been achieved with alternative regimens, such as EMA-CO, which contain VP-16,[3, 76, 83] (see appendix).

The EMA-CO regimen consits of two parts. Course one is given on days 1 and 2; course two is given on day 8. Course one may require an overnight hospital stay; course two does not. Under certain circumstances, the stay can be reduced to 1 night every 2 weeks.[3] These courses are usually given on days 1 and 2, 8, 15 and 16, 22 etc., and the intervals should not be extended without good reason (see Appendix).

If central nervous system metastases are present, the prognosis is poor, and a multlimodal therapy is often necessary (see page 74).

As previously mentioned, more than 90% of the patients with malignant GTN achieve complete and sustained remission when appropriate therapy is administered.[40] Unfortunately, patients who develop brain metastases do not share this favorable prognosis. The low response rates, with survival rates ranging from 18–50%, have been attributed to diagnostic delay, decreased responsiveness of the tumor to chemotherapy in this location (blood-brain barrier), and unexpected, fatal, intracerebral hemorrhage.[46, 50, 72, 80]

Most authorities agree that patients with brain metastases need combination chemotherapy. The role of radiotherapy in the management of brain metastases is more controversial. Physicians who recommend radiotherapy, contend that irradiation of intracerebral choriocarcinoma not only can prevent intracranial haemorrhage, but may also have a tumoricidal effect. Arguments against the use of radiotherapy center around survival rate data, demonstrating that tumors in this location can be eradicated by chemotherapy alone.[46]

Weed et al. treated 23 patients with brain metastases with brain irradiation and chemotherapy. Seven of 11 patients (64%) who presented initially with evidence of brain lesions were successfully treated, but only three of 12 patients (25%) who developed brain lesions while undergoing systemic chemotherapy (or while in remission) survived.[79, 80] Whole-brain radiation therapy in combination with systemic chemotherapy has been successful in patients with brain involvement, but there has been little interest in intrathecal therapy in the U.S.

Bagshawe recommended intrathecal methotrexate for CNS lesions, especially as prophylaxis for all patients with pulmonary metastases or "high-risk" disease.[1, 8] Intrathecal methotrexate (dose = 12.5 mg) is given with each systemic dosage of methotrexate. When brain metastases are detected, the dosage of MTX in the EMA-CO regimen is increased to 1 gm/m² in conjunction with folinic acid (30 mg every 12 hours for 3 days) starting 32 hours after the start of treatment.[3, 66] In this treatment protocol, radiotherapy is not used in first-line management.

Most patients with liver metastases have extensive disease and a poor prognosis. The management of hepatic metastases is particularly challenging because of acute bleeding. Whole-liver radiation, together with combination chemotherapy and a selective hepatic artery embolization, have been proposed to control the hemorrhage.[35, 40, 75] If a patient's tumor is resistant to systemic chemotherapy, hepatic artery infusion of chemotherapeutic agents may induce remission.

Only two-thirds of the patients with "high-risk" GTN achieved remission; however, this number has increased in recent years.[40] A multimodal approach to this disease, with the use of intensive combination chemotherapy and radiotherapy, and surgery, where indicated, has resulted in cure rates of over 80% for patients with "high-risk" metastatic GTN.[3, 8, 19, 51] The use of the WHO prognostic scores helped to identify a group of patients (score > 7) who are at the highest risk of recurrence and need intensive combination chemotherapy.[34, 76] Factors responsible for treatment failures in patients with "high-risk" GTN are: presence of extensive disease at the time of diagnosis, lack of appropriate aggressive initial treatment, and drug resistance.[51]

▪ Radiation Therapy

Brain metastases: Whole-brain radiation therapy in combination with systemic chemotherapy has been successful in patients presenting with brain involvement.[53, 73, 79] About 50% of patients are curable with such a multimodal therapy. Radiation therapy (30–36 Gy) is given simultaneously with the initiation of combination chemotherapy. Because irradiation is thought be hemostatic and tumoricidal, the combination of these two modalities may be the therapy of choice. Long-term side effects of radiation therapy such as brain necrosis, mental dysfunction, or the occurrence of a secondary malignant tumor (glioblastoma) are rare.[6]

Liver metastases: The use of radiation therapy for liver metastases is controversial. Hammond et al.[39] proposed a dose of 20 Gy over 10 days to reduce the risk of liver hemorrhage. However Wong et al.[83] reported on 15 patients with liver metastases, treated by chemotherapy alone, without any liver hemorrhage. The side effects of whole liver irradiation can be substantial.

▨ Hormones

In the treatment of GTN, hormone therapy is not indicated. Since a new pregnancy during the follow-up period can greatly confuse the clinical assessment and management, effective contraception is mandatory during the entire interval of gonadotropin follow-up. A Gynecologic Oncology Group study concluded that oral contraceptives are the preferred method of contraception after evacuation of a hydatidiform mole.[22]

▨ Follow-up Management

Follow-up of Hydatidiform Mole

After evacuation of a molar pregnancy, patients should be monitored by weekly beta-hCG levels (see Fig. **5**). Using the highly sensitive and specific serum beta-hCG RIA, Morrow et al.[56] constructed a normal postmolar pregnancy hCG regression curve, based on weekly determinations in patients undergoing spontaneous titer remission, that may be used as reference value during follow-up (see Fig. **5**).

While serial beta-hCG titers are the most important part of surveillance of patients with hydatidiform mole, other studies are helpful as well. A gynecologic examination is necessary 1 and 4 weeks after evacuation (uterine size, adnexal masses, metastases in the genital tract). Normally, titer remission occurs spontaneously within 14 weeks (see Fig. **5**). If the regression is

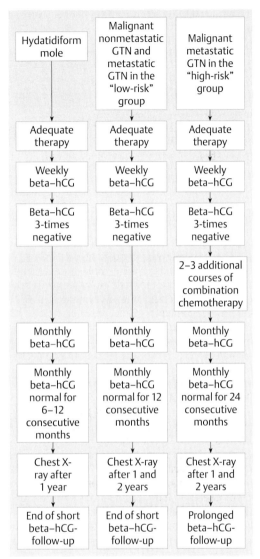

Fig. **6** Follow-up of GTN: As described in the text, recommendations for follow-up vary from institution to institution. The presented flow chart only represents a proposal, and individualization is often necessary

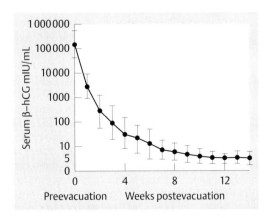

Fig. **5** Normal regression curve of beta-hCG after molar evacuation (reprinted with permission from Morrow CP et al., 1977)

normal, the beta-hCG titers should be monitored for 6 consecutive months; if not, beta-hCG values are obtained for 12 months before the patient is released from medical supervision (see Fig. **6**). Contraception should be started early in the follow-up period.[43] The preferred method of contraception after evacuation of a hydatidiform mole is the use of oral contraceptives.[22]

Table **8** Indication for treatment during postmole follow-up

1. Tissue diagnosis of choriocarcinoma
2. Serum beta-hCG values rising for 2 weeks
3. Serum beta-hCG values on a plateau for 3 weeks or more (> 500 mIU/ml)
4. High beta-hCG levels (> 20000 mIU/ml) more than 4 weeks after evacuation
5. Persistently elevated beta-hCG levels 6 months after evacuation
6. Presence of metastasis
7. Significant elevation of serum beta-hCG values after reaching normal levels
8. Postevacuation hemorrhage not due to incomplete evacuation

The risk of developing a malignant GTN after evacuation of hydatidiform mole is quite high. Goldstein et al.[30, 31] reported an incidence rate of 14.7% nonmetastatic and 4% metastatic GTN. Lurain et al.[52] found 19.2% postmolar GTN, 3% were metastatic. The indications for initiating treatment during postmole follow-up are shown in Table **8**.[9, 21, 52, 56, 84] For the treatment of a persistent mole, the choice of treatment depends on which treatment group the patient belongs to (see Figs. **3** and **4**).

Follow-up of Malignant GTN

All patients with malignant nonmetastatic and metastatic GTN in the "low-risk" group should be monitored by a weekly measurement of hCG titers until they are normal for 3 consecutive weeks. When beta-hCG titers are normal, monthly beta-hCG titers should be determined until levels are normal for 12 consecutive months. Effective contraception during the entire interval of beta-hCG follow-up is essential (see Fig. **6**).

Patients with "high-risk" metastatic disease are monitored with weekly measurement of beta-hCG titers until they are normal for 3 consecutive weeks. Then monthly beta-hCG titers are required until they are normal for 24 consecutive months, because patients are at increased risk for late recurrence (see Fig. **6**). Before that, 2–3 additional treatment courses are given. Patients with placental site trophoblastic tumor should have a long-term follow-up, including indefinite monitoring of serum beta-hCG (see page 70). Some authors recommend monitoring all patients at 6-months intervals indefinitely, although it is rare for a patient to develop recurrent disease more than 1 year after remission.[5]

Pregnancy after Chemotherapy for GTN

A large number of successful pregnancies have been reported in patients whose reproductive organs were retained, despite exposure to drugs that have teratogenic potential.[31, 65a, 78a] These patients had no increase in fetal congenital anomalies, stillbirths, prematurity, or major obstetrical problems. A slightly increased risk of spontanous first and second-trimester abortion was reported (19.7%).[31] The year of required contraception may help damaged ova to degenerate.

Recurrent Disease

▓ Diagnostic and Surgical Procedures

Surgery may play an important role in the cure of patients with recurrent or resistant GTN. It may be necessary to eradicate persistent disease in the uterus if all evidence of metastatic disease has disappeared and if the beta-hCG remains elevated despite repeated chemotherapy. As previously mentioned (see pages 70–71), vaginal pulmonary, hepatic, or cerebral metastases may require surgical treatment (excision of resistant tumor foci).

▓ Chemotherapy

The best choice of salvage chemotherapy for an individual patient depends on the regimen first used and the patient's medical status. There is no indication for single-agent chemotherapy in this patient population. Cis-platinum and etoposide are the most active new agents for the treatment of resistant GTN (Fig. **4**). If drug resistance occurs, other regimens with combination chemotherapy with or without radiation therapy or surgery are required. Respectable salvage data have been reported for different regimens. The EMA-CO regimen (etoposide, methotrexate. Actinomycin D, cyclophosphamide, vincristine) is currently not only considered the regimen of choice in most "high-risk" patients, but also one of the most effective treatments for drug-resistant patients.[16, 58] Salvage with vincristine, bleomycin, cis-platinum,[59, 61] and vinblastine, bleomycin, cis-platinum (VBP; [24, 33, 68, 75]) were also reported. Since Newlands and Bagshawe[60] have reported on the use of etoposide: VP-16, bleomycin, methotrexate;[83] VP-16, actinomycin D, cis-platinum,[78] and VP-16, bleomycin, cis-platinum[81] have been shown to be active in recurrent disease.

▓ Radiation Therapy

In case of brain or liver metastases, radiotherapy together with combination chemotherapy can help to improve the remission rate of recurrent GTN (see Fig. **4**).

▓ Hormones

The importance of careful follow-up with the beta-hCG cannot be overemphasized. As a therapeutical modality, hormones have not been used in GTN.

▓ Follow-up Management

In Figure **6**, the follow-up management for GTN is shown, which also applies to recurrent disease. Only by careful follow-up and with the use of beta-hCG titers, can early recurrence be detected and adequate treatment started. Especially after a recurrence, an indefinitive follow-up is mandatory.

Current Research

▓ Ongoing Clinical and Basic Research Efforts

Compared to other malignancies, GTN has been studied less in regard to tumor aneuploidy. Martin et al. studied DNA content as a prognostic index in GTN and found that aneuploidy identifies a "high-risk" group of molar pregnancies and may represent those that have undergone malignant transformation.[54] Future efforts are required in the field of cytogenetic studies and flow cytometric measurement of nuclear deoxyribonucleic acid content. Studies on oncogenes are ongoing. One of the most important goals in the field of chemotherapy for GTN is to define the most dose-intensive VP-16-containing combina-

tion regimen for "ultrahigh-risk" patients. Another important question is whether bleomycin and/or cis-platinum should be included in the treatment protocols for patients who are at this time treated by Bagshawe's EMA-CO regimen. Surwit[76] favors clinical trials that compare the EMA-CO regimen with a regimen that is similarly designed, but deletes actinomycin-D, allowing higher dosages of VP-16, and replaces vincristine and cytoxan, given on day 8, with VP-16 and cis-platinum. Therefore, large, cooperative, randomized trials are required. Other therapy modalities, such as photodynamic therapy, are under investigation. Photodynamic therapy uses light-activated compounds, such as hematoporphyrins, to produce cytotoxic effects after illumination. High success rates of photodynamic therapy in human choriocarcinoma have been shown in an animal model,[17] and clinical trials with photodynamic therapy now appear justified. Understanding the mechanisms involved in methotrexate resistance in human choriocarcinoma cells is incomplete and fragmentary. Complete elucidation is essential for the modification and design of dosing schedules. The mechanisms elucidated in animal models have provided the avenues of research to be explored in human choriocarcinoma cells.[67] Some mechanisms are known, such as impaired cell membrane uptake and gene amplification of dihydrofolate reductase.[42] Further investigations in the field of methotrexate and multidrug resistance are required. Furthermore, there is a need to establish an in vitro model for testing new drugs in recurrent disease.[47a] However, the most interesting research relates to the immunobiology of the disease.

Appendix: Treatment Protocols, Including Dosages, Schedules, Side Effects, Complications, and Monitoring Requirements

I. Chemotherapy for nonmetastatic and "low-risk" metastatic GTN:

1. Methotrexate 0.4 mg/kg i.v. or i.m. every day ×5 days; repeat every 12–14 days (7–9-day window)
2. Methotrexate 1 mg/kg i.m. days 1, 3, 5, 7; folinic acid 0.1 mg/kg i.m. days 2, 4, 6, 8; repeat every 15–18 days (7–10-day window)

3. Actinomycin-D 10–13 μg/kg i.v. every day × 5 days; repeat every 12–14 days (7–9-day window)
4. Actinomycin-D 1.25 mg/m² i.v.; repeat every 14 days

Monitoring requirements:

- Complete blood count,
- Platelet count,
- SGOT (= serum glutamic oxaloacetic transaminase),
- BUN
- In general it seems safe to proceed when the total leukocyte count is in excess of 2000/mm³ and the platelet count is in excess of 100 000/mm³.

Side effects:

Methotrexate: Stomatitis, mucositis, myelosuppression (frequent but with standard clinical doses generally mild to moderate; nadir: 1–2 weeks followed by rapid recovery), occasionally diarrhea, transient elevation of liver function tests, alopecia

Actionmycin-D: The major toxicity is myelosuppression (nadir at 3 weeks; thrombocytopenia may be profound and may precede leukopenia). Nausea and vomiting are moderate to severe, alopecia is moderate, substantial mucositis only when large doses are given.

II. Combination chemotherapy for "high-risk" GTN

There have been different MAC-regimens described. They consist of methotrexate (± Folinic acid), actinomycin D and chlorambucil or cyclophosphamide and are given every 14–21 days.

1. "MAC"
   Methotrexate 0.3 mg/kg i.m. or i.v., day 1–5
   Actinomycin-D 8–10 μg/kg i.v., day 1–5
   Chlorambucil 0.2 mg/kg p.o., day 1–5

2. "MAC"
   Methotrexate 0.3 mg/kg i.m. or i.v., day 1–5
   Actinomycin-D 8–10 μg/kg i.v., day 1–5
   Cyclophosphosphamide 3–5 mg/kg i.v., day 1–5

3. "MAC"
   Methotrexate 1.0 mg/kg i.m., days 1, 3, 5, 7
   Folinic acid 0.1 mg/kg i.m., days 2, 4, 6, 8
   Actinomycin-D 12 μg/kg i.v., days 1–5
   Cyclophosphamide 3 mg/kg i.v., days 1–5

4. EMA-CO

Course 1: EMA
Day 1   Etoposide (VP-16)   100 mg/m² i.v. infusion in 250 mL saline over 30 min
         Actinomycin-D   0.5 mg i.v. push
         Methotrexate   100 mg/m² i.v. push
                             200 mg/m² i.v. infusion over 12 h
Day 2   Etoposide   100 mg/m² i.v. infusion in 250 mL saline over 30 min
         Actinomycin-D   0.5 mg i.v. push
         Folinic acid   15 mg i.m. every 12 h, 4 doses beginning 24 h after starting methotrexate

Course 2: CO
Day 8   Vincristine   1.0 mg/m² i.v. push
         Cyclophosphamide   600 mg/m² i.v. in saline

Monitoring requirements:

- Complete blood count,
- Platelet count,
- Liver and renal function tests

Side effects:
The toxicity is significantly greater to combination chemotherapy than to single-agent treatment. Toxic reactions are similar to those listed for methotrexate and actinomycin D. Additional complete alopecia occurs and myelosuppression is sometimes severe. Nausea and vomiting can be moderately severe. Vincristine may cause neurotoxicity. Cis-platinum needs to be given with forced diuresis to avoid nephrotoxicity. Bleomycin has potential pulmonary toxicity. Etoposide (VP-16) leads to myelosuppression which may be dose limiting. The main drawback of etoposide is the marked but reversible alopecia that is induced in almost all patients.

References

1. Athanassiou A, Begent RHJ, Newlands ES, Parker D, Rustin GJS, Bagshawe KD. Central nervous system metastases of choriocarcinoma: 23 years' experience at Charing Cross Hospital. 1983; Cancer 52:1728.
2. Bagshawe KD. Risk and prognostic factors in trophoblastic neoplasia. Cancer. 1976; 192:1373.
3. Bagshawe KD. Treatment of high risk choriocarcinoma. J Reprod Med. 1984; 29:813.
4. Bagshawe KD. Treatment of trophoblastic tumors. Recent results. Cancer Res. 1977; 62:192.
5. Bagshawe KD. Choriocarcinoma. Acta Oncological. 1992; 1:99–106.
6. Barnes AE, Liwnicz BH, Schellhas HF, Astshuler G, Aron BS, Lippert WA. Case report. Successful treatment of placental choriocarcinoma metastatic to brain followed by primary brain glioblastoma. Gynecol Oncol. 1982; 13:108.
7. Barter JF, Soong SJ, Hatch KD, Orr JW Jr, Patridge EC, Austin JM Jr, Shingleton HM. Treatment of non-metastatic gestational trophoblastic disease with oral methotrexate. Amer J Obstet Gynecol. 1987; 5:166.
8. Begent RHJ, Bagshawe KD. The management of high-risk choriocarcinoma. Semin Oncol. 1982; 9:198.
9. Berkowitz RC, Goldstein DP, Bernstein MR, Sablinska B. Subsequent pregnancy outcome in patients with molar pregnancy and gestational trophoblastic tumors. J Reprod Med. 1987; 32:680.
10. Berkowitz RS, Goldstein DP, Bernstein MR. Methotrexate infusion and folinic acid in primary therapy of nonmetastatic gestational trophoblastic tumors. Gynecol Oncol. 1990; 36:56–59.
11. Berkowitz RS, Goldstein DP, Bernstein MR. Methotrexate with citrovorum factor rescue as primary therapy for gestational trophoblastic disease. Cancer. 1982; 50:2024–2027.
12. Berkowitz RS, Goldstein DP, Bernstein MR. Modified triple chemotherapy in the management of high-risk metastatic gestational trophoblastic tumors. Gynecol Oncol. 1984; 19:173.
13. Berkowitz RS, Goldstein DP. Pathogenesis of gestational trophoblastic neoplasms. Pathobiol Annu. 1981; 11:391.
14. Berkowitz RS, Goldstein DP, Bernstein MR. Modified triple chemotherapy in the management of high-risk metastatic gestational trophoblastic tumors. Gynecol Oncol. 1984; 19:173.
15. Berkowitz RS, Goldstein DP. Methotrexate with citrovorum factor rescue for non-metastatic gestational trophoblastic neoplasms. Obstet Gynecol. 1979; 54:725–728.
15a. Berkowitz RS, Goldstein DP, Bernstein MR. Ten year's experience with methotrexate and folinic acid as primary therapy for gestational trophoblastic disease. Gynecol Oncol 1986; 23:111–118.
16. Bolis G, Bonazzi C, Landoni F et al. EMA/CO regimen in high-risk gestational trophoblastic tumor (GTT). Gynecol Oncol. 1988; 31:439–444.
17. Brand E, Choi HS, Braunstein GD, Grundfest WS, Lagasse LD. Photodynamic therapy of human choriocarcinoma transplanted to hamster cheek pouch. Gynecol Oncol. 1989. 34:289–293.
18. Brewer JI, Eckman TR, Dolkart RE et al. Gestational trophoblastic disease. A comparative study of the results of therapy in patients with invasive mole and with choriocarcinoma. Am J Obstet Gynecol. 1971; 109:335.
19. Curry S, Blessing J, DiSaia P, Soper J, Twiggs L. A prospective randomized comparison of methotrexate, actinomycin D, and chlorambucil (MAC) versus modified Bagshawe regimen in "poor-prognosis" gestational trophoblastic disease (Abstract). Gynecol Oncol. 1987; 26:407.
20. Curry SL, Blessing JA, DiSaia PJ et al. A prospective randomized comparison of methotrexate, dactinomycin and chlorambucil versus methotrexate, dactinomycin, cyclophosphamide, doxorubicin, melphalan, hydroxyurea, and vincristine in "poor-prognosis" metastatic GTD: a GOG study. Obstet Gynecol 1989a; 73:357–362.
21. Curry SL, Hammond CB, Tyrey L, Creasman WT, Parker RT. Hydatidiform mole. Diagnosis, management, and long-term follow-up of 347 patients. Obstet Gynecol. 1975; 45:1.
22. Curry SL, Schlaerth JB, Kohorn EI, Boyce JB, Gore H, Twiggs LB, Blessing JA. Hormonal contraception and trophoblastic sequelae after hydatidiform mole (a Gynecologic Oncology Group study). Am J Obstet Gynecol. 1989b; 160:805–811.
23. Dessau R, Rustin GJS, Dent J, Paradinas FJ, Bagshawe KD. Surgery and chemotherapy in the management of placental site tumor. Gynecol Oncol. 1990; 39:56–59.
24. DuBeschter B, Berkowitz RS, Goldstein DP, Bernstein M. Vinblastine cisplatin and bleomycin as salvage therapy for refactory high risk metastatic gestational trophoblastic disease. J Reprod Med. 1989; 34:189–192.
25. Duboc-Lissoir J, Seizig S, Schlaerth JB, Morrow DP. Metastatic gestational trophoblastic disease: a comparison of prognostic classification. Gynecol Oncol. 1992; 45:40–45.
26. Eckstein RP, Paradinas FJ, Bagshawe KD. Placental site trophoblastic tumour (trophoblastic pseudotumor): A study of four cases requiring hysterectomy including one fatal case. Histopathology 1982; 6:211–226.
27. Eckstein RP, Russell P, Firedlander ML, Tattersall MHN, Bradfield A. Metastasising placental site trophoblastic tumour: A case study. Human Pathol 1985; 16:632–636.
28. Edwards JL, Makez AR, Bagshawe KD. The role of thoracotomy in the management of pulmonary metastases of gestational choriocarcinoma. Clin Oncol. 1975; 1:329.
29. Goldstein DP, Berkowitz RS, Bernstein MR. Management of molar pregnancy. J Reprod Med. 1981; 26:208.

30. Goldstein DP, Berkowitz RS, Cohen SM. The current management of molar pregnancy. Curr Prob Obstet Gynecol. 1979; 3:1.

31. Goldstein DP, Berkowitz RS. Gestational trophoblastic neoplasms. Clinical principles of diagnosis and management. Philadelphia: WB Saunders; 1982.

32. Goldstein DP. The chemotherapy of gestational trophoblastic disease. Principles of clinical management. JAMA. 1972; 220:209.

33. Gordon A, Kavanagh J, Gershenson D, Saul P, Copeland L, Stringer A. Cisplatin, Vinblastine, and Bleomycin combination chemotherapy in resistant gestational trophoblastic disease. Cancer. 1986; 58:1407–1410.

34. Gordon AN, Gershenson DM, Copeland LJ, Stringer CA, Morris M, Wharton JT. High-risk metastatic gestational trophoblastic disease: Further stratification into two clinical entities. Gynecol Oncol. 1989; 34:54–56.

35. Grumbine FC, Rosenhein NB, Brereton HD, Kaufman SL. Management of liver metastases from gestational trophoblastic neoplasia. Am J Obstet Gynecol. 1980; 137:959.

36. Hammond CB, Borchert LG, Tyrey L, Creasman WT. Treatment of metastatic trophoblastic disease: Good and poor prognosis. Am J Obstet Gynecol. 1973; 115:451.

37. Hammond CB, Hertz R, Ross GT, Lipsett MB, Odell WD. Primary chemotherapy for nonmetastatic gestational trophoblastic neoplasms. Am J Obstet Gynecol. 1967; 98:71.

38. Hammond CB, Parker TR. Diagnosis and treatment of trophoblastic disease. Obstet Gynecol. 1970; 35:132.

39. Hammond CB, Soper JT. Poor-prognosis metastatic gestational trophoblastic neoplasia. Clin Obstet Gynecol. 1984; 27:228.

40. Hammond CB, Weed JC Jr, Currie JL. The role or operation in the current therapy of gestational trophoblastic disease. Am J Obstet Gynecol. 1980; 136:844.

41. Hertz R. Lewis JL, Lipsett MB. Five years' experience with chemotherapy of metastatic choriocarcinoma and related trophoblastic tumors in women. Am J Obstet Gynecol. 1961; 82:631.

42. Hilgers RS, Newlands ES, Hoffman R, Mitchell H, Bagshawe KD. Correlation of plasma methotrexate concentration with human chorionic gonadotropin in therapeutic response to low-dose methotrexate-citrovorum factor in low-medium-risk gestational trophoblastic tumors. Gynecol Oncol. 1991; 41:117–122.

43. Ho PC, Wong LC, Ma HK. Return of ovulation after evacuation of hadatidiform moles. Am J Obstet Gynecol. 1985; 153:638.

44. Homesley H, Blessing J, Rettenmaier M, Major F, Twiggs L. Single agent weekly methotrexate therapy in the treatment of nonmetastatic gestational trophoblastic disease (Abstract). Gynecol Oncol. 1987; 26:414.

45. Jones WB, Lewis JL Jr. Treatment of gestational trophoblastic disease. Am J Obstet Gynecol. 1974; 120:14.

46. Jones WB. Gestational trophoblastic disease: What have we learned in the past decade? Am J Obstet Gynecol. 1990; 162:1286–1295.

47. Köchli OR, Sevin BU, Benz J, Petru E, Haller U. Gynaekologische Onkologie. Berlin, Heidelberg, New York: Springer; 1991.

47a. Köchli OR, Schaer GN, Sevin BU, Perras JP, Schenk V, Rodriguez M, Untch M, Steren A, Haller, U. In vitro chemosensitivity of paclitaxel and other chemotherapeutic agents in malignant gestational trophoblastic neoplasms. Anticancer Drugs. 1995; 6:94–100.

48. Lawler SD. Some comments on the epidemiology, aetiology and genetics of gestational trophoblastic disease. Takagi S, Friedberg V, Haller U, Knapstein PG, Sevin BU, ed. Gynecologic Oncology, Surgery and Urology. Tokyo: Central Foreign Books Ldt; 1987.

49. Li M, Hertz R, Spencer DB. Effects of methotrexate therapy upon choriocarcinoma and chorioadenoma. Proc Soc Exp Biol Med. 1956; 93:361.

50. Liu TL, Deppe G, Chang QT, Tan TT. Cerebral metastatic choriocarcinoma in the people's Republic of China. Gynecol Oncol. 1983; 15:166.

51. Lurain JR, Brewer JI, Torok EE, Halpern B. Gestational trophoblastic disease. Treatment results at the Brewer Trophoblastic Disease Center. Obstet Gynecol. 1982; 60:354.

52. Lurain JR, Brewer JI, Torok EE, Halpern B. Natural history of hydatidiform mole after primary evacuation. Am J Obstet Gynecol. 1983; 145:591.

53. Lurain JR, Brewer JI. Treatment of high-risk gestational trophoblastic disease with methotrexate, actinomycin D and cyclophosphamide chemotherapy. Obstet Gynecol. 1985; 65:830.

54. Martin DA, Sutton GP, Ulbright TM, Sledge GW, Stehman FP, Ehrlich CE. DNA content as prognostic index in gestational trophoblastic neoplasia. Gynecol Oncol. 1989; 34:383–388.

55. Maymon R, Maymon BB, Shulman A, Pomeranz M, Bahrly C. Placental site trophoblastic tumors (trophoblastic pseudotumors): Pathology and clinical importance. Obstet Gynecol Surv. 1990; 10:654–656.

56. Morrow CP, Kletsky OA, DiSaia PJ, Townsend DE, Mishell DR, Nakamura RM. Clinical and laboratory correlates of molar pregnancy and trophoblastic disease. Am J Obstet Gynecol. 1977; 128:424.

56a. Mortakis AE, Braga CA. "Poor prognosis" metastatic gestational trophoblastic disease: the prognostic significance of the scoring system in predicting chemotherapy failures. Obstet Gynecol. 1990; 76:272–277.

57. Mutch DG, Soper JT, Baker ME, Bandy LC, Cox EB, Clarke-Pearson DL, Hammond CB. Role of computed axial tomography of the chest in staging patients with nonmetastatic gestational trophoblastic disease. Obstet Gynecol. 1986; 68:348.

58. Newlands ES, Bagshawe KD, Begent RHJ, Rustin GJS, Holden L. Developments in chemotherapy for medium- and high-risk patients with gestational trophoblastic tumours (1979–1984). Br J Obstet Gynaecol. 1986; 93:63.

59. Newlands ES, Bagshawe KD. Activity of high-dose cis-platinum in combination with vincristine and methotrexate in drug-resistant gestational choriocarcinoma. Br J Cancer. 1979; 40:943.

60. Newlands ES, Bagshawe KD. Antitumour activity of the epipodophyllin derivative VP16-213 (Etoposide: NSC-141540) in gestational choriocarcinoma. Eur J Cancer. 1980; 16:401.

61. Newlands ES. New chemotherapeutic agents in the management of gestational trophoblastic disease. Semin Oncol. 1982; 9:239.

62. Osathanondh R, Goldstein DP, Pastorfide GB. Actinomycin D as the primary agent for gestational trophoblastic disease. Cancer. 1975; 36:863.

63. Petrilli ES, Twiggs LB, Blessing JA, Teng NNH, Curry S. Single-dose actinomycin D treatment for non-metastatic gestational trophoblastic disease. Cancer. 1987; 60:2173.

64. Ross GT, Goldstein DP, Hertz R, Lipsett MB, Odell WD. Sequential use of methotrexate and catinomycin D in the treatment of metastatic choriocarcinoma and related trophoblastic diseases in women. Am J Obstet Gynecol. 1965; 93:223.

65. Ross GT, Stolbach LL, Hertz R. Actinomycin D in the treatment of methotrexate-resistant trophoblastic disease in women. Cancer Res. 1962; 22:1015.

65a. Ross GT. Congenital anomalies among children born of mothers receiving chemotherapy for gestational trophoblastic neoplasms. Cancer. 1976; 37:1043–1047.

66. Rustin GJ. Tophoblastic tumours (Abstract). Third biennial meeting of the international gynecologic cancer society. Cairns. 1991:100.

67. Sakai KS, Wake N, Fujino T, Yasuda T, Kato H, Fujimoto S, Fujinaga K. Methotrexate-resistant mechanisms in human choriocarcinoma cells. Gynecol Oncol. 1989; 34:7–11.

68. Schlaerth JB, Morrow CP, Depetrillo AD. Sustined remission of choriocarcinoma with cis-platinum, vinblastine and bleomycin after failure of convential combination drug therapy. Am J Obstet Gynecol. 1980; 136:983.

69. Schlaerth JB, Morrow CP, Nalick RH, Gaddis O. Single-dose actinomycin D in the treatment of postmolar trophoblastic disease. Gynecol Oncol. 1984; 19:53.

70. Smith EB, Weed JC Jr, Tyrey L, Hammond CB. Treatment of nonmetastatic gestational trophoblastic disease: Results of methotrexate alone versus methotrexate-folinic acid. Am J Obstet Gynecol. 1982; 144:88.

71. Smith JP, Chemotherapy in gynecologic cancer: Malignant trophoblastic tumors. Clin Obstet Gynecol. 1975; 18:113.

72. Song H, Yia Y, Wu B, Wang Y. 20 years' experience in chemotherapy of choriocarcinoma and malignant mole. Chin Med J [Engl]. 1979; 92:677.

73. Soper J, Hammond C. Role of surgery therapy and radiotherapy in gestational trophoblastic disease. J Reprod Med. 1987; 32:663–668.

74. Sung HC, Wu PC, Yang NY. Reevaluation of 5-fluorouracil as single therapeutic agent for gestational trophoblastic neoplasms. Am J Obstet Gynecol. 1984; 150:69.

75. Surwit EA, Hammond CB. Treatment of metastatic trophoblastic disease with poor prognosis. Obstet Gynecol. 1980; 55:565.

76. Surwit EA. Management of high-risk gestational trophoblastic disease. J Reprod Med. 1987; 32:657–662.

77. Szulman AE, Surti U. The clinicopathologic profile of the partial hydatidiform mole. Obstet Gynecol. 1982; 59:597.

78. Theodore C. Azab M, Droy J et al. Treatment of high risk gestational trophoblastic disease with chemotherapy combination containing cisplatin and etoposide. Cancer. 1989; 64:1824–1818.

78a. Walden PA, Bagshawe KD. Reproductive performance of women successfully treated for gestational trophoblastic tumors. Am J Obstet Gynecol. 1976; 125:1108–1114.

79. Weed JC Jr, Hammond CB. Cerebral metastatic choriocarcinoma: Intensive therapy and prognosis. Obstet Gynecol. 1980; 55:89.

80. Weed JC Jr, Woodward Kt, Hammond CB. Choriocarcinoma metastatic to the brain: Therapy and prognosis. Semin Oncol. 1982; 9:208–212.

81. Willemse P, Aalders J, Bouma J, Sleijfer D. Chemotherapy-resistant gestational trophoblastic neoplasia treated successfully with cisplatin, etoposide, and bleomycin. Obstet Gynecol. 1980; 71:438–440.

82. Wong LC, Choo YC, Ma HK. Methotrexate with citrovorum factor rescue in gestational trophoblastic disease. Am J Obstet Gynecol. 1985; 152:59.

83. Wong LC, Choo YC, Ma HK. Primary oral etoposide therapy in gestational trophoblastic disease: an update. Cancer. 1986; 58:14.

84. World Health Organization scientific group on gestational trophoblastic disease. Gestational trophoblastic disease. Geneva (692): Technical report WHO; 1983.

5 Uterine Cervix

M. Höckel and P. G. Knapstein

Primary Disease

▨ General

Although incidence and mortality rates of invasive cervical cancer have declined during recent decades in Western countries, this tumor entity is still important in gynecologic oncology. At present, cervical cancer is diagnosed yearly in approximately 8 out of 100 000 women in the United States, ranking fourth in gynecologic malignancies after breast, endometrial, and ovarian cancer. The current annual death rate is about 3 in 100 000 women, surpassed only by breast and ovarian cancer.[13] In underdeveloped countries, cancer of the uterine cervix is the second most frequent malignant disease in women.

It is believed that cervical cancer is a progression from intraepithelial neoplasia, and therefore cytologic screening programs may have profound effects on the morbidity and mortality of this disease. A variety of factors influencing the risk for a woman to develop cervical cancer has been identified from epidemiologic studies, including age, participation in cancer-screening programs, socioeconomic status, number of male sexual partners (including their female sexual partners), age at first coitus, infection with sexually transmitted diseases (especially human papilloma virus [HPV]), long-term cigarette smoking, multiparity, reduced immune competence, and a diet low in carotene and vitamin C. Prenatal exposure to diethylstilbestrol may be linked to the rare clear cell-adenocarcinoma of the cervix in young women. Although subject to intense investigation, the cause(s) and molecular mechanisms of carcinogenesis and tumor progression of cervical cancer are far from being clear to date.

Malignant disease of the uterine cervix appears in a variety of histologic types, which are summarized in Table **1**. Squamous cell carcinoma is by far the most frequent cervical neoplasm, followed by endocervical adenocarcinoma and adenosquamous carcinoma, which are all believed to arise from malignant transformation of the reserve cell at the basal layer of the cervical epithelium.

After developing the ability to penetrate through the basement membrane, cervical neoplastic cells invade the cervical stroma. The disease may extend locally to the vagina, uterine corpus, parametria, pelvic wall, bladder, and rectum. Regional lymphatic spread is determined by the topographic anatomy of the pelvic lymphatic system, including the parametrial obturator, external/internal/common iliac, and presacral lymph nodes (see Figures **1** and **2**, page X). In cases of pelvic lymph node involvement, higher lymphatic stations, such as the periaortic and scalene node regions, may contain tumor metastases. Hematogenous metastases are rare and usually occur relatively late in the

Table **1** Histologic classification of malignant diseases arising in the uterine cervix
(According to refs. 138, 523)

Squamous cell carcinoma
    Large cell keratinizing
    Large cell nonkeratinizing
    Small cell nonkeratinizing

Adenocarcinoma
    Endocervical-type
    Endometrioid
    Clear cell
    Serous
    Mesonephric
    Intestinal-type

Adenosquamous carcinoma
    Glassy cell carcinoma

Adenocarcinoma with carcinoid features

Small cell carcinoma

Adenoid carcinoma

Adenoid cystic carcinoma

Other malignant tumors
    Melanoma
    Sarcoma
    Lymphoma

disease course. The most common sites for distant metastases (except lymph nodes) are the abdomen, liver, lungs, and bones. There is evidence that adenocarcinomas exhibit a somewhat different pattern of tumor spread compared to squamous cell carcinomas, with a higher incidence of infiltration of the corpus uteri and periaortic lymph node metastasis in early stages.[112]

Diagnosis and Staging

Adequate diagnostic workup to determine the type and extent of the cervical neoplasia includes the patient's history and a thorough physical examination. Visible gross tumor should be punch biopsied for histologic investigation. Otherwise, cytologic smears (unless bleeding) and colposcopy should precede site-directed biopsies, conization, or dilatation and curettage. In locally advanced cervical tumors, cystoscopy and rectosigmoidoscopy are mandatory. The standard radiographic studies are chest film and intravenous pyelography. A barium enema is justified if infiltration of the rectosigmoid colon is suspected. The highest yield of noninvasive diagnostic information concerning the periaortic lymph nodes is obtained from a CT scan, whereas extracervical tumor extension in the pelvis is best evaluated by MRI in combination with a

Table **2**   Staging of carcinoma of the uterine cervix

Primary Tumor		
AJC	FIGO (1995, Montreal Modifications)	
TX		Primary tumor cannot be assessed
T0		No evidence of primary tumor
Tis		Carcinoma in situ
T1	I	Cervical carcinoma confined to uterus (extension to corpus should be disregarded)
T1A	IA	Preclinical invasive carcinoma, diagnosed by microscopy only
T1A1	IA1	Measured invasion of stroma < 3.0 mm in depth and no wider than 7.0 mm
T1A2	IA2	Measured invasion of stroma > 3.0 mm and < 5.0 mm and no wider than 1.0 mm
T1B	IB	Clinical lesions confined to the cervix or preclinical lesions greater than IA
T1B1	IB1	Tumor < 4 cm diameter
T1B2	IB2	Tumor > 4 cm diameter
T2	II	Cervical carcinoma invades beyond uterus but not to pelvic wall or to the lower third of vagina
T2A	IIA	No obvious parametrial invasion
T2B	IIB	Obvious parametrial invasion
T3	III	Cervical carcinoma extends to the pelvic wall and/or involves lower third of vagina or causes hydronephrosis or nonfunctioning kidney
T3A	IIIA	Tumor involves lower third of the vagina, no extension to pelvic wall
T3B	IIIB	Tumor extends to pelvic wall or causes hydronephrosis or nonfunctioning kidney
T4	IVA	Tumor invades mucosa of bladder or rectum and/or extends beyond true pelvis Presence of bullous edema is not sufficient evidence to classify a tumor T4
SGO Microinvasive Carcinoma		
TIA	IA	Depth of invasion up to 3 mm from the base of epithelium without lymphatic vascular space involvement

Regional Lymph Nodes		
Regional lymph nodes include paracervical, parametrial, hypogastric (obturator), common, internal and external iliac, presacral, and sacral nodes.		
NX		Regional lymph nodes cannot be assessed
N0		No regional lymph node metastases
N1		Regional lymph node metastases

Distant Metastases		
MX		Presence of distant metastases cannot be assessed
M0		No distant metastases
M1	IVB	Distant metastases, including periaortic lymph node metastases

bimanual rectovaginal examination. The useful-ness of transvaginal or transrectal sonography is currently under investigation. Standard labora-tory studies consist of complete blood count, blood chemistry for liver and kidney functions, and urine analysis. Pretherapeutic determination of squamous-cell associated antigen (SCC), carcinoembryonic antigen (CEA), CA-125, urinary gonadotropin fragment (UGF), and prolactin (PRL) as potential tumor markers may aid the follow-up later on.

Accurate clinical tumor staging according to the Fédération Internationale de Gynécologie et d'Obstétrique (FIGO) recommendations or the American Joint Committee on Cancer (AJC) TNM system is a prerequisite for the evaluation of the overall treatment results. The current clinical staging criteria are listed in Table **2**. To enable the comparison of treatments, the FIGO staging system does not allow the integration of the pre-therapeutic findings of lymphograms, CT, MRI, laparoscopy, or laparotomy. Only the classifi-

cation of FIGO stage IA requires pathologic assessment. In the Unites States, the Society of Gynecologic Oncologists' (SGO) definition of microcarcinoma of the uterine cervix is used instead of the FIGO criteria (Table **2**).

Several studies have demonstrated profound differences between clinical staging and surgical and pathological findings.[498] Nevertheless, it has not yet been proven that surgical staging, includ-ing periaortic lymphadenectomy and scalene-node biopsy, has any impact on patient sur-vival.[266] The incidence of locoregional lymph node metastases and distant metastases in re-lation to the clinical tumor stage is represented in Table **3**. The probability of nodal spread also cor-relates with tumor size and depth of stromal infiltration for FIGO stage I and II tumors.

The determination of prognostic factors has been the topic of numerous previous and current studies on cervical cancer. A detailed list of fac-tors that have been shown to influence treatment outcome, disease-free, or overall survival is given

Table **3**   Tumor dissemination in primary cancer of the uterine cervix

FIGO stage	Pelvic N⊕[a] (%)	Periaortic N⊕[a] (%)	M⊕[b] (%)
IA1 SGO Micro	0	0	0
IA2	3 (0 – 13)	<1	<1
IB	18 (9 – 31)	7 (0 – 29)	4 (2 – 8)
IIA	25 (20 – 50)	11 (0 – 23)	6 (4 – 16)
IIB	31 (20 – 50)	19 (7 – 33)	10 (8 – 15)
IIIA, B	45 (36 – 50)	30 (17 – 43)	14 (9 – 18)
IVA	60 (55 – 67)	40 (33 – 67)	18 (17 – 19)

Incidence of periaortic N ⊕ in case of pelvic N ⊕: ~35%
Incidence of scalene N ⊕ in case of periaortic N ⊕: 10 – 35%
Incidence of M ⊕ in case of periaortic N⊕: ~ 50%

For FIGO stage IA – IIB tumors

Size (sq mm)	Depth of invasion (mm)	Tumor-cervix quotient[c]	Pelvic N⊕[a] (%)
< 100	< 5	–	<1
100 – 900	5 – 15	< 40	19 – 25
> 900 – 1800	> 15 – 30	> 40 – 80	35 – 44
> 1800	> 30	> 80	62 – 67

[a] Lymph node metastases evaluated from surgical treatment or surgical staging.
[b] Distant metastases (except periaortic lymph node metastases) evaluated from follow-up data of patients with local control.
[c] According to refs. 58, 59.
The data are based on refs. 37, 45, 57, 61, 138, 147, 177, 212, 286, 325, 344, 372, 374, 422, 443, 449, 469, 525

in Table **4**. For the evaluation of any risk factor in cancer of the uterine cervix, the following considerations should be recognized: (a) several prognostic factors may be relevant only for defined subsets of patients, tumor, or treatment forms; (b) the majority of prognostic factors have not been studied in a prospective manner with sufficiently large patient cohorts; (c) weighted combinations of prognostic factors appear to be superior in predicting the disease course than the use of single features; (d) as long as the clinical benefit of any alternate primary treatment or adjuvant therapy has not been demonstrated, the importance of prognostic factors is limited to stratify patients in clinical trials, and for patient information.

To date, FIGO stage, tumor size/volume, depth of cervical stromal infiltration invasion beyond the cervix (parametria, vagina), metastatic potential exhibited as lymphatic vascular space involvement, and number, size, and location (pelvic vs. periaortic) of lymph node metastases are the most valid features of tumor biology and prognosis.

Surgery

At the end of the 19th century, the surgical treatment of cancer of the uterine cervix was either radical abdominal hysterectomy (the Wertheim operation) or radical vaginal hysterectomy (the Schauta operation) without lymphadenectomy. Due to the success of radiation therapy with radium, operative treatment became less popular during the first 4 decades of this century. A reappraisal of surgical treatment after World War II was strongly promoted by Joe Meigs. He extended the radicality of the original Wertheim abdominal approach and included complete pelvic lymphadenectomy consistent with the goal of classic surgical oncology, i.e., the eradication of all locoregional tumor, which is achieved by resection of the neoplasm with wide margins and removal of the locoregional lymph nodes. There is no dispute that the Wertheim–Meigs operation is appropriate for FIGO stages I and IIA tumors. Sufficient data now exist that justify the treatment of those FIGO IA cancers that belong to the SGO definition of microcarcinomas with simple vaginal or abdominal hysterectomy or conization, loop diathermy, since the risk for metastasis and local recurrence is zero in these early cancers

that invade the cervical stroma by less than 3 mm and do not show lymphatic vascular involvement.

The various surgical techniques of the classic Wertheim–Meigs operation are described in detail elsewhere.[21] The extent of radicality of resecting parts of the endopelvic fascia related to the uterine cervix (sacrouterine ligaments, cardinal ligaments, vesicocervical ligaments) and vagina may be adapted to the size and penetration depth of the tumor as described by Piver and others.[370] However, although widely practiced to lower the risk of perioperative and postoperative complications, this tailored surgical approach has not been shown to be advantageous compared to operative techniques that aim at dissecting the parametria directly at the pelvic wall. Burghardt et al. showed the possibility of missing lymph nodes in the lateral parametria if left in situ.[59] The parametrial scars may also increase the risk of local recurrence by harboring surviving tumor cells. However, to avoid postoperative functional bladder and rectum disturbances, it is mandatory to follow the surgical anatomy carefully and spare the vegetative nerves of the pelvic plexus in the lower parts of the parametria.

The current concept of surgical treatment of cervical cancer assumes a therapeutic effect of the locoregional lymphadenectomy, necessitating the complete removal of the obturator, external, internal, common iliac, as well as the presacral lymphatic tissues. If pelvic lymph node metastases are detected by frozen section investigation intraoperatively, the lymph node dissection should include the periaortic region. The primary upper limit for periaortic lymphadenectomy in cervical cancer is the aortic insertion of the inferior mesentery artery. If metastases are found in this region as well, lymph node dissection may proceed to the renal veins. Primary periaortic lymph-node dissection is advocated in bulky (≥4 cm diameter) stage IB2 and IIA squamous cell carcinomas, in stage IB and IIA adenocarcinomas, and in all stage IIB carcinomas.

In premenopausal women salpingo-oophorectomy is not part of the surgical treatment. The benefit of transposing the ovaries lateral higher into the upper abdomen, to keep them out of the field of potential postoperative pelvic radiation, has been questioned recently because of potential loss of function, cyst formation, and pain associated with this procedure in about half

Table **4**   Prognostic factors in cancer of the uterine cervix

Prognostic factor	Comments	References
Host features		
Poor performance state	General disadvantage	449
Poor nutritional state	General disadvantage	334
Age	Advanced stage: young age (< 35 yrs) disadvantage	36, 94, 125, 263, 430
	Early stage: young age advantage	392, 459, 462
	Not confirmed by others	73
Pregnancy	Disadvantage in advanced stages	170, 173, 270, 326
	Not confirmed by others	88, 441
Anemia	Disadvantage for radiation therapy	63, 120, 187, 230, 510
Uremia	Disadvantage for radiation therapy	449
Fever	Disadvantage for radiation therapy	231, 496
Microvascular pathology	Disadvantage for radiation therapy	191
Smoking	Possible disadvantage for radiation therapy	
Cancer of the cervical stump	Disadvantage in adenocarcinomas	87, 154
Immunologic staging system	Higher score[a] possibly disadvantageous	367
Natural killer cell activity	Low activity coincides with tumor dissemination (small study)	504
Gross and microscopic tumor features		
FIGO stage	Disadvantage with increasing stage	211, 541
Tumor size/volume	Disadvantage with increasing size/volume	10, 11, 23, 58, 59, 99, 100, 212, 372, 380, 415, 501
Depth of invasion	Disadvantage with increasing infiltration depth of	
	cervical stroma in FIGO stage I A, B, II A, B tumors	100, 212
	endometrium in FIGO stage I B, II A, B tumors	310, 331, 353
	parametrium in FIGO stage I B, II A, B, III B tumors	256, 282
	vagina in FIGO stage II A tumors	137, 271
Histologic type	Small cell carcinomas disadvantageous	307, 499
	Disadvantages with glassy cell carcinomas, if not treated with surgery and radiation	431
	Inconsistent results with adenocarcinomas and adenosquamous carcinomas	30, 405, 486, 500
Histologic grade	Inconsistent results in squamous cell carcinomas	90, 148, 164, 402, 405, 471, 523
	Higher grades disadvantageous in adenocarcinomas	95, 210, 398, 399
Tumor stromal responses	Lymphoplasmacytic response advantageous	24, 157, 451
	Eosinophilic response disadvantageous	37
Intralesional resection margin	Disadvantage in surgically treated FIGO stage I A – II B tumors	59, 60, 69, 125, 269
Lymphatic vascular involvement	Associated with lymph node metastases	50, 126, 145, 322
	Inconsistent results in case of negative nodal status	24, 50, 69, 100, 486

Table 4   (contd.)

Prognostic factor	Comments	References
Gross and microscopic tumor features		
Pelvic lymph node metastases	Disadvantage with increasing number of positive nodes, bilateral location, and size of node metastasis Site of metastases probably of no influence	11, 38, 100, 372, 475, 486, 487 24, 117, 212, 213, 368 147, 172
Periaortic lymph node metastases	Further disadvantage compared to pelvic lymph node Indicate systemic spread in approximately 50% of the cases with early disease	21, 37, 45, 57, 286, 325, 374, 381, 422, 525
Cell/molecular biological tumor features		
Ploidy	Inconsistent results	116, 221, 222, 237, 307, 426, 466, 494, 541
Proliferation markers	S + G2M phases: inconsistent results	466, 541
Gene expression	HPV-DNA: inconsistent results	158, 221, 222, 246, 294, 411, 493, 513, 529
	c-myc oncogene: possible disadvantage	216
	HER-2/neu oncogene: possible disadvantage	34
	uPA[b]: possible disadvantage	467
	EGF-receptor: possible disadvantage	360
	MHC class I[c]: possible disadvantage	82
	Steroid receptors. inconsistent results	93, 209, 245
Intrinsic radiosensitivity	Higher SF2[d] values indicate reduced curability by radiation	524
Pathobiological tumor features		
Tumor oxygenation	Low pO_2 disadvantageous in advanced stages treated by radiation ± chemotherapy	201, 203
Interstitial pressure	High interstitial pressure possible disadvantageous with radiotherapy	414
Multiple parameter scores		
Malignancy grading system (MGS)	Inconsistent results	39, 89, 464, 465, 541
FIGO stage, size, MGS, ploidy	Predictive of lymph node metastases in FIGO stages I B, II A tumors	219

---

[a]   Score generated from the immunological variables CD4 + lymphocytes, CD4/CD8 ratio, natural killer cells, concanavalin A—induced suppressor index, circulating immune complexes.
[b]   uPA: urokinase-type plasminogen activator.
[c]   MHC: major histocompatibility complex.
[d]   SF2: surviving fraction at 2 Gy.

of the cases after irradiation.[15] Likewise, ovarian transposition without subsequent pelvic irradiation led to cyst formation in 24% compared to 7.4% of patients without transposition.[71]

The collective treatment results and the rates of major complications of surgical treatment of the uterine cancer are compiled in Table **5**.

▨ **Radiation Therapy**

Both squamous cell and adenocarcinoma of the cervix are moderately radiation sensitive tumors. However, due to the topographic anatomy of the cervix and the local tumor spread, a relatively high radiation dose can be safely applied to the primary tumor, thus rendering cervical carcinoma one of the neoplasms most successfully treated by radiation therapy.

Radiation therapy of cervical cancer goes back to the beginning of this century. With the use of intracavitary radium-226 devices, three techniques (the Stockholm, Paris, and Manchester methods) gained world-wide acceptance (for review see ref. 418). To eliminate the considerable radiation exposure to the treatment staff using these methods, afterloading applicators

were developed in the 1950s and 1960s. The Henschke[182] and Fletcher-Suit[468] applicators, using radium-226 or cesium-137, have been most widely used and are still applied today in various modifications.

External-field irradiation of the pelvis has been added to brachytherapy to sterilize potential lymph node metastases. The early orthovoltage machines have been replaced by cobalt-60 and high-energy electron accelerators, which produce photons with megaelectron voltage energies that reach the deep pelvic structures without significant dose reduction, but are only partly absorbed by the skin. Thus even very adipose patients can be treated, and skin tolerance to the radiation therapy is no longer a limiting factor.

Present standard schemes for the primary radiation treatment of cervical cancer, which have been evaluated by long-term follow-up of large patient cohorts, are given elsewhere.[300, 301, 354] Except for stage IA carcinomas, which are controlled by brachytherapy alone, treatment consists of whole-pelvis teletherapy in combination with brachytherapy tailored to the stage and volume of the tumor. The goal of whole-pelvis

Table **5**   Results and complications of radical abdominal hysterectomy and locoregional lymph node dissection for cancer of the uterine cervix

FIGO stage	5-year survival rate (%)	References
	Unweighted means (range)	
IA2	97 (95 – 100)	443, 452, 489, 503, 518, 176, 251, 423
IB	84 (67 - 96)	9, 19, 40, 56, 59, 76, 97, 137, 194, 239, 279, 305, 327, 341, 379, 474, 491, 502
IB bulky[a b]	74 (70 – 79)	12, 44, 409
IIA	78 (72 – 88)	59, 137, 474
IIB[b]	60 (44 – 77)	59, 133, 519
IVA (bladder infiltration)	30	309

Treatment-related mortality rate: 1% (0.5 – 2%); Refs: 177, 355, 449
Complications necessitating surgical repair: 5% (2 – 7%); Refs: 32, 314, 325, 327
Complications with long-term morbidity: 3% (1 – 5%)

---

[a] Tumor size ≥ 4 cm.
[b] Patients receiving postoperative adjuvant irradiation included.

teletherapy of 45–50 Gy is the eradication of small tumor deposits in the pelvic–lymphatic system, shrinkage of the initial tumor mass, and partial restoration of cervical and vaginal anatomy, allowing for the proper insertion of the brachytherapy applicators. With the addition of intracavitary brachytherapy, a pear-shaped target volume is generated in the central pelvis, delivering 75–85 Gy (in bulky tumors up to 90 Gy) to the reference point A.[75] In case of parametrial tumor extension or macroscopic pelvic lymph-node metastases, additional teletherapy fields with central shielding are applied to the lateral pelvis, increasing the local dose to 60 Gy. The tolerance doses of the pelvic hollow organs (i.e., small bowel 45 Gy, rectosigmoid 65 Gy, bladder 70 Gy) should not be exceeded.

The treatment results and complications of standard primary irradiation therapy of cervical cancer are given in Table **6**. Analysis of these data reveals excellent local control for early-stage/small-volume cervical cancers and impressive stage-dependent cure rates compared to other malignancies. However, local control in advanced and bulky disease is still unsatisfactory. Failure to achieve local control with radiation therapy results in an ominous situation, since treatment for local recurrence—if possible at all—is very difficult, and the risk of developing distant metastases is high.[469] To improve local control in advanced disease, new irradiation techniques and means for radiosensitization have been investigated.

New Irradiation Techniques

The fixed A and B reference points for intracavitary brachytherapy according to the Manchester system may lead to underdosage of large and overdosage of small cervical tumors. The Créteil method uses a plastic cervicovaginal moulage, individually shaped according to the patient's anatomy, and claims to avoid these shortcomings.[366] Other centers have designed applicators, allowing CT or MRI aided dosimetry,[242, 438, 521] and are exploring 3-D treatment planning.[512] The reduction of late radiation complications without loss of therapeutic gain is the subject of another area of research, which is directed towards computer assisted optimization of dosimetry[259] and applicator shielding.[277, 311, 528]

Table **6**   Results and complications of primary radiation therapy for cancer of the uterine cervix

FIGO stage	5-year survival rate (%)	References
	Unweighted means (range)	
IA2	98 (96–100)	163, 355
IB	84 (72–92)	106, 128, 175, 193, 233, 244, 248, 255, 265, 312, 352, 379
IB bulky[a]	64 (60–78)	81
IIA	74 (70–89)	193, 233, 244, 352
IIB	62 (56–69)	128, 162, 233, 299, 349
III	34 (25–64)	128, 162, 233, 312, 404
IVA	27 (18–34)	233, 257, 309

Treatment-related mortality rate: < 1%
Grade 2[b] complications: 10% (6–13%); Refs: 193, 254, 312, 350, 386
Grade ≥ 3[b] complications: 10% (6–15%); Refs: 233, 355

[a]   Tumor size ≥ 4 cm.
[b]   According to the Radiation Therapy Onology Group/European Organization on Research and Treatment of Cancer score.

HDR-Brachytherapy

The introduction of high-dose rate (HDR) brachytherapy with iridium-192 and cobalt-60 sources created the possibility of drastically reducing treatment times and radioactive source dimension. Much higher precision in applying an anatomically defined target volume by brachytherapy appeared to be possible. On the other hand, the theoretical radiobiological comparison of HDR with low-dose rate (LDR) treatments by Liversage[280] revealed that high fractionation of HDR brachytherapy is necessary to obtain biological isoeffects with LDR treatment. For example, a LDR regimen of 60 Gy delivered in 72 hours would need 18 fractions for replacement by HDR therapy. Moreover, the oxygen enhancement effects, i.e., the factor by which oxygen increases the radiosensitivity of tumor cells, is somewhat lower for LDR irradiation, supporting the use of this treatment form in the mostly hypoxic cervical cancers. Because of these theoretical considerations, HDR brachytherapy for cervical cancer was not favored by U.S. radiation oncologists until recently.[139] However, in Europe and Asia, HDR treatment has been clinically studied for the last two decades. Recent radiobiological estimations suggest that the results of LDR brachytherapy are equivalent to about five fractions of HDR brachytherapy, if appropriate applicators and packing are used.[53, 54, 92]

Initial trials with HDR brachytherapy, in which optimal fractionation schemes were not applied, led to significantly more severe late complications. Meanwhile empiric clinically feasible fractionation schemes, in combination with teletherapy, have been evaluated in larger studies, showing that the results of HDR therapy are indeed comparable to conventional LDR therapy.[5, 6, 166, 447, 450] For review see Ref. 139.

Interstitial Brachytherapy

Transperineal–interstitial brachytherapy may improve local control and suvical in patients with stage III cervical cancer, poor cervicovaginal geometry, or cancer of the cervical stump.[388, 390, 444, 473] Prempree[391] reported in a study with 49 cases of stage IIIB cervical cancer, a 5-year survival rate of 65% and a local control rate of 84%. Aristizabal et al.[17] obtained local control in 75% of stage IIIB and 40% of stage IVA patients at a mean follow-up of 23 months. The rate of severe complications was considerably higher than with intracavitary brachytherapy (18% vs. 8%). No advantage of transperineal–interstitial brachytherapy could be demonstrated for stage IIB cervical cancer.[18] Considering the high incidence of distant failures and local complications, other authors also question the therapeutic benefit of interstitial–intracavitary brachytherapy in advanced disease.[14, 140] The afterloading perineal templates of Syed–Neblet ("Transperineal Parametrial Butterfly"[124]) and Martinez ("MUPIT",[302]) have been widely used. Recent modifications of the implant treatment[119] and of the templates[52, 204, 266] may enable safer clinical application.

Periaortic Field Irradiation

The problem of including the periaortic region in the treatment field of definitive radiation therapy of cervical carcinoma is unsolved.[144] Initial trials that delivered up to 60 Gy to the para-aortic region found excessive treatment-related morbidity and mortality, mostly due to radiation damage of the small bowel.[525] After limiting the para-aortic dose to 45–50 Gy, the rate of severe complications declined to 5–20%.[91, 374, 381]

The reported results[45, 91, 171, 416, 417, 449] indicate that extended (periaortic) field irradiation with 45–50 Gy may be beneficial in cases of bulky stage IB, IIA, and IIB disease, without evidence of macroscopic para-aortic nodal metastases, as evaluated by lymphangiogram of CT examination.

Particle Irradiation

Particle irradiation is another new tool in radiation oncology. The lethal effect of photon irradiation on cells is significantly influenced by tissue oxygenation and cell cycle phase. One feature of particle irradiation is a higher linear energy transfer (LET) compared to photon irradiation, which means that most cell damage after irradiation is lethal and relatively independent of oxygen tension and cell cycle.[531, 532] Moreover, due to different dose distribution patterns, smaller treatment volumes for a given target volume are irradiated. A clinical benefit from this very costly modality in the treatment of cervical cancer has not been shown so far.

Fast neutrons have high LET characteristics, but are similar to photons in dose distribution. Fast neutron beams have been used in phase II and III studies for the treatment of cervical cancer. Until now no definitive therapeutic gain could be obtained with either pelvic neutron-beam therapy or brachytherapy with the fast neutron emitting radioisotope californium 252.[142, 296, 297, 303, 304, 313]

Modified Fractionation Schemes

Based on empirical data, the standard fractionation scheme for photon irradiation is 2 Gy/day 5 days per week. From a radiobiological and tumor-biological standpoint, modified fractionation patterns may improve the overall result of radiotherapy in certain clinical situations.[118, 533] Whereas hyperfractionation may reduce late complications of radiotherapy, and accelerated fractionation should be more effective in rapidly growing tumors or tumors with high potential for rapid regrowth, accelerated hyperfractionation may combine both potential benefits.[85] Initial nonrandomized studies with these altered fractionation schemes have been performed in gynecologic malignancies and appear to confirm the theoretical expectations.[192, 250, 514] A phase I/II study of carcinoma of the cervix in clinical stages IB, II and III by the Radiation Therapy Oncology Group has been initiated. The trial evaluates a total dose of 60 Gy to the parametria delivered in 50 fractions of 1.2 Gy twice daily, followed by intracavitary brachytherapy.[85] Split-course irradiation, e.g., a 2-week interruption of radiotherapy after 25–30 Gy, may improve patient tolerance during the treatment. However, a trial comparing this modality with conventional noninterrupted treatment in pelvic malignancies including 107 patients with cervical carcinoma by Parsons et al.,[343] paradoxically revealed a higher rate of late gastrointestinal complications in the split-course group. Local control and survival were similar in both groups.

Radiosensitization

Although there are major intratumoral and intertumoral variations in oxygenation, about half of locally advanced cervical cancers exhibit significant amounts of tissue areas with less than half-maximum radiosensitivity.[199, 201, 203] Pronounced tumor hypoxia is regarded as the major reason for decreased local response to radiotherapy observed in anemic patients with cervical cancer.[63, 120, 439, 510] Blood transfusions to raise the Hb levels above 12 g/dl have been shown to improve irradiation results, at least in patients with acute anemia.[187] Consequently, means to increase tumor oxygenation have been investigated in order to yield better results with radiotherapy for cervical cancer. One approach that has been studied in a series of trials is the application of hyperbaric oxygen. The overall results of these studies are equivocal. Some trials found slight therapeutic improvement; others did not detect any benefits, only increased morbidity.[29, 180] A therapeutic gain using hyperbaric oxygen in radiotherapy of cervical cancer was only obtained with lower than conventional fractionation schemes[33] and severely anemic patients.[108] Primary well-oxygenized tumors and reoxygenation during fractionated radiotherapy may diminish the beneficial effect of hyperbaric oxygen in cases not selected with regard to intratumoral pO_2.

The use of electron-affinic chemical compounds, which should sensitize cells to radiation through fixation of the radicals in the DNA by oxidation, has been proposed as another means to reduce hypoxia-related radioresistance. 2-nitroimidazole compounds (e.g., misonidazole) have been found to be potent hypoxic cell radiosensitizers in animal experiments. In addition, these substances are metabolized under anaerobic conditions to cytotoxic drugs, which may enhance the lethal effects on hypoxic cells. Following phase I, II, and III trials including carcinoma of the cervix by the Radiation Therapy Oncology Group,[273, 363, 517] the Gynecologic Oncology Group performed a randomized trial of hydroxyurea versus misonidazole as an adjuvant to radiation therapy in advanced primary carcinoma of the cervix.[461] Until now, no convincing evidence could be supplied by the clinical trials that misonidazole improves the results of radiotherapy in cervical cancer. Because of the dose-limiting neurotoxicity of the compound, the achievable tumor concentration of the sensitizer may be too low to be effective. At present, two new 2-nitroimidazole derivatives with less toxicity (SR 2508 and Ro-03-8799) and different application schemes are being tested in phase I studies.[80]

One of the first nonhypoxic radiosensitizers used in cervical cancer patients was hydroxyurea. It is presumed that this compound is cytostatic to cells in S-phase, leading to cell synchronization in the G1-phase.[361] G1-phase cells are more radiosensitive than S-phase cells. Moreover, hydroxyurea may also interfere with the repair of cells after sublethal radiation damage.[453] Several prospective clinical trials demonstrate an improvement in survival in patients with advanced primary carcinoma of the cervix treated with hydroxyurea and irradiation compared to irradiation alone.[206, 207, 240, 371, 373, 375, 377] The hydroxyurea treatment produced more short-term side effects in terms of gastrointestinal and bone marrow toxicity, but no increase in late complications.

▨ Chemotherapy

Squamous cell carcinoma of the uterine cervix is moderately chemosensitive. Consequently, chemotherapy as the sole treatment modality cannot be regarded as curative, only palliative. The effectiveness of cytotoxic therapy is determined by the rate and duration of complete and partial responses defined by the International Union Against Cancer (UICC). Side effects are graded according to the World Health Organization (WHO) scale, ranging from one to five.[527]

Cisplatin, is currently the most active single drug that shows response rates of up to 30% and response durations of 4–6 months with few severe complications in untreated locally advanced primary cancer of the uterine cervix.[46] Other cytotoxic drugs that show some activity against squamous cell carcinoma of the cervix include platin analogs (carboplatin), alkylating agents (cyclophosphamid, ifosfamid, and mitolactol), antibiotics (doxorubicin, epirubicin, bleomycin, and mitomycin C), antimetabolites (5-fluorouracil, methotrexate), alkaloids (vincristine, vindesine) and hexamethylmelamine.

According to recent studies, cisplatin combinations appear more effective in untreated locally advanced primary tumors, attaining response rates of 80–100%, with complete responses in 20–40% (Table 7). In most of these trials, chemotherapy has been given as pretreatment before surgery or radiation ("neoadjuvant"), not allowing for evaluation of the duration of the response. Moreover, only small patient numbers have been studied, and no randomization with respect to cisplatin alone has been carried out.

Chemotherapy is seemingly less effective in adenocarcinoma of the cervix, with maximum single-agent response rates of 20% obtained with cisplatin.[233] Cisplatin, doxorubicin, and etoposide combination chemotherapy is currently the most potent cytotoxic regimen in small cell cancer of the cervix, with a reported response rate of 57% in small trials.[110, 275, 315]

Regional Chemotherapy

Although based on sound theoretical considerations, an advantage of regional intra-arterial chemotherapy over systemic application could not be clinically proven for the treatment of locally advanced primary cancer of the uterine cervix.[185, 333] Using sophisticated, interventional-radiologic techniques, selective placement of catheters into the hypogastric or uterine arteries is possible, allowing prolonged tumor cell exposure to the anticancer drug during continuous infusion.[537] However, this does not necessarily result in a higher cytotoxicity. For cis-platinum, it was recently demonstrated that the increment in intratumoral drug concentration obtained by the i.a. route compared to i.v. treatment is probably too small to be of clinical significance.[506] Regional chemotherapy offers the advantage of fewer systemic side effects; however, local tissue injury resulting in inflammatory pain and even necrosis can be considerable. Whereas 100% response rates have been reported in untreated locally advanced primary disease with intra-arterial cis-platin-based combination chemotherapy, the results of other groups are less optimistic.[215, 235, 345] Because of the low numbers of patients enrolled in these studies and the lack of randomized trials, evaluation of this modality is not possible at present.

An unconventional chemotherapeutic approach has been carried out by Shafik,[445] who demonstrated impressive response rates in advanced cervical cancer with injection of methotrexate into the anal submucosa. In previous studies, this author showed the existence of two to six hemorrhoidal veins, which transmit the blood unidirectionally from the hemorrhoidal venous plexus to the urinary bladder, vagina, and uterus. Arterial chemoembolization with microencapsulated anticancer drugs in the treatment of cervical cancer needs further evaluation.[234]

Table **7**   Results of cisplatin-based cytotoxic therapy on untreated locally advanced squamous cell cancer of the uterine cervix

Agents	Dose i.v. mg/m^2	Response rate n/N^a (%)	Grade > 3 toxicity rate^b (%)	References
Cisplatin	50	31/150 (21)		46
Cisplatin	100	52/166 (31)		
Cisplatin	5 × 20	32/128 (25)		
Cisplatin 5-Fluorouracil	100 1000 × 5	98/113 (87)	11	342
Cisplatin Mitomycin C	50 10	13/17 (77)	6	101
Cisplatin Bleomycin	40 × 5 15 × 4	23/26 (88)	8	338
Cisplatin Methotrexate Bleomycin	60 – 75 100 – 300 ·15 – 30	16/24 (67)	0	195
Cisplatin Vincristine Bleomycin	50 1 25 × 3	68/74 (92)	0	315
Cisplatin Mitomycin C Vincristine Bleomycin	50 10 1 10 (U.i.m.)	28/28 (100)	0	110, 275

^{a} Number of patients responding/number of patients treated.
^{b} Except nausea/vomiting and alopecia.

Combined Treatment Modalities

Numerous multimodality treatment concepts in cancer of the uterine cervix have been designed to achieve improvements in (I) the local control of bulky and advanced stage disease and (II) the prevention of distant metastases.

Multimodality regimens that have been explored or that are currently being studied include combinations of

- surgery and radiation,
- surgery and chemotherapy,
- radiation and chemotherapy, and
- surgery, radiation, and chemotherapy.

The rationale for the different treatment combinations in terms of the modified Steel and Packham concept,[460] and an analysis of the current clinical results will be provided in the following sections.

Surgery and Radiation

Radiation can be applied before, during, or after surgery. Combining the two locoregional treatments permits targeting of the same region of tumor growth. "Debulking" of macroscopic tumor may improve response to subsequent radiation therapy. Likewise, preoperative radiotherapy could improve operability of a tumor. Intraoperative radiation enables protection of normal tissues. Unfortunately, the two treatment modalities are not free of complications; indeed, their combination may potentiate side effects significantly. Moreover, utilizing radiation for primary treatment significantly reduces the treatment options and survival of the patient when she develops locoregional tumor recurrence.

Radiation before Surgery

Bulky (> 4 cm diameter) stage I B and II A cervical cancers exhibit a 10–12% probability for central recurrence after irradiation as well as a higher incidence of distant metastases when compared to smaller tumors of the same stage.[81] Similar reduced local-control rates and increased probability of distant metastases have been found in stage I B/II A cervical carcinomas with either isthmic stromal or endometrial extension, which is most often seen in adenocarcinomas. In both situations, parts of the primary tumor may be located outside the optimal isodose lines. These patients could potentially be undertreated by radiotherapy alone, and thus have been regarded as candidates for a combined radiation and surgery approach. The combination of radical hysterectomy with locoregional lymphadenectomy after full-dose primary radiation therapy is associated with a median severe complication rate of about 20%.[4, 86, 217, 348] Complications are significantly fewer if the radicality of either the radiation therapy or the surgery is reduced. Two regimens have been evaluated in clinical studies:

(a) brachytherapy followed by radical hysterectomy and locoregional lymphadenectomy; and
(b) definitive combined telebrachytherapy followed by extrafascial hysterectomy.

Einhorn et al.[117] reported improved 5-year survival rates for young patients (younger than 40 years) with stage I B cervical cancer after combined surgery and brachytherapy compared to radiotherapy alone (96% vs. 81%), whereas stage II A patients had poorer outcomes with the combined treatment (66% vs. 74%). Likewise, other studies showed that extrafascial hysterectomy performed 6 weeks after completion of definitive irradiation improves the therapeutic results of bulky stage I B/II A tumors and early stage adenocarcinomas.[115, 141, 324, 428, 429] However, the application of a higher irradiation dose without hysterectomy led to comparable results.[351] A significant benefit of these combined modality approaches could not be detected in several other trials.[12, 60, 81, 184, 268] In summary, a small advantage of radiation therapy followed by surgery in this subset of patients may be obtained; however, this has not been unequivocally demonstrated.

Radiation after Surgery

Several studies address the value of locoregional lymphadenectomy before definitive irradiation.[111, 266, 382] The radiobiological background for this treatment approach is the relationship between tumor size and radiation dose necessary for tumor control. To sterilize micrometastases of a moderately radiosensitive tumor like cancer of the cervix requires a radiation dose of 45–50 Gy, whereas more than 60 Gy may be necessary to cure macroscopic lymph node metastases. Therefore, resection of lymph node metastases prior to irradiation could reduce the macroscopic tumor burden of locoregional lymphatic spread to microscopic levels with a higher chance of local control. Although Downey et al.[111] provided evidence in favor of that treatment approach in a recent trial comparing the 5-year survival rates of patients with negative lymph nodes, microscopic metastases, resected, and non-resected macroscopic nodal metastases, no prospective randomized study at present answers this question definitively.

The importance of periaortic lymphadenectomy and subsequent extended field irradiation is also not clear at present. Several studies with treatments consisting of radical hysterectomy, periaortic lymphadenectomy, and postoperative extended-field irradiation demonstrated that up to 50% of patients with positive periaortic lymph node metastases with stage I B and II A cervical cancers survived 5 years.[91, 286, 421] From these and other studies[37, 57, 323, 325] it can be concluded that positive periaortic lymph node metastases do not necessarily indicate systemic spread, and these patients may have the chance to be cured in case of local control. The combination of transperitoneal lymph node dissection and extended-field irradiation significantly increases radiation-induced bowel complications. A severe complication rate of 19%, including one treatment-related death, was reported in a recent study of 21 patients.[91] However, no studies answer the question, if retroperitoneal approaches (which may be less radical) lead to superior results, or if preradiation periaortic lymphadenectomy has an effect on survival at all. In locally advanced disease (FIGO stages III and IVA) and in cases with bulky periaortic disease it is unlikely that lymphadenectomy preceding definitive irradiation will improve the overall poor prognosis.

One of the most controversial issues in the treatment of cervical cancer to day is the relevance of postoperative radiation after radical hysterectomy.

Traditionally, adjuvant irradiation following radical surgery has been given to patients with FIGO stage IB and IIA tumors in the presence of one or more risk factors, such as lymph node metastases, lymphatic vascular space involvement, bulky tumor, advanced infiltration of the cervical stroma, parametrial, vaginal, or endometrial extension, or close resection margins. The predictive value of these tumor features in significantly reducing the 5-year survival rate in surgically treated stage IB/IIA tumors is well established (Table **8**).

Radiation is usually administered as 45–50 Gy whole-pelvis teletherapy, with or without a brachytherapy boost delivered to the vaginal apex. The combined treatment leads to a mean increase in the rate of severe complications from 2–6% in the surgery-only group, to 12–14% in the combined treatment group.[44, 317] After benefits were reported in initial trials, retrospective studies with larger patient cohorts could not confirm a significant improvement in 5-year survival with adjuvant radiotherapy. However, postoperative adjuvant radiation apparently results in a prolonged recurrence-free interval and a reduced incidence of local recurrences. A shift in location of the clinically detectable pelvic recurrences from the pelvic wall to a more central site seems to be another consequence of postoperative whole-pelvis teletherapy. More patients in the irradiated group present with distant metastases without detectable locoregional recurrent disease.[44, 77, 126, 127, 169, 247, 319, 406, 457, 482]

One of the most important goals in treatment of early cancer of the uterine cervix is to clarify the role of postoperative adjuvant radiation therapy for surgically treated high-risk tumors in randomized controlled prospective trials, and to define subsets that indeed benefit from the combined treatment.

A recent report on patients with glassy cell carcinomas[285] suggests that the combined treatment is associated with a significant 5-year survival advantage compared to surgery alone (87% vs. 45%). Nevertheless, prospective confirmation is warranted.

A role for postoperative brachytherapy of the vaginal vault following radical hysterectomy of early stage cervical cancer has not been established. It has been suggested that patients without lymph node metastases, but with deep stromal penetration, may be candidates for this approach.[365] However, the area of anatomic scar tissue after radical hysterectomy by far exceeds the vaginal vault brachytherapy treatment volume. Central recurrences at the vaginal apex are infrequent following radical hysterectomy. Indication for postoperative vaginal brachy-

Table **8** 5-year survival rates of patients with surgically treated FIGO stage IB/IIA cancers of the uterine cervix according to various prognostic factors

Factor	Number of patients	Percent 5-year survival
Lymph nodes		
Negative	1233	90
Positive	227	46
Lymphatic vascular space		
Negative	572	88
Positive	545	64
Tumor size		
≤4 cm	203	91
>4 cm	100	64
Stromal invasion		
Superficial	331	90
Deep (>10 mm or >50%)	91	70

(Modified from ref. 492)

therapy might be a close vaginal resection margin or in situ carcinoma in the resected vaginal cuff.

Concomitant Surgery and Radiation

The concept of intraoperative radiation therapy (IORT) had alraedy been developed in the 1920s with orthovoltage photon therapy.[530] However, the full advantage of IORT first became possible with the evolution of electron beam technology. This modern IORT was pioneered by Japanese radiotherapists in the 1970s.[1, 2, 3] Today, several centers have established facilities for IORT.[79, 153, 165, 539] In principle, IORT improves the therapeutic ratio of radiation because: (a) the target volume of radiation can be most accurately defined by surgical exploration; (b) the tumor can be surgically reduced to microscopic disease prior to radiation; and (c) radiosensitive vital organs can be surgically displaced out of the treatment field during irradiation. IORT can be administered only in a single fraction of up to 25 Gy; therefore it is mostly used as a boost in addition to external beam radiation and brachytherapy. However, since the radiobiological equivalence of the radiation dose applied as IORT is regarded two to three times the radiation dose of conventionally fractionated photons,[539] IORT might be curative alone, especially in combination with preceding debulking surgery, when only microscopic tumor has to be treated by irradiation. IORT appears to be suitable for the treatment of the para-aortic region and the lateral pelvic side wall in advanced cancer, since the most sensitive organs within these treatment fields, i.e., small bowel, rectosigmoid, ureters, and bladder can be surgically displaced.

Preliminary results of a few phase I/II IORT trials have now been published.[98, 143, 152, 539] Delgado et al.[98] treated 16 patients with advanced primary cervical carcinomas (FIGO stages II B, III B and IV A—11 of them with positive para-aortic nodes) with IORT, external beam, and brachytherapy. Eight patients were still living (two of them with disease) 10 to 36 months after surgery. The most important complications were femoral motor weakness and leg edema. No wound healing or gastrointestinal complications occurred. Controlled studies with more patients and longer follow-up periods are necessary for the evaluation of IORT in advanced primary cervical carcinoma.

Surgery and Chemotherapy

Chemotherapy can be applied for the treatment of cervical cancer either preoperatively or postoperatively. The combination of the locoregional and systemic therapy permits time sequencing, whereby side effects may be minimized, without reducing the therapeutic benefits.

Preoperative Chemotherapy

The rational for preoperative ("induction," "neoadjuvant") chemotherapy is the potential elimination of micrometastases and the reduction of the primary tumor mass (downstaging) to attain operability of locally advanced disease.[132] Kim et al.[241] treated 35 patients with bulky carcinomas of the uterine cervix (tumor diameter ≥ 4 cm) FIGO stages IB, IIA, B with one to five courses of a cisplatin, vincristine, and bleomycin combination, followed by radical surgery. They concluded that induction chemotherapy is effective in reducing tumor volume and stage and might also eliminate lymph node metastases, thus facilitating surgery. Similar results have been attained by other researchers using various cisplatin-based combination regimens either systemically or regionally.[110, 146, 249, 338] Induction chemotherapy followed by radical surgery was well tolerated without increasing short-term complications of the locoregional treatment. Although the initial outcome may look promising in small studies with short follow-ups, the results of prospective randomized trials must be awaited for evaluation of this combined treatment.[243, 338]

Shortcomings of this approach may result from the delay of effective treatment if the tumor does not respond to chemotherapy; development of chemoresistance and radioresistance; and an increase in metastatic potential. Not responding to neoadjuvant chemotherapy has been found to be a strong prognostic factor indicating poor survival in cervical cancer.[337]

Postoperative Chemotherapy

The possibility of reducing the incidence of distant metastasis and locoregional recurrences of early stage cancers with poor prognosis by adjuvant chemotherapy after radical surgery is currently being investigated in large multi-institutional studies. Patients whose tumors exhibit one or several poor prognostic factors, such as locoregional lymph node metastases, lymphatic vascular space involvement, deep cervical stromal or parametrial invasion, tumor size ≥4 cm, or small cell histologic type are randomized against control groups receiving radiotherapy or no adjuvant treatment.

Radiation and Chemotherapy

Advanced stage cervical cancer treated by standard radiation therapy exhibits high locoregional and distant failure rates. The combination of radiotherapy and chemotherapy offers potential therapeutic advantages based on theoretical considerations. Within the locoregional treatment compartment, potential supra-additive tumor cell kill may be achieved by synergistic interactions between irradiation and chemotherapy at the level of the tumor cells and their microenvironment.[420, 460] Radiosensitization through chemotherapy may be exerted by a variety of mechanisms, including cell cycle synchronization, reduced capacity for the repair of sublethally damaged cells, and increased reoxygenation.[31, 65, 479] However, the relevant biologic mechanism of radiation-chemotherapy interactions are poorly understood at present, rendering clinical approaches mostly empirical, and in particular, making late complications unpredictable.[362, 421, 488]

Sequential Chemo- and Radiotherapy

Regimens that have been investigated in FIGO stage IIB–IVA tumors apply chemotherapy preceding pelvic irradiation using conventional fractionation schemes.[41, 123, 135, 144, 150, 321, 342, 345, 369, 425, 434, 477, 511] Initial chemotherapy of advanced stage tumor is claimed to provide more favorable conditions for radiotherapy through shrinkage of the tumor mass, cell cycle synchronization, and reoxygenation. The addition of chemotherapy, either preceding or following radiation, should also eradicate systemic micrometastases. The majority of these studies have a phase I and II character with mostly small patient numbers and a follow-up period of less than 5 years (Table **9**). Chemotherapeutic agents used were cis-platinum, bleomycin, vinblastine, cyclophosphamide, methotrexate, mitomycin C, 5-fluorouracil, and adriamycin either a single substances or in combination with standard doses. Chemotherapy

was administered i.v., except in the trials of Falappa et al.[123] and Patton et al.[345], which used intra-arterial therapy. One to six courses of chemotherapy in 3–4 week cycles were given prior to standard percutaneous/intracavitary radiotherapy. Patients with periaortic lymph node involvement were treated with periaortic field irradiation as well. Initial complete response rates using the combined modality were 30–65%. Studies with posttreatment surveillance periods of more than 2 years could not demonstrate significant benefits in survival with small patient numbers. Survival rates after 2 to 3 years were in the range of 20–50%. However, Park et al.[345] reported an exceptionally high 5-year survival rate of 69% for stage III and IV disease that was claimed to be significantly improved compared to a historical control group. A recent communication of Sardi[434] on a prospective randomized study comparing radiotherapy alone versus sequential chemotherapy and radiotherapy, demonstrated a significant 3-year disease-free survival benefit with the latter group for stage IIB (61% vs. 79%) and stage IIIB (35% vs. 59%) lesions. On the contrary, Tattersall et al.[477] could not demonstrate an advantage in 5-year survival with a randomized trial comparing sequential chemoradiotherapy and radiotherapy alone for locally advanced cervical cancers. There was a trend toward reduced distant metastases but higher local recurrences in the combined treatment group. A potential shortcoming of sequential chemoradiotherapy may be the induction of higher tumor proliferation rates by the cytotoxic treatment. The accelerated repopulation of tumor cells could then lead to failure of the subsequent radiation therapy. Nonfatal myelodepression, diarrhea, nausea, and vomiting were the most common early side effects. However, Friedlander et al.[135] reported one potential treatment-related death, three deaths due to intercurrent diseases, and the development of respiratory distress syndrome during posttreatment pelvic surgery in 18 patients treated by chemotherapy followed by radiation. Patton et al.,[345] using intra-arterial cis-platinum and bleomycin, as well as intravenous vincristine, noted a treatment-related mortality of 7%. Few data are available on late complications, which appear to be more frequent here than after treatment with standard radiotherapy. Continuation of chemotherapy after irradiation was not feasible in several instances.[511] This was observed

Table **9** Sequential chemoradiotherapy for locally advanced cancer of the uterine cervix

Investigation	No. of evaluable patients	FIGO stages	Drugs	No. of courses preradiation	Radiation therapy	Complete respones	Actuarial DFS	Severe complications		Survival comparison to controls
								early	late	
Friedlander et al. 1984	18	IIB, III	CDDP, VBL, BLM	3	Standard	50%	40%/16 mth	NR	NR	–
Goldhirsch et al. 1986	16	IIIB	CDDP, MTC, BLM	2	Extended field	NR	19%/28 mth	19%	19%	–
Muss et al. 1987	11	IIIB, IVA	CDDP	6	Extended field	27%	27%/21mth	9%	NR	–
Volterraini et al. 1990	23	II, III	CDDP, BLM	3	Standard (+ extended field)	57%	48%/38 mth	5%	NR	–
de la Garza et al. 1987	20	IIB–IBA	CDDP, EPI, CYC	2–8	Standard	55%	NR	NR	NR	–
Patton et al. 1991	46	(IIB), III, IVA	CDDP, BLM i.a., VCR i.v.	1–3	Standard	NR	30%/60 mth	20–30% 7% treatment-related deaths	15%	–
Sardi et al. 1991	29 27	IIB, IIIB	CDDP, VBL, BLM	3	Standard	NR	79%/36 mth 59%/36 mth	NR	NR	p < 0.05 p < 0.05
Park et al. 1991	46	III, IVA	CDDP/5-FU CDDP, CYC, ADR	2–3	NR	NR	69%/60 mth	NR	NR	p < 0.01
Tattersall et al. 1992	34	IIB–IVA	CDDP, VBL, BLM	3	Standard	65%	47%/60 mth	NR	NR	n.s.

ADR, adriamycin, doxombicin; BLM, bleomycin; CDDP, cisplatin; CYC, cyclophosphamide; EPI, epimbicin; 5-Fu, 5-fluorouracil; MTC, mitomycin C; VBL, vinblastine; VCR, vincristine; DFS, disease-free survival; NR, not reported; n.s., not significant.

Table **10** Concomitant chemoradiotherapy for locally advanced cancer of the uterine cervix

Investigation	No. of evaluable patients	FIGO stages	Drugs	Radiation therapy	Complete responses	Actuarial DFS	Severe complications		Survival comparison to controls
							early	late	
John et al. 1990	38	IIB–IVA	CDDP,	Standard	NR	63%/25 mth	47%	NR	–
Nguyen et al. 1991	38	IB–IVA	5-FU, MTC	Standard	80%	47%/48 mth	24%	11%	–
Roberts et al. 1991	67[a]	IIB–IVA	CDDP, 5-FU	Standard	85%	22%/60 mth	9%	13%	–
Drescher et al. 1992	10	I–IVA + periaortic metastases	5-FU	Extended field	90%	15%/24 mth	20%	NR	–
Thomas et al. 1984	27	IB–IVA	5-FU, MTC	Split course (+ extended field)	74%	59% (4–24 mth)	3%	11% (1 death)	–
Evans et al. 1987	14	II–IVA	5-FU, MTC	Standard	NR	70%/26 mth	12%	8%	–
Choo et al. 1986	20	IIB–III	CDDP	Standard	NR	80%/10–34 mth	NR	NR	n.s.
Potish et al. 1986	29	IB–IVA	CDDP	Extended field	76%	61%/30 mth	no	10%	n.s.
O'Reilly et al. 1986	15	IIIB–IVA	CDDP	Standard	NR	46%/3–30 mth	NR	NR	–
John et al. 1987	10	IIB–IVA	5-FU, MTC,	Standard	100%	80%/6–37 mth	no	10%	–
Wong et al. 1989	39	IIB–III	CDDP	Standard	74%	51%/42–72 mth	no	8%	n.s.
Roberts et al. 1989	21	IB–III	5-FU, CDDP	Split course	86%	48%/17 mth	no	10%	–
Runovicz et al. 1989	43	I bulky–IVB	CDDP	Standard	91%	84%/12 mth	no	7%	–
Kersh et al. 1989	44[b]	II–IVA	5-FU, MTC	Standard	73%	51%/29 mth	5%	5%	–

[a] 11 pts. with vaginal/vulvar carcinomas.
[b] 8 pts. with vaginal carcinomas.

Table **10**   (contd.)

Investigation	No. of evaluable patients	FIGO stages	Drugs	Radiation therapy	Complete responses	Actuarial DFS	Severe complications		Survival comparison to controls
							early	late	
Kuske et al. 1989	15	IIB–IVA	5-FU, CDDP	Standard	NR	53%/12–36 mth	NR	NR	–
Goolsby et al. 1968	22	IIB–IVA	5-FU	Standard	NR	55%/6–69 mth	27%	18%	–
Ludgate et al. 1988	38	IIB–IVA	MTC, 5-FU	Standard (+ extended field)	80%	68%/5–36 mth	8%	8%	p < 0.01 only for stage IIB historical controls
Malfetano and Keys 1991	13	IB–IIIB + periaortic metastases	CDDP	Extended field	100%	67%/25–67 mth	no	NR	–
Heaton et al. 1990	20	II–IVA	5-FU, CDDP	Hyperfract. split course (+ extended field)	66%	53%/12–76 mth	no	10%	–

For abbreviations see Table 9.

in GOG protocol #59, which was designed to compare postirradiation cisplatinum-based chemotherapy with no further treatment, for patients with carcinomas of the cervix metastatic to high common iliac and/or periaortic lymph nodes.[51]

Concomitant Chemotherapy and Radiotherapy

Numerous studies have been carried out investigating the clinical effect of concomitant chemotherapy and radiotherapy for advanced cervical cancer.[72, 74, 113, 122, 156, 178, 225, 227, 229, 238, 262, 278, 287, 289, 292, 293, 329, 336, 347, 383, 394, 408, 412, 413, 424, 481, 490, 535]

Most of these studies are of phase I–II type and involve only small or medium-sized patient cohorts (Table **10**). Generally, standard combined irradiation techniques of tele/brachytherapy, with or without periaortic extended field irradiation, have been performed. In a few trials, radiotherapy was administered as a split course with a 10 to 14-day break. Hyperfractionated irradiation was used by Heaton et al.[178] The chemotherapeutic agents given concomitantly with irradiation in these trials, either single or in combination (i.e., cis-platinum, 5-fluorouracil, mitomycin C), are stated to be radiosensitizers in addition to their direct cytotoxic effects on cervical cancer cells.

The reported preliminary clinical data are promising with respect to initial complete response rates which range from 70–100%. Fifty to eighty percent of the patients were free of disease at short follow-up of approximately 2 years. In terms of clinical results, no combined regimen can be claimed to be superior to others at the present time. However, long-term surveillance studies[329, 413, 535] show a high incidence of local and distant tumor recurrence in the patients who responded initially. Up to now, no long-term benefit of concomitant chemoradiotherapy is apparent in patients with locally advanced cancer of the uterine cervix. Short-term side effects were similar to those reported for sequential chemoradiotherapy. Life-threatening acute complications and treatment-related deaths were occasionally seen. Late complications could not be fully assessed to date. Again, as with the sequential mode, higher treatment-related morbidity must be expected compared to radiation therapy alone.

The clinical importance of chemoradiotherapy of cervical cancer will have to await long-term results of prospective randomized multicenter trials, which are currently under way.

Surgery, Radiation, and Chemotherapy

The combination of the three classic antitumor treatments has been studied in various sequencing schemes in small nonrandomized trials.[41, 123, 408, 421] Sardi et al.[435] presented the actuarial survival data of patients with bulky FIGO stage IB squamous cell carcinomas prospectively randomized to treatment with three courses of induction chemotherapy (cisplatin, vincristine, bleomycin) followed by radical hysterectomy and locoregional lymph node dissection and subsequent adjuvant whole-pelvis radiation with 50 Gy (n = 74), versus surgery and radiotherapy without neoadjuvant chemotherapy (n = 72). Three patients of the neoadjuvant group and six control patients received definitive radiation instead of surgery and adjuvant radiation because they were determined to be inoperable at staging laparotomy. Patients with tumors larger than 60 mL as measured by pretherapeutic ultrasound did significantly better: Their 4-year survival probability was 88% compared to 60% in the control group. Toxicity was stated as not severe. The lower survival in the retrospective control may be misleading due to small patient numbers. In addition, the incidence of pelvic recurrence was unusually high. Thus, more mature results are necessary to evaluate the benefit of the three-modality therapy in cancer of the uterine cervix.

▮ Current Treatment Concepts

The FIGO stage distribution and stage-related therapy modalities of a large patient cohort with cancer of the uterine cervix recruited worldwide are published in the FIGO Annual Report on treatment results of gynecological cancers.[358] The data obtained for patients treated in 1979 to 1981 are compiled in Table **11**.

The treatment suggestions for cervical cancer outlined in this section are made on the basis of a review of the literature, which was introduced above and the experiences of the University of Mainz Medical Center. The proposed treatment algorithms are shown in Figures **1–5**.

Table **11**   Stage distribution and corresponding treatment modalities of 23 804 patients with cancer of the uterine cervix treated 1979–1981 at 114 institutions published in the Annual Report (Ref. 358)

FIGO stage	Percent of all patients treated with			
	RT	Surgery	RT + Surgery	All treatments
I	10	13	13	36
II	22	2	8	32
III	22	< 1	1	23
IV	4	< 1	< 1	4
NR	–	–	–	5

Except for certain special situations, i. e., very old age, pregnancy, cancer of the cervical stump, specific histologic types, and inadequate treatment, a general treatment scheme based on FIGO stage and established prognostic factors can be followed.

Stage IA

FIGO stage IA carcinomas can be safely treated conservatively by simple abdominal or vaginal hysterectomy in women who have completed childbearing, or by conization and close surveillance in women wanting to preserve fertility if the SGO criteria for microinvasive carcinoma (see Table **2**) are met. Otherwise, radical hysterectomy and pelvic lymphadenectomy should be performed (Fig. **1**). If the operative treatment carries a high risk because of other preexisting diseases, intracavitary radiation therapy is the alternative treatment.

Stages IB and IIA

Although radiotherapy and surgery are equivalent in 5-year survival, we regard surgery as the therapy of first choice in early-stage disease, i.e., FIGO stages IB and IIA (Fig. **2**), since a properly performed radical hysterectomy and locoregional lymphadenectomy involves a smaller treatment volume and has less side effects in terms of disturbed functional anatomy than primary pelvic radiation. Ovarian function and elasticity, as well as secretory function of the vagina are preserved only with surgical treatment. The radiation-induced stem cell loss in the whole pelvic compartment is thought to lead to more long-term unfavorable effects than the surgical removal of the upper third of the vagina, uterus, parametria, and the locoregional lymphatic tissue.

We recommend performing a complete parametrial resection, which corresponds to the type III radical hysterectomy classification by Piver et al.[370] since we believe that the parametrial stumps are the most common sites of local recurrences in surgically treated cervical cancers. Likewise, the pelvic lymphadenectomy should be as thorough as possible. Periaortic lymph node dissection is added primarily if high-risk factors are present, i.e., bulky ≥ 4 cm diameter tumors, adeno-, adenosquamous and

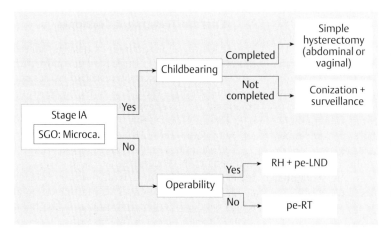

Fig. **1**   Treatment algorithm for FIGO stage IA cancer of the uterine cervix
ca = carcinoma
LR/HR = low risk/high risk
c/p = clinical/postoperative
pe = pelvic; pa = periaortic
RH = radical hysterectomy
LND = lymphadenectomy
RT = radiation therapy
ChT = chemotherapy
LVS = lymphatic vascular space
CT = computer tomography
⊗ = consider participation in a prospective randomized trial

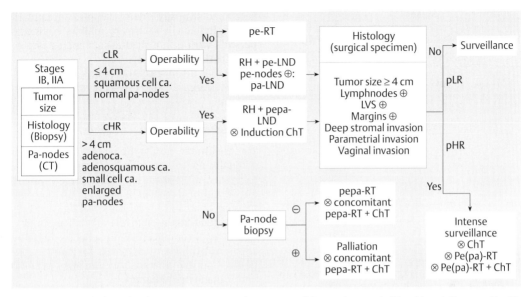

Fig. 2   Treatment algorithm for FIGO stages I B and II A cancer of the uterine cervix (For abbreviations see Fig. **1**)

small cell carcinomas, and enlarged periaortic lymph nodes as determined on CT scan. If a frozen section investigation demonstrates pelvic lymph node metastases, periaortic lymphadenectomy is carried out independent of the above-mentioned features. Radiotherapy is applied in early stage disease if operability is not given. Whole-pelvis teletherapy and intracavitary brachytherapy treatment doses are planned with respect to tumor volume according to the radiation techniques published elsewhere.[354] A periaortic field extension, with a total dose of 45 Gy, is made in all cases that otherwise would be treated by primary periaortic lymph node dissection, but where gross periaortic metastasis ist not evident. However, a treatment dilemma will become evident in inoperable patients with enlarged periaortic lymph nodes histologically proven to contain metastatic disease by CT-guided fine-needle biopsy. As bulky periaortic disease cannot be controlled by percutaneous radiotherapy without fatal side effects, these patients can only be treated palliatively, despite the early FIGO stage.

Multimodality treatments in early stage cervical cancer should be applied only in conjunction with multi-institutional prospective randomized trials. In clinically high-risk patients,

induction chemotherapy prior to radical surgery or concomitant chemoradiotherapy are currently being investigated.

If surgically treated patients exhibit one or several of the risk factors derived from the histologic investigation of the removed specimen, i.e., tumor size ≥ 4 cm, parametrial or deep stromal invasion, positive resection margins, lymph node metastases, or lymphatic vascular space involvement, participation in adjuvant chemotherapy, adjuvant radiotherapy, or adjuvant chemoradiotherapy trials is suggested. During the first 2 years, the postoperative surveillance of these patients should be intensified to detect local recurrences early, thus increasing their chance to be salvaged.

Stages II B, III and IV

Locally advanced (FIGO stages II B, III and IV) disease without evidence of distant metastases or gross periaortic lymph node metastases are currently treated by primary radiation (Fig. **3**). Higher pelvic doses of radiation (up to 85 Gy at point A and 60 Gy at point B) or extended field techniques may be administered accepting an increased complication rate for a better chance to cure a patient. However, patients have practically no survival potential in case

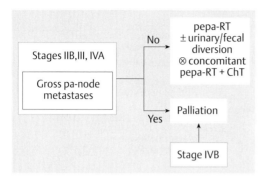

Fig. 3   Treatment algorithm for FIGO stages IIB, III and IV cancer of the uterine cervix (For abbreviations see Fig. 1)

of treatment failure. If major distortion of the cervicovaginal anatomy by tumor or stricture is evident, interstitial brachytherapy may be more effective than intracavitary techniques. Adequate urinary and fecal diversion is necessary before initiation of radiation therapy in case of a tumor-associated urinary and fecal fistula, respectively. Obstruction of the ureter should be managed by insertion of a pig-tail catheter or percutaneous nephrostomy, unless residual renal function cannot be demonstrated.

Patients without gross periaortic or distant disease may be randomized for concomitant

chemoradiotherapy trials. Palliative treatment with systemic chemotherapy may be offered to patients with established distant metastases or bulky periaortic disease.

Several distinct circumstances in the treatment of cervical cancer deserve special considerations.

Advanced age

The treatment results in elderly patients are generally poor, even in early stage disease.[73] In early stage disease, the surgical treatment should not be withheld in favor of radiation therapy only because of advanced age if the patient is otherwise in good condition to tolerate radical surgery. The surgical complication rate appears not to be significantly higher compared to younger patients, and the therapeutic outcome may be better than with radiation.

Pregnancy

Invasive cervical cancer is detected during pregnancy with a reported incidence of 0.002–0.04%.[49, 454] The diagnosis of early invasive carcinoma by Pap smear, colposcopy, and directed punch biopsy may be more difficult due to pregnancy-induced anatomical changes. Since up to half of the patients are asymptomatic and vaginal bleeding or discharge may be mis-

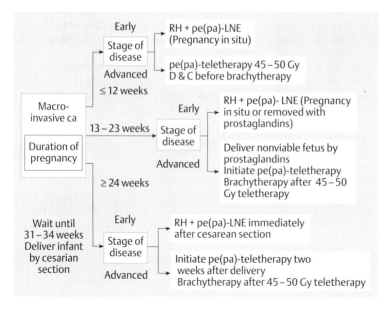

Fig. 4   Treatment algorithm for invasive cervical cancer in pregnancy (For abbreviations see Fig. 1)

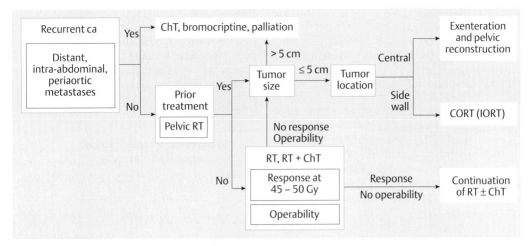

Fig. 5   Treatment algorithm for pelvic recurrences of cervical cancer (For abbreviations see Fig. 1)

interpreted as induced by pregnancy, the diagnosis of malignancy may be delayed.

Divergent opinions have been published regarding optimal treatment of cervical cancer in pregnancy.[161, 167, 170, 252, 270, 290, 326, 330, 436, 454, 484]

If cone biopsy reveals a microcarcinoma (FIGO stage IA_1, SGO definiton) expectant management with monthly Pap smears and colposcopy is advocated. Therapeutic recommendations for cases of tumor extension no longer consistent with microcarcinoma are outlined in Figure **4**. Unless the fetus is viable at the time of the diagnosis of the malignancy (before the 23rd week of gestation), termination of pregnancy is justified if the patient agrees; otherwise pregnancy is allowed to continue until the 31st to 34th week to achieve fetal pulmonary maturity, and the baby is delivered by cesarian section. Early stage (FIGO stages IA_2 [SGO: nonmicro], IB, IIA) cervical cancer should be treated with radical hysterectomy ("radical cesarian hysterectomy") and pelvic and periaortic lymphadenectomy adhering to the same criteria as in the nonpregnant state. Radical hysterectomy is performed with the pregnancy in situ in the first trimester or after delivering the nonviable fetus or the (premature) infant through a transabdominal hysterotomy. Participation in adjuvant treatment studies is not influenced by the postpregnancy state.

Patients with advanced-stage disease should receive radiation therapy. In the first trimester, initial teletherapy will usually result in abortion. If not, dilatation and curettage should be carried out before insertion of the brachytherapy applicator, or at an earlier time if uterine hemorrhage occurs. In more advanced pregnancies, the uterus may be evacuated by abdominal hysterotomy before or after external radiation if the fetus is not viable (less than 23 weeks old), or by cesarean section before radiation if the infant has a good chance of survival. In the second postoperative week, teletherapy is initiated. Brachytherapy is scheduled about 5 weeks later, when the risk of inducing uterine sepsis by the intrauterine insertion is minimized. Radiation therapy planning with respect to dose distribution, inclusion of a periaortic field, and the combination with concomitant chemotherapy is independent of pregnancy.

The reported data on treatment outcome and survival do not allow definitive conclusions about the importance of pregnancy as an independent prognostic factor. Stage for stage, no clear difference in survival between cervical cancer in the pregnant and nonpregnant patient has been demonstrated. Delaying treatment by up to 4 months to reduce the hazards of prematurity for the infant, and even vaginal delivery through a cervix carrying an advanced stage malignant disease, could not be unequivocally associated with poorer results.

Cancer of the Cervical Stump

Supracervical hysterectomy is rarely performed today. "True cervical-stump cancers" arise in a cervix after supracervical hysterectomy. By definiton, at least 2 years must have passed between the time of subtotal hysterectomy and the detection of the malignancy. Present series report an incidence of "true cervical-stump cancers" of approximately 1–2%.[308, 357, 534] While the prognosis of coincident cervical-stump cancer that existed unrecognized at the first time of supracervical hysterectomy is worse, the 5-year survival of "true stump cancers" is similar to that of cervical carcinoma with an intact uterus, when compared stage for stage and established risk factors.[256, 357, 432, 530, 534] However, one study found a significantly less favorable outcome in adenocarcinomas of the cervical stump, compared to equal stage adenocarcinomas of the intact uterus or squamous cell carcinoma of the cervical stump.[154] Definitive radiation treatment of the cervical stump using combined tele-brachytherapy produces relatively high rates of severe late complications ranging from 10–50%.[253, 357, 530] Radiation-induced late morbidity involves the bladder, rectosigmoid, and vaginal vault and is caused by the lack of the uterine body as radioprotector. As a consequence, early (stage IA–IIA) cancers of the cervical stump should be optimally treated with radical surgery despite potential difficulties due to adhesions and some distortion of the anatomy. Otherwise, treatment principles are the same as outlined in Figures **1–3**.

Nonsquamous Cell Cancer of the Uterine Cervix

It is still controversial wheter there is a difference between the overall prognosis of squamous cell carcinoma and adenocarcinoma. The established differences in continuous and metastatic spread between the cervical cancer subtypes have been taken into consideration in the treatment algorithm of Figure **2**.

Some of the rare histologic types are, however, associated with a remarkably poorer outcome: glassy cell carcinoma, which is a poorly differentiated adenosquamous carcinoma, adenoid cystic carcinoma, and small cell carcinomas. A recent report from Lotocki et al. (1992) on 32 patients with glassy cell carcinoma claimed that the therapeutic outcome of this biologically aggressive tumor could be markedly improved by bidmodal treatment with radical surgery and radiotherapy[285] compared to surgery

alone (87% vs. 45% in FIGO stage IB, 85% vs. 50% in stage II). No data are available demonstrating treatment-related differences in the other rare, poor prognostic histologic subtypes. Sarcomas, lymphomas, and the melanomas arising primary or secondarily in the cervix should be treated on an individual basis according to their known biological tumor features.

Invasive Carcinoma Treated by Simple Hysterectomy

If in a simple hysterectomy specimen, minimal invasive cancer of the uterine cervix (≤ 3 mm invasion depth, no lymphatic vascular space involvement) with clear resection margins is detected, no further treatment is necessary. Prompt secondary treatment is mandatory, however, in case of greater tumor extension. One possibility is reoperation, removing the loco-regional lymph nodes, parametria, and vaginal cuff (radical parametrectomy); otherwise post-operative radiation therapy should be initiated. Postoperative radiation combines whole pelvis and parametrial split-field teletherapy as well as vaginal ovoid and possibly interstitial brachytherapy, tailored to the potential residual tumor following inadvertent simple hysterectomy.[160, 190, 355] Most studies investigating the outcome of inadvertent hysterectomy followed by definite surgical or radiation therapy could not find significant differences in survival compared to adequate primary treatment either by radiotherapy or radical surgery. However, treatment results, when adjusted by stage and established prognostic factors, were poorer if the salvage treatment was delayed and in cases of adenocarcinomas.[96, 114, 160, 190, 288, 339, 356] Severe complication rates after simple hysterectomy followed by salvage treatments are significantly higher than those of appropriate primary radiation or radical surgery.

▪ Follow-up Surveillance

Traditionally, patients are seen for posttreatment surveillance at 3-month intervals for the first 2 years, every 6 months during the next 3 years, and once yearly thereafter—although this timing may vary. Patients are questioned regarding recurrence-related symptoms and examined by supraclavicular, abdominal, inguinal palpation, speculum inspection, Pap-smear, and bimanual rectovaginal palpation. Besides detection of recurrences, posttreatment surveillance is aimed at diagnosing therapy-related complications and secondary malignancies. If findings are negative, it is most important to reassure the patient, to reduce her anxiety, and help her live a normal life. Despite the uncertainties in patients treated with irradiation, cervicovaginal cytology is an important diagnostic tool.[446] However, equivocal opinions exist with regard to other diagnostic tests. Intravenous pyelograms and chest films were shown to be of benefit for routine use in a study by Photopulos et al.,[364] but the value of both procedures as a routine diagnostic tool was questioned by Shingleton and Orr.[499] Other conventional tests for detection of recurrent carcinoma of the cervix, such as barium enema, cystoscopy, proctoscopy, and bone scan are without clinical foundations in the asymptomatic patient. Computerized tomography (CT), and more recently magnetic resonance imaging (MRI), are presently the most powerful radiologic tools used to detect pelvic recurrences.[131, 437] Although not yet proven by clinical trials, MRI may be superior in the pelvis, whereas investigating the para-aortal lymph node chain is still the domain of CT.[25] Both diagnostic studies—in particular MRI—are expensive and time consuming and their ability to detect early (< 2 cm diameter) recurrences is unproven. Therefore, these methods should not be used for routine surveillance but should be restricted to patients with symptoms and/or pathological findings by palpation. The value of tumor markers in posttreatment surveillance is under investigation. The two most important markers are squamous cell carcinoma antigen (SCC), which is expressed in about half to two-thirds of squamous cell carcinomas of the cervix, and CA 125, which is found in similar frequency in cervical adenocarcinomas.[272, 328] Transrectal fine needle aspiration cytology has been shown to aid the diagnosis of persistent and recurrent disease.[443a]

Recurrent Disease

▨ General

About one-third of all cervical cancers persist or relapse. Disease is defined as persistent if tumor is detected 6–12 months after cessation of therapy. Tumor biology, lesion size, and treatment modality of the primary tumor dictate the incidence, time course, and site of the recurrent disease. The prognostic factors, with regard to the incidence of tumor recurrence, were discussed in the section on primary cancer of the cervix. Seventy to eighty percent of all recurrences are diagnosed within 2 years after treatment. Relapses after 5 years of survival without evidence of disease occur in about 5% of patients. After 10 years, the rate of recurrences drops to less than 1%.[393, 497] A recent prospective surgicopathological study in patients with stage IB squamous cell carcinoma of the cervix revealed tumor size, positive lymphatic vascular spaces, and depth of tumor invasion as independent prognostic factors for the length of the disease-free interval.[100] Fuller et al.[137] reported a median time for relapse of 22 months in node-negative and of 10 months in node-positive patients managed surgically for stage IB and IIA cervical carcinomas. The size of the largest lymph node in patients with pelvic lymph node metastasis has also been found to be a predictor of the disease-free interval.[213] There is evidence that the median time of recurrence is shorter in patients treated surgically than in patients receiving primary or adjuvant radiation therapy. Shingleton and Orr[449] reported median disease-free intervals of 1 year for patients treated surgically and 1.3 years for patients treated by primary radiation in a patient cohort matched for tumor size. Although comparison between surgery and primary irradiation treatments may be hampered by the inaccuracy to determine lesion size in radiated patients, other studies with cervical cancer stage IB and IIA matched for stage, tumor size, number, and location of positive lymph nodes, also found shorter median times of recurrence in the surgery-only group, compared to the adjuvant irradiation group.[77, 126]

Numerous reports have addressed the sites of recurrent cervical carcinomas with respect to patient, tumor, and treatment characteristics. Adenocarcinomas of the cervix have usually been included in most studies with squamous cell carcinomas. Recent investigations confirm the similarities between both histological types with respect to rates of recurrence and survival.[154] However, differences in distribution of distant metastases are obvious.[112] The relapse pattern of a large homogeneous patient cohort treated with definitive irradiation is presented by the Mallinckrodt Institute of Radiology.[349, 458] Similar figures have been reported from other radiation centers.[346] Upon summarizing these data, it can be calculated that about 45% of all patients relapsing after radiation therapy show distant recurrence only at initial diagnosis, 33% distant and pelvic recurrence, and 22% pelvic recurrence only (Table **12**). The impact of local failure on the incidence of distant recurrence in cervical cancer patients treated by irradiation is remarkable.[469]

Relapse pattern after surgical therapy of cervical cancers stages IB, IIA, and IIB can hardly be compared with the irradiation data, as most postsurgical studies are based on a smaller number of patients who are, in addition, usually selected with respect to prognostic factors. Patients with less favorable prognostic factors were mostly treated with adjunctive radiation as well. Nevertheless, surgical therapy of stages IB and IIA tumors tends to result in more pelvic failures and fewer distant metastases at initial diagnosis of recurrence (Table **13**). Postoperative adjuvant irradiation of stage IB and IIA patients after adequate surgery, i.e., radical hysterectomy and pelvic lymphadenectomy, results in a shift of the failure from the pelvis to distant sites with apparently no effect on the overall failure rate.

Overall, the location of recurrences within the pelvis at initial diagnosis is central in about 25–40% of patients and at the side wall in 60–75% of patients. Several studies could not detect a relationship between pelvic relapse location and treatment (if adequate), stage, tumor size, histologic type, grade, and nodal status.[77, 236, 283, 318, 349, 520] Contrary to these findings, Thomas and Dembo[482] state that tumors of node-positive patients tend to recur at the lateral pelvic

side wall, whereas pelvic relapses in node negative patients are mostly located centrally. Higher rates of central recurrences are also reported for barrel-shaped stage IB/IIA cervical cancer treated with definitive radiation or with suboptimal radical surgery.[115, 502]

The prognosis of recurrent cervical cancer is poor. Studies on unselected treated patients reveal 5-year survival rates of approximately 5%.[66, 78, 159, 174, 318, 502, 520] Median survival time in patients treated with second line therapy depends on the relapse-free period and the site of recurrence. Sommers et al.[458] observed a median survival time of 9 months for patients with a relapse-free period of less than 36 months, and 22.5 months if time between treatment and diagnosis of recurrence was more than 36 months. Krebs et al.[258] reported median survival times of 11 months for central recurrences, 8 months for side-wall disease, and 4 months for distant metastases in patients who had been treated primarily by radical hysterectomy and pelvic lymph node dissection for stage IB–IIB cancer of the cervix and by various therapies for the recurrent disease. A similar trend in postrecurrence survival was found in an investigation from Look and Rocereto.[283] Other researchers could not find a relationship between the site of recurrence and the median survival time.[62] Without therapy, 5-year survival rates of 1% and median survival times of 5 months are reported.[458] In a study of Evans et al.,[121] all patients suffering from unresectable locoregional recurrent cancer of the cervix were dead within 15 months if untreated. Autopsy findings in patients who died of persistent or recurrent cervical carcinoma demonstrated

Table **12**   Patterns of failure in cancer of the uterine cervix treated with primary radiation therapy

FIGO stage	Percent of all treated patients relapsing			
	Pelvis only	Pelvis and distant	Distant only	References
IB	1	7	8	458
	1	4	5	220
IIA	2	15	17	458
	3	3	13	220
IIB	10	11	15	458
	4	9	21	220
III	15	24	19	458
	13	9	18	220
IVA	17	61	17	458

Table **13** Patterns of failure in cancer of the uterine cervix treated with radical hysterectomy and locoregional lymphadenectomy

FIGO stage	Percent of all treated patients relapsing			
	Pelvis only	Pelvis and distant	Distant only	References
I B	11	2	6	520
	6	3	4	62
	8	5	3	269
	5	0	6	247
	7	3	5	482
II A, B	8	NR	15	520
	14	NR	17	62
	11	NR	16	269

a shift to a higher percentage of extrapelvic disease from about 50% in 1948/1949[181] to about 80% in 1967,[22] obviously due to earlier detection and better local control of the primary tumor by improved treatment techniques. Nevertheless the cause of death is pelvic disease in more than half of the patients.

▨ Diagnosis

Presently, most recurrences are detected following the occurrence of symptoms and only few are diagnosed through postsurveillance examinations before symptoms occur. Symptoms suggestive of pelvic recurrence include vaginal bleeding or discharge; flank, pelvic, or leg pain, and lower extremity swelling. Treatment-related changes in the pelvis may make diagnosis difficult. Following surgical therapy, pelvic infection, hematoma, lymphocyst, ovarian cyst, and scarring may interfere with early tumor detection. Lymphocysts and hypertrophic scars can persist and may even enlarge for more than a year. Late effects of radiation therapy in the pelvis including fibrosis and atrophy ("frozen pelvis"), necrosis, vaginal obliteration, fistula formation, and pelvic infection may render diagnosis of small recurrences impossible. Another problem with posttreatment surveillance of patients after radiation therapy results from radiobiological effects in the tumor itself. Proliferating cells need up to three duplication times to be killed by therapeutic irradiation. Therefore, macroscopic tumor regression after cessation of radiation therapy may not be complete for months although clonogenic malignant cells are no longer persistent. Difficulties also arise with cytologic testing. Depending on the time interval between treatment and cytologic evaluation, interpretation of the specimen may be difficult due to radiation changes on normal epithelium or malignant cells, which may render a precise diagnosis impossible.[298] Radiation-induced microvascular changes can mimic colposcopic criteria of malignancy. Only biopsy material can make the correct diagnosis. If symptoms or clinical findings suggest recurrence, early histologic confirmation is mandatory. Cervical biopsies and curettages for central recurrence may be hampered by complete obliteration of the upper vagina in irradiated patients. Vaginal biopsies for abnormal cytology or mucosal lesions in the irradiated patient carry the risk of fistula formation which must be weighed against the potential benefits. Transvaginal or transrectal needle biopsies have a high diagnostic yield with minimal morbidity in patients with clinically suspected recurrences without mucosal lesions.[284, 443a] For masses located higher in the pelvis and periaortic region, CT-directed percutaneous aspiration biopsies are appropriate. Pelvic and periaortic masses may also be aspirated under ultrasound guidance.[35] In case of ureteral obstruction, leg edema, pelvic, or sciatic pain, without malignant cytology on needle biopsy, explorative laparotomy may be necessary to discriminate between early recurrence and treatment-related causes.

If a pelvic recurrence is confirmed, diagnostic workup for distant metastases i.e., chest film, liver scan, or bone scan is warranted. The value of scalene lymph node biopsy is equivocal in patients without enlarged aortic or supraclavicular nodes.

Surgery

Surgery alone can be appropriate treatment for central pelvic recurrences after radiation without evidence of distant metastases. In very rare instances of radiation failure, when a small recurrent tumor is confined to the uterus, total or radical hysterectomy will suffice for complete tumor removal. Superficially growing recurrent cervical cancer in the vagina, which is generally indistinguishable from a second primary vaginal cancer, can be treated by partial or total vaginectomy. However, in most cases of central recurrent disease, pelvic exenteration is necessary to achieve local tumor control. Pelvic exenteration was introduced into gynecologic oncology in 1948 by Alexander Brunschwig.[56] This major operation includes resection of the bladder and/or the rectum en bloc together with a radical hysterectomy and vaginectomy. Exenteration is classified as "supralevator" if the caudal resection plane is located above the levator ani muscle, and as "infralevator" if the resection extends below the levator ani plane.[291] Vulvectomy may also be included in the resection. If other anatomic structures, such as parts of the pelvic bones, major blood vessels, or small and large bowel are removed as well, the exenteration is usually not curative ("extended"). Periaortic and pelvic lymphadenectomy is performed for explorative reasons if the corresponding lymph nodes had not been resected during primary treatment or metastases are suspected intraoperatively. The benefits and complications of pelvic exenteration have been reported in several large series since the technique was introduced.[291] Whereas the 5-year survival rates for central pelvic recurrences of cervical cancer remained unchanged in the range of 25–50% (obviously depending on the selection criteria), the treatment-related mortality could be reduced from 23% in the first report by Brunschwig to 5–10% or less within the last decades. Sophisticated perioperative support, improved surgical techniques, and the use of omentum and muscle flaps to reconstruct the pelvic floor have decreased the excessive early and late complication rates to 30–50%. Various new developments in surgical reconstruction of the bladder, bowel, vaginal, and vulvoperineal

functions assist the postexenteration patient in achieving psychosexual adjustment and an acceptable quality of life.[249] The magnitude of the therapeutic efforts associated with prolonged rehabilitation, as well as the fact that median survival after incomplete resection of the recurrent cervical cancer by exenterative surgery is only about 3 months, demand that the treatment goal of pelvic exenteration be curative. Palliative indications must be rare exceptions. The present criteria for locally recurrent cervical cancer to be treated with exenteration for cure are (a) central pelvic location without infiltration of the pelvic wall, i.e., the existence of a surgical free space between recurrent tumor and pelvic wall; (b) no para-aortic lymph node metastases; and (c) no intraperitoneal tumor spread. Pelvic lymph node metastasis lowers the 5-year survival rate to 10% or less. Multiple, large, or bilateral pelvic lymph-node metastases are no longer compatible with cure as is hydronephrosis. The prognostic significance of adhering small bowel infiltrated by recurrent tumor is still under debate but considered high risk for treatment failure. Advanced age, reduced mental status, extreme obesity, and debilitated health are contraindications for pelvic exenterations. The high treatment costs should also be considered; however, this issue is beyond the scope of this chapter.

Radiation Therapy

Patients with recurrent carcinoma of the cervix are regarded as candidates for radiation therapy if the disease is located in the pelvis and the primary treatment has been surgical. Radiation techniques for surgical failures in the pelvis usually consist of megavoltage external-beam irradiation of the whole pelvis with midpelvis doses between 40 and 60 Gy. Additional boost radiation, either by reduced field teletherapy or intravaginal brachytherapy, is tailored to the site of recurrent disease, attaining tumor doses of up to 100 Gy.[63, 102, 136, 224, 258, 385] The reported 5-year survival rates range from 4% to 40% in small patient series, obviously depending on the selection criteria. The mean 5-year survival rates of these studies are 34% for central disease and 16% for side-wall disease. The higher salvage rate for central disease is obviously due to the high portion of vaginal recurrences in this group, which have probably been detected at a lower tumor mass due to bleeding as a symptom.[224]

Median survival time is 11–42 months for central recurrences and 8–12 months for pelvic side-wall recurrences. In contrast to these results, Potter et al.[385] could not find differences in radio-curability with regard to location of pelvic recurrences in their study of 32 patients treated with radiation therapy for surgical failure. Histologic grade and type, as well as disease-free interval after primary treatment, also had no influence. In case of pelvic failure after external beam or combined radiation, conventional radiation techniques are no longer adequate to achieve local control since the whole pelvis does not tolerate a second tumoricidal radiation dose.[70, 261] Earlier studies reported overall 5-year survival rates between 9% and 27% with conventional reirradiation techniques, i.e., external beam and/or intracavitary brachytherapy.[320] However, more recent reports no longer support these findings. Keetell et al.[236] found only four of 145 patients (3.1%) with recurrent cervical cancer after radiation therapy, which had been reirradiated with conventional techniques, surviving 5 years. In the series reported by Jones et al.,[228] consisting of 53 initially irradiated patients who were reirradiated for recurrent pelvic disease, only one patient was alive 3.5 years after therapy and none survived for 5 years. The corresponding 5-year survival rates in the study by Sommers et al.[458] were 4% for patients receiving external reirradiation and 0% for those retreated by external irradiation and intracavitary brachytherapy. The better re-irradiation results in the early studies may be due to the less-effective initial radiation treatment, which led to a higher occurrence of limited central disease and allowed a higher percentage of curative secondary irradiation procedures.

If recurrent disease occurs very late, i.e., more than 10 years following irradiation treatment, the chance to survive for 5 or more years appears to be better. Prempree et al.[389, 393] reported on three of ten reirradiated patients living longer than 5 years without disease and another three patients living without evidence of disease for 2.5 years and longer.

Successful reirradiation of small central pelvic recurrences with interstitial brachytherapy techniques have been reported from several centers.[261, 332, 395, 401] Because of the steep decline in radiation dose with interstitial therapy, the treatment volume is minimal for a given tumor target. Whereas radium-226 and gold-198 seeds with poor geometric distribution were used earlier, re-

cent interstitial irradiation techniques mainly employ permanent iodine-125 or temporary iridium-192 implants. Implantation is performed either transperineally, guided by a template, or through laparotomy. Although the total number of patients treated with these methods is still very low, local control rates of more than 50% are claimed with projected 5-year survival rates of 20–46%.

While the rate of severe late complications for pelvic irradiation of surgical failures is less than 10%, and treatment-related mortality is less than 1%[136], complication rates for reirradiation of recurrent tumors following prior radiation therapy are much higher. Severe complication rates of up to 33% are reported if second potentially curative irradiation doses are applied within 5 years after primary treatment.[228, 236, 387]

Complication rates of reirradiation seem to be lower in cases with late or very late recurrences in the preirradiated pelvis.[343] New interstitial implant techniques may also lower grade III late complications of reirradiation. Puthawala et al.[395] found 15% serious complications in their series of 40 patients. When evaluating these numbers, it must be considered that the overall prognosis in pelvic recurrences is poor. Most of the patients die before late radiation complications can develop.

Although the value of palliation of pelvic recurrences of cervical carcinoma by irradiation or reirradiation has been advocated by several authors,[228, 236, 495] it is difficult to demonstrate objective benefits. Lower back, hip and leg pain, and vaginal bleeding are sometimes regarded as indications for palliative irradiation treating only a small treatment volume and using hypofractionation.

Chemotherapy

Chemotherapy as a sole modality has been applied in recurrent cervical carcinoma for treatment of locoregional, as well as systemic disease. Cytotoxic substances that are active in primary cervical cancer have also been used for the treatment of recurrent or metastatic disease (Table **14**).

Contrary to the results in untreated locally advanced primary disease, no significant differences between cisplatin alone and cisplatin combinations were found in several randomized studies.[25, 47, 70, 188, 376, 378, 419, 479, 516] Response rates were in the range of 30–40% with median

Table **14**   Results of cisplatin-based cytotoxic therapy in locally recurrent and metastatic squamous cell cancer of the uterine cervix

Agents	Dose i.v. mg/m^2	Response rate n/N^a (%)	Median response duration (months)	Grade > 3 toxicity rate^b (%)	References
Cisplatin	50	13/34 (38)	NR	NR	191,480
Cisplatin	50 – 100	24/79 (32)	6	24	419
5-fluorouracil	1000 × 5				47
Cisplatin	20 × 5	10/17 (53)	8	12	43
Bleomycin	30				
Cisplatin	60 – 75	11/36 (27)	NR	0	195
Methotrexate	100 – 300				
Bleomycin	15 – 30				
Cisplatin	50 – 75	13/69 (19)	12	20	455
Mitomycin C	10 – 15				189
Bleomycin	15 – 20				
Cisplatin	50	51/98 (52)	10	20	400
Ifosfamid	5000			(one death)	64
Bleomycin	30				260
Cisplatin	50	12/54 (22)	7	NR	8
Mitomycin C	10				
Vincristine	1				
Bleomycin	10				

^{a} Number of patients responding/number of patients treated.
^{b} Except nausea/vomiting and alopecia.

response durations of 3–6 months and median survival of 5–9 months. Hoskins et al.[195] obtained response rates of 27% in recurrent disease compared to 67% in primary cancer of the cervix with cis-platinum, methotrexate, and bleomycin combination chemotherapy. In previously irradiated sites, only 9% of the patients with recurrent carcinoma responded. In general, recurrent, persistent, or gross metastatic disease represent advanced disease, with a high probability for the tumor to have developed multidrug resistance. In addition, a bulky tumor mass is associated with a lower growth fraction of tumor cells and a larger portion of clonogenic nonproliferating cells; both lead to reduced susceptibility to chemotherapy.[103, 151] Low pO$_2$ regions, which are more frequent in recurrent tumors (Höckel et al., unpublished results), reduce the sensitivity of tumor cells toward most cytotoxic drugs.[410, 478] Even if all tumor cells are senstive to a chemotherapeutic regimen, insufficient tumor perfusion due to high intratumoral–interstitial pressure prevent adequate drug transport and complete tumor cell death by chemotherapy.[218] These effects are especially pronounced in recurrent or persistent pelvic tumors following surgical or irradiation treatments that have resulted in fibrotic or fibroatrophic tumor beds. Moreover, the application of full courses of chemotherapy in patients with recurrent cervical carcinoma may be hampered by reduced renal function associated with ureteral obstruction and by a compromised bone marrow reserve in case of prior irradiation.

Although suggested, it has not been shown unequivocally that chemotherapy has an impact on survival in metastatic cancer of the uterine cervix.[509] Nevertheless, anecdotal reports on long-term survival of patients with distant, in particular periaortic and lung metastases after chemotherapy, have been published.[7, 378, 384, 507]

Reported data are scarce with respect to second-line chemotherapy. Wheelock et al.[526] recently demonstrated that the cytotoxic combination of bleomycin, vincristine, and mitomycin C is ineffective as second-line chemotherapy against recurrent cervical cancer after failure of cis-platinum as first-line treatment.

Attempts to improve the clinical results of chemotherapy for pelvic recurrences by regional arterial perfusion techniques did not show the expected results to date.[68, 235, 226, 316, 472] Superselective perfusion of pelvic tumors that recur after surgical or radiation therapy is rarely possible because of the treatment-related alterations in pelvic vascular anatomy.

In vitro sensitivity testing may be of value in selecting patients who would or would not benefit from chemotherapy because of primary resistant tumor cells.[79, 340] An approach using programmed chemotherapy for recurrent cervical carcinoma has been suggested by some authors.[20, 335] This involves the use of one drug to enrich or synchronize a fraction of cells within a phase of the cell cycle when another drug exhibits an optimal cytotoxic effect.[26] Cycle phases can be monitored in tumor tissue biopsies by flow cytometric techniques to obtain the most precise timing for drug administration. Until now a clinical breakthrough by this laborious method could not be achieved.

▪ Combined Treatment Modalities

Surgery and Radiation

The CORT Procedure

Based on tumor and radiobiological considerations, Höckel et al. have introduced the combined operative and radiotherapeutic treatment (CORT) approach[197, 198, 200, 202] for recurrent gynecologic malignancies infiltrating the pelvic wall. The operative part consists of (a) surgically defining the extent of disease; (b) R_1 tumor resection; (c) implantation of guiding tubes for afterloading brachytherapy of the tumor bed at the pelvic wall; (d) pelvic wall plasty with either muscle, myocutaneous, and greater omentum flaps, and (e) individualized pelvic reconstructive surgery. Radiotherapy is performed as preoperative teletherapy of the pelvis and postoperative brachytherapy via implanted tubes. In case of previous pelvic irradiation, tube-guided brachytherapy is applied exclusively. It is suggested that the CORT concept synergistically combines surgical and radiation treatment to improve the therapeutic ratio between tumor control and tissue tolerance in the pelvis. Higher local radiation doses can be applied compared to conventional methods in cases of prior surgery, and reirradiation with

locally controlling doses is possible even after previous primary or adjuvant radiation. Surgical tumor resection is performed with the goal of leaving only a microscopic residuum at the pelvic wall. By R_1 resection of the tumor, a significantly lower radiation dose is necessary to achieve tumor control.[536] Due to the intraoperative placement of afterloading tubes for brachytherapy directly on the tumor bed and because of the steep dose decline of interstitial irradiation, the treatment volume for a given tumor target is minimized. One rationale for using tissue flaps to cover the tumor bed is to create a protective distance between the guide tubes at the pelvic wall and the radiointolerant hollow pelvic organs. The radiation dose to the mucosa of these organs is thereby reduced to 15% or less. The pelvic wall plasty is also thought to reduce the risk of pelvic infection and abscess formation, which could lead to significant postoperative morbidity and mortality, and would strongly reduce the antitumor radiation effects.[231] Moreover, pelvic wall plasty is regarded as a surgical means of therapeutic angiogenesis,[205] compensating for the radiation-induced microvascular compromise of the pelvic wall tissues. The transfer of well-vascularized nonirradiated tissue with high angiogenic potential to the preirradiated pelvic wall should improve its radiotolerance. Therapeutic angiogenesis of the tumor bed by the pelvic wall plasty may also increase the radiosensitivity of residual hypoxic tumor through reoxygenation.

From 1989 to 1993; 37 patients with postirradiation recurrent gynecologic malignancies of the pelvic wall were treated with CORT and studied in a prospective trial at the University of Mainz. Twenty-two patients had recurrent cervical cancers infiltrating the pelvic wall. No patient died from the treatment. Seven patients developed complications necessitating surgical intervention. At a median follow-up of 20 months (range 3–45 months), 11 patients (50%) progressed in the pelvis and/or recurred distantly. Four-year survival probability according to the Kaplan–Meier method was 40%. During the same period, 13 patients comparable in age, recurrence-free interval, recurrent tumor size, and history of pelvic radiation and with central recurrences from cancer of the uterine cervix were treated by exenteration alone. Survival of these patients with central relapses was similar to the patients with pelvic wall recurrences.

According to the Cox proportional hazards model, recurrent tumor size and patient age influenced survival but not relapse location.

Intraoperative Radiation Therapy (IORT)

The basis of intraoperative radiation therapy was described in the chapter on primary cervical carcinoma. Because of its proposed improved therapeutic ratio, IORT has also been used for the treatment of locally recurrent cervical carcinoma not resectable with tumor-free margins, such as periaortic and pelvic side-wall disease. Several small studies of IORT in recurrent cervical carcinoma have been published.[67, 98, 109, 143, 539] The data do not allow appropriate evaluation of this combined modality treatment for recurrent cervical cancer at present.

Chemotherapy and Radiation

A few studies on chemoradiotherapy for advanced primary cervical carcinoma also included recurrent disease.[178, 262, 267, 481] For a critical evaluation of this treatment concept, its methodological variations, and reported results, the reader is referred to the corresponding chapter in the primary disease section. Patient numbers treated with chemoradiotherapy for recurrent cervical carcinoma—either sequentially or concomitantly—are generally too small to draw conclusions on the effect of this combined modality treatment compared to radiation alone.

However, a recent report from Thomas et al.[483] noted a 5-year survival probability of 45% in patients with surgical failures treated with concomitant chemoradiation. Thirty-one out of 40 patients had recurrent cervical cancers infiltrating the pelvic side wall. Disease was biopsy proven in 85%.

The radiation regimen consisted of whole-pelvis teletherapy, delivering a tumor dose of 53 Gy, followed by a cesium application into the vaginal vault or an external boost of radiation to a smaller volume. One to three courses of 5-fluorouracil (1000 mg/m^2) were given by continuous intravenous infusion for 3–4 days during teletherapy. Serious late bowel complications occurred in five patients (12%) being fatal in one patient who presented with tumor progression at that time.

■ Current Treatment Strategies

An algorithm suggested for the treatment of recurrent cervical cancer is shown in Figure **5**. The demonstration of distant, intra-abdominal, or periaortic metastases with or without local pelvic disease renders recurrent cervical cancer incurable. Likewise, large-volume local disease, recurrent after radiation therapy, is associated with such a high probability of distant metastasis that long-term survival is extremely rare even after complete surgical resection by exenterative procedures. Our own series investigated 35 patients with locally recurrent cancer of the uterine cervix, treated with exenteration for central disease, and CORT in case of pelvic-wall infiltration. The study revealed a 4-year survival probability for tumors with a diameter of more than 5 cm of 10%, compared to 64% for tumor sizes up to 5 cm in diameter. Multivariate Cox regression analysis confirmed local tumor volume as the most significant predictive parameter of survival. It must be decided on an individual basis whether chemotherapy (which may prolong survival for a few months) should be applied or not. The anecdotally reported antiproliferative effect of bromocriptine is probably mediated through the inhibition of autocrine prolactin production, which has been recently detected in a subset of cervical carcinomas.[168, 208]

The individualized surgical and/or radiotherapeutic treatment of single-site distant metastases, as well as palliative treatment of recurrent cervical cancer symptoms, such as pain, hemorrhage, urinary and bowel fistulas or obstruction, thrombosis, sepsis, uremia, etc. are beyond the scope of this text.

Individualized radiation or concomitant radiochemotherapy could be the first treatment option for surgical failures. If radiation has already been applied or pelvic irradiation for recurrences does not show any response at 45–50 Gy, exenterative surgery should be offered in case of central pelvic disease and general operability of the patient. The CORT procedure now expands the indication for pelvic exenteration to pelvic side-wall disease recurring or progressing after radiation, which has been regarded so far as a contraindication. IORT can only apply a single radiation dose to the tumor bed at the pelvic wall, whereas CORT allows fractionation and higher cumulative doses. However, the therapeutic effectiveness of CORT and

IORT in controlling pelvic side-wall disease has not been compared in controlled studies. Likewise, no prospective trials have been performed comparing radiotherapy alone, concomitant radiochemotherapy, or exenterative surgery and CORT, as treatments for local surgical failures.

Future Prospects

Current research in basic and clinical oncology, with respect to novel concepts and modalities to treat solid tumors, focuses on four topics: (a) reduction of radicality in the treatment of early primary tumors without compromising long-term survival; (b) improvement in locoregional control of advanced and recurrent local disease; (c) more effective prevention of systemic disease in patients whose tumors are locally controlled; and (d) improved palliation of gross systemic disease.

Predictive Assays

To securely reduce local treatment radicality in early stage cancer of the uterine cervix, biologic tumor parameters predicting the invasive and metastatic potential of the individual neoplasm must be detectable before treatment. One important step toward this goal has been to define microinvasive carcinomas that can be treated adequately with conization or simple hysterectomy, if the patient wishes to maintain fertility.

Jakobsen et al. (1990) established a score derived from FIGO stage, tumor size, DNA index, and malignancy grade score (MGS) to predict lymphatic tumor spread in FIGO stage IA_2, IB and IIA tumors.[219] MGS[463] considers eight histopathologic parameters of a tumor biopsy, i.e., growth pattern, cell type, nuclear polymorphism, mitotic activity, mode of invasion, depth of invasion, vascular invasion, and plasmolymphocytic cellular response in the tumor periphery. This score has been prospectively evaluated. A subset of patients with practically no risk of lymph node metastases was selected, which could have been treated with conization, simple hysterectomy, or vaginal radical hysterectomy instead of the traditional Wertheim–Meigs operation, without loss of therapeutic efficacy. Future research may identify molecular-biologic tumor parameters,

which can be determined within a clinical setting from pretreatment biopsy material and allow unbiased estimates of the invasive and metastatic potential.

To obtain local control in patients with advanced or recurrent cancer of the uterine cervix, newer treatment modalities such as hyperthermia, photodynamic therapy, and immunotherapy are being explored.

For locally advanced and recurrent disease without tumor dissemination, which is traditionally treated with radiation, pretherapeutic assessment of radiocurability will become an important future prospect. The radiosensitivity of solid tumor depends not only on the intrinsic properties of the tumor cells, but is also significantly influenced by extrinsic factors of the host mediated through the microenvironment of tumor growth. A variety of assays for intrinsic radiosensitivity, tumor cell repair capacity, normal tissue response, as well as the determination of tumor cell kinetics and ploidy are currently under investigation for their importance as predictive assays in radiation therapy.[524]

Höckel et al. have shown that microenvironmental tumor oxygenation measured with a computerized polarographic needle electrode histograph is the most powerful predictor of survival and recurrence-free survival in locally advanced primary cancer of the uterine cervix, treated with standard radiation with or without preceeding chemotherapy.[199, 201, 203] Intratumoral pO_2 histography enables pretherapeutic selection of low pO_2 tumors as candidates for modified treatment approaches, such as radiation concomitant with carbogen or hyperbaric oxygen breathing, hypoxic cell sensitization, or hyperthermia.[27, 80, 186] Another therapeutic option to be investigated in locally advanced low pO_2 cervical cancers, may be extended radical surgery, including exenterative procedures and CORT[198, 202] in case of pelvic side-wall involvement.

Hyperthermia

Heating mammalian cells to 43°C and above results in a certain degree of cell killing, possibly due to denaturation of chromosomal proteins and membrane damage. Sensitivity of cells to hyperthermia varies greatly with the cell type. Generally, tumor cells are more thermally sensitive than normal cells, although temperature-resistant mutants can be obtained after thermal shock, either by induction or selection. Thermal resistance also depends on the cell cycle phase: the S-phase is most sensitive and the G1-phase most resistant to hyperthermic treatment. Hypoxic, nutritionally deprived, low pH cells are somewhat more heat sensitive.[105] Besides direct cell killing, hyperthermia induces profound changes in tissue perfusion, which may secondarily lead to lethal cell damage. Tumor microvasculature seems to be more sensitive to heating than normal tissue vasculature.[505]

As cell-killing characteristics between hyperthermia and photon-electron irradiation are complementary—both radioresistant S-phase cells and hypoxic cells are radiosensitized by heating—the combination of these treatment modes may offer significant therapeutic gain in cancer therapy. Nevertheless, many problems must be solved empirically, such as the optimal temperature and the sequence for applying hyperthermia and irradiation. Precise temperature control is critical.[232] The possibility that hyperthermia may increase local complications, as well as the metastatic potential also has to be taken into consideration.[231]

Hyperthermia alone, as well as combined hyperthermia and radiotherapy, is presently being investigated as a new treatment form for persistent and recurrent cervical cancer. Regional hyperthermia is applied either by radiofrequency current via perineal interstitial needles or with an annular array of electromagnetic wave applicators. Several feasibility studies have been published on a variety of malignant diseases, recurrent or persistent, after multimodal primary treatment, including some gynecologic tumors.[196, 264, 359, 396, 397, 433, 440, 448] Surwit et al.[470] applied interstitial thermoradiotherapy in 12 patients with recurrent cervical cancer following primary or adjuvant irradiation. Three patients had complete responses of 15, 8, and 3 months duration; partial responses were noted in six patients. Two severe complications (rectovaginal fistulas) occurred. Since heating also enhances the cytotoxicity of many (but not all) chemotherapeutic agents, the combined use of hyperthermia and chemotherapy might lead to a therapeutic improvement. With respect to the application of thermochemotherapy for cervical carcinoma, only anecdotal and phase I studies have been published.[214] Although the first clinical studies support the general projections deduced from basic tumor biology, a benefit of hyperthermia used alone or in combination with radiation or cytotoxic drugs in cervical cancer has yet to be proven.

Photodynamic Therapy

The cytotoxic mechanism of this novel treatment approach is the photoactivation of hematoporphyrin derivatives, which are selectively concentrated in the tumor tissue after systemic application. Photoactivation by means of visible light generated by laser systems leads to the formation of single oxygen radicals with a high potency to destroy the tumor vascularization and tumor cells themselves, supposedly by membrane damage. Presently the major technical problem of photodynamic therapy is the delivery of high light intensities to the treated tissue. Therefore, superficially located sites have mostly been studied with this treatment modality. However, more deeply seated tumors may be illuminated by interstitial glass fiber implants. Photodynamic therapy has been applied with phase I/II studies in a small number of recurrent cervical cancers after radiation.[84, 274, 407, 515] The role of this new modality as salvage treatment remains to be established.

Immunotherapy/Biological Response Modifiers

Means to stimulate the immune response of the host against malignant disease are referred to as immunotherapy. The target of the stimulated immune response is usually the tumor cell but may also be the tumor vasculature. Increased knowledge of the biology of the tumor and the host's immune system, and the development of advanced biochemical, molecular, and cell biological technology have led to a broad spectrum of immunotherapeutic approaches in experimental clinical oncology. Earlier methods of active immunotherapy involved either the injection of unspecific immunostimulants such as BCG (Bacillus Calmette Guérin) or specific tumor antigens. Although successful in animal experiments and initial clinical studies, large randomized prospective studies could not confirm benefits of nonspecific immunotherapy using systemic BCG for primary, as well as adjuvant treatment, in cervical carcinoma.[107] In addition to classic immunotherapy, a variety of sophisticated new treatment forms have recently been designed using autologous immune cells and/or biologic response modifiers. One reason for the typically weak immune response of the host against the tumor is believed to be the dominant action of T suppressor cells. Therefore, immuno-therapeutic strategies are aimed at either selectively reducing T suppressor cells, or increasing the number of T helper cells.

A number of biologic response modifiers have also been found to be either antiprolifera-tive/cytotoxic for tumor cells or for the tumor vasculature, and/or to activate the immune response against the malignant disease. Since these substances are available by large-scale production with recombinant gene technologies, a large number of clinical studies have been performed administrating biologic response modifiers into tumor patients. In general, systemic toxicity prevented a major breakthrough in antineoplastic therapy by this approach. However, there is some evidence that biologic response modifiers may improve therapeutic effects if used together with other treatment modalities such as chemotherapy or radiation.[281, 442, 522] Another use of biologic response modifiers is to reduce hematopoetic complications of cytotoxic chemotherapy with colony-stimulating factors. It remains to be demonstrated if any of these approaches will be of benefit in the treatment of cervical cancer.

Prevention and Palliation of Systemic Disease

The impact of systemic chemotherapy in conjunction with conventional regimens as adjuvant treatment of patients whose tumors may be locally controlled, but bear a high risk of distant relapses, is awaited from the large multicenter studies recently initiated. Based on these results, new systemic therapies need to be investigated, which may also include novel biological anti-metastatic approaches.[179]

Finally, new concepts for the palliation of gross systemic disease with acceptable side effects must be studied. These may involve anti-angiogenic therapy or approaches interfering with tumor cell proliferation.[42, 129, 130, 487]

References

1. Abe M, Takahashi M, Yabumoto E, Onoyama Y, Torizuka K. Techniques, indications and results of intraoperative radiotherapy of advanced cancers. Radiology. 1975; 116(3):693–702.

2. Abe M, Takahashi M, Yabumoto E, Adachi H, Yoshii M, Mori K. Clinical experiences with intraoperative radiotherapy of locally advanced cancers. Cancer. 1980; 45:40–48.

3. Abe M. Intra-operative radiotherapy: The Japanese experience. J Radiat Oncol Biol Phys. 1981; 7:863–868.

4. Adcock L. Radical hysterectomy preceded by pelvic irradiation. Gynecol Oncol. 1979; 8:152–163.

5. Akine Y, Arimoto H, Ogino T, Kajiura Y et al. High-dose-rate intracavitary irradiation in the treatment of carcinoma of the uterine cervix: Early experience with 84 patients. Int J Radiat Oncol Biol Phys. 1988; 14:893–898.

6. Akine Y, Tokita N, Ogino T et al. Dose equivalence for high-dose-rate to low-dose-rate intracavitary irradiation in the treatment of cancer of the uterine cervix. Int J Radiat Oncol Biol Phys. 1990; 19:1511–1514.

7. Alberts DS, Martimbeau PW, Surwit EA, Oishi N. Mitomycin-C, bleomycin, vincristine, and cis-platinum in the treatment of advanced, recurrent squamous cell carcinoma of the cervix. Cancer Clin Trials. 1981; 4:313–316.

8. Alberts DS, Kronmal R, Baker L. Phase II randomized trial of cisplatin chemotherapy regimens in the treatment of recurrent or metastatic squamous cell cancer of the cervix: A Southwest Oncology Group study. J Clin Oncol. 1987; 5:1791–1795.

9. Allen HH, Collins JA. Surgical management of carcinoma of the cervix. Am J Obstet Gynecol. 1977; 127:741–744.

10. Alvarez RD, Soong SJ, Kinney W. Identification of prognostic factors and risk groups in patients found to have nodal metastasis at the time of radical hysterectomy for early stage squamous carcinoma of the cervix. Gynecol Oncol. 1989; 35:130–131.

11. Alvarez RD, Potter M, Soong S-J et al. Rationale for using pathologic tumor dimensions and nodal status to subclassify surgically treated stage IB cervical cancer patients. Gynecol Oncol. 1991; 43:108–112.

12. Alvarez RD, Gelder M, Gore H, Soong S, Pathridge E. Radical hysterectomy in the treatment of patients with bulky early stage carcinoma of the cervix uteri. Surg Gynecol Obstet. 1993; 176:539–542.

13. American Cancer Society: Cancer Statistics, 1991. CA. 1991; 41:1.

14. Ampuero F, Doss L, Khan M, Skipper B, Hilgers R. The Syed-Neblett interstitial template in locally advanced gynecological malignancies. Int J Radiat Oncol Biol Phys. 1983; 9:1897–1903.

15. Anderson B, LaPolla J, Turner D, Chapman G, Buller R. Ovarian transposition in cervical cancer. Gynecol Oncol. 1993; 49:206–214.

16. Angel C, DuBeshter B, Lin JY. Clinical presentation and management of stage I cervical adenocarcinoma: A 25 year experience. Gynecol Oncol. 1992; 44:71–78.

17. Aristizabal SA, Valencia A, Surwit E, Hevezi J. Treatment of locally advanced cancer of the cervix with transperineal interstitial irradiation. Am J Clin Oncol. (CCT) 1983; 6:645–650.

18. Aristizabal SA, Woolfitt B, Valencia A, Ocampo G, Surwit E, Sim D. Interstitial parametrial implants in carcinoma of the cervix stage II-B. Int J Radiat Oncol Biol Phys. 1987; 13:445–450.

19. Artman LF, Hoskins W, Bibro MC. Radical hysterectomy and pelvic lymphadenectomy for stage IB carcinoma of the cervix: Twenty-one years' experience. Gynecol Oncol. 1987; 28:8–13.

20. Averette HE, Weinstein GD, Ford Jr JH, Girtanner RE, Hoskins WJ, Ramos R. Cell kinetics and programmed chemotherapy for gynecologic cancer. I. Squamous-cell carcinoma. Am J Obstet Gynecol. 1976; 124:912–923.

21. Averette HE, Nguyen HN, Donato DM et al. Radical hysterectomy for invasive cervical cancer. Cancer. 1993; 71:1422–1437.

22. Badib AO, Kurohara SS, Webster JH, Pickren JW. Metastasis to organs in carcinoma of the uterine cervix. Influence of treatment on incidence and distribution. Cancer. 1968; 21:434–439.

23. Baltzer J, Koepcke W. Tumor size and lymph node metastases in squamous cell carcinoma of the uterine cervix. Arch Gynecol. 1979; 227:271.

24. Baltzer J, Lohe KJ, Koepcke W. Histological criteria for the prognosis in patients with operated squamous cell carcinoma of the cervix. Gynecol Oncol. 1982; 13:184.

25. Bandy LC, Clarke-Pearson DL, Silverman PM, Creasman WT. Computed tomography in evaluation of extrapelvic lymphadenopathy in carcinoma of the cervix. Obstet Gynecol. 1985; 65:73–76.

26. Barranco SC, Luce SK, Romsdahl MW, Humphrey RM. Bleomycin as a possible synchronizing agent for human tumor cells in vivo. Cancer Res. 1973; 33:882–887.

27. Barthelink H, Overgaard J. Tumor hypoxia. Radiother Oncol Suppl. 1991; 20:1–157.

28. Barter JF, Soong SJ, Hatch KD, Orr JW, Shingleton HM. Diagnosis and treatment of pulmonary metastases from cervical carcinoma. Gynecol Oncol. 1990; 38:347–351.

29. Bates TD. The treatment of stage 3 carcinoma of the cervix by external radiotherapy and high-pressure oxygen. Br J Radiol. 1969; 42:266–269.

30. Beecham JB, Halvorsen T, Kolbenstvedt A. Histologic classification, lymph node metastases, and patient survival in stage IB cervical carcinoma. An analysis of 245 uniformly treated cases. Gynecol Oncol. 1978; 6:95.

31. Belli JA, Piro AJ. The interaction between radiation and adriamycin damage in mammalian cells. Cancer Res. 1977; 37:1624–1630.

32. Benedet JL, Turko M, Boyes DA. Radical hysterectomy in the treatment of cervical cancer. Am J Obstet Gynecol. 1980; 137:254–262.

33. Bennett MB. The treatment of stage III squamous carcinoma of the cervix in air and hyperbaric oxygen. Br J Radiol. 1978; 51:68.

34. Berchuck A, Rodriguez G, Kamel A. Expression of epidermal growth factor receptor and HER-2/neu in normal and neoplastic cervix, vulva, and vagina. Obstet Gynecol. 1990; 76:381–387.

35. Berkowitz RS, Leavitt Jr T, Knapp RC. Ultrasound-directed percutaneous aspiration biopsy of periaortic lymph nodes in recurrence of cervical carcinoma. Am J Obstet Gynecol. 1978; 131:906–908.

36. Berkowitz RS, Ehrmann RL, Lavizzo-Mourey R, Knapp RC. Invasive cervical carcinoma in young women. Gynecol Oncol. 1979; 8:311–316.

37. Berman ML, Keys H, Creasman W, DiSaia P, Bundy B, Blessing J. Survival and patterns of recurrence in cervical cancer metastatic to periaortic lymph nodes. Gynecol Oncol. 1984; 19:8–16.

38. Berman ML, Bergen S, Salazar H. Influence of histological features and treatment on the prognosis of patients with cervical cancer metastatic to pelvic lymph nodes. Gynecol Oncol. 1990; 39:127–131.

39. Bichel P, Jakobsen A. Histopathologic grading and prognosis of uterine cervical carcinoma. Am J Clin Pathol. 1985; 8:247–254.

40. Blaikley JB, Ledermann M, Pollard W. Carcinoma of the cervix at Chelsea Hospital for Women, 1935–1965: Five-year and 1-year results of treatment. J Obstet Gynaecol Br Commonw. 1969; 76:729–740.

41. Blake PR, Lambert HE, MacGregor WG, O'Sullivan JC, Dowdell JW, Anderson T. Surgery following chemotherapy and radiotherapy for advanced carcinoma of the cervix. Gynecol Oncol. 1984; 19:198–203.

42. Bloch A. Induced cell differentiation in cancer therapy. Cancer Treat Rep. 1984; 68:199–205.

43. Bloch B, Nel CP, Kriel A, Atad J, Goldberg G. Combination chemotherapy with cisplatin and bleomycin in advanced cervical cancer. Cancer Treat Rep. 1984; 68:891–893.

44. Bloss JD, Berman ML, Mukhererjee J et al. Bulky stage IB cervical carcinoma managed by primary radical hysterectomy followed by tailored radiotherapy. Gynecol Oncol. 1992; 47:21–27.

45. Blythe JG, Hodel KA, Wahl TP, Baglan RJ, Lee FA, Zivnuska FR. Para-aortic node biopsy in cervical and endometrial cancers: Does it affect survival? Am J Obstet Gynecol. 1986; 155:306–314.

46. Bonomi, P, Blessing JA, Stehman FB. Randomized trial of three cisplatin dose schedules in squamous cell carcinoma of the cervix: A gynecologic oncology group study. J Clin Oncol. 1985; 3:1079–1085.

47. Bonomi, P, Blessing JA, Ball H, Hanjani P, DiSaia PJ. A phase II evaluation of cisplatin and 5-fluorouracil in patients with advanced squamous cell carcinoma of the cervix: A gynecologic oncology group study. Gynecol Oncol. 1989; 34:357–359.

48. Boronow RC. Should whole pelvic radiation therapy become past history? A case for the routine use of extended field therapy and multimodality therapy. Gynecol Oncol. 1991; 43:71–76.

49. Boutselis JG. Intraepithelial carcinoma of the cervix associated with pregnancy. Obstet Gynecol. 1972; 40:657–666.
50. Boyce JG, Fruchter RG, Nicastri AD. Vascular invasion in stage I carcinoma of the cervix. Cancer. 1984; 53:1175–1180.
51. Brady LW, Markoe AM, DeEulis T, Lewis Jr GC. Gynecology: Combined radiotherapy and chemotherapy in gynecologic oncology. Int J Radiat Oncol Biol Phys. 1988; 14:5203–5209.
52. Branson AN, Dunn P, Kam KC, Lambert HE. A device for interstitial therapy of low pelvic tumors–the Hammersmith perineal hedgehog. Br J Radiol. 1985; 58:537–542.
53. Brenner DJ, Hall EJ. Fractionated high dose-rate versus low dose-rate regimens for intracavitary brachytherapy of the cervix. II. Equivalent regimens for combined brachytherapy and external irradiation. Int J Radiat Oncol Biol Phys. 1990; 18:1407–1413.
54. Brenner DJ, Hall EJ. Fractionated high dose rate versus low dose rate regimens for intracavitary brachytherapy of the cervix. I. General considerations based on radiobiology. Br J Radiol. 1991; 64:133–141.
55. Brinton LA, Hoover RN. Epidemiology of Gynecologic Cancers. In: Gynecologic Oncology. Hoskins HJ, Perez CA, Young RC, eds. Philadelphia: Lippincott; 1992:3–26.
56. Brunschwig A, Barber HRK. Surgical treatment of carcinoma of the cervix. Obstet Gynecol. 1966; 27:21–29.
57. Buchsbaum HJ. Extrapelvic lymph node metastases in cervical carcinoma. Am J Obstet Gynecol. 1979; 133:814–824.
58. Burghardt E, Pickel H. Local spread and lymph node involvement in cervical cancer. Obstet Gynecol. 1978; 52:138–145.
59. Burghardt E, Pickel H, Haas J, Lahousen M. Prognostic factors and operative treatment of stages IB to IIB cervical cancer. Am J Obstet Gynecol. 1987; 156:988–996.
60. Burke TW, Hoskins WJ, Heller PJ. Prognostic factors associated with radical hysterectomy failure. Gynecol Oncol. 1987; 26:153–159.
61. Burke TW, Heller PB, Hoskins WJ, Weiser EB, Nash JD, Park RC. Evaluation of the scalene lymph nodes in primary and recurrent cervical carcinoma. Gynecol Oncol. 1987; 28:312–317.
62. Burke TW, Hoskins WJ, Heller PB, Shen MC, Weiser EB, Park RC. Clinical patterns of tumor recurrence after radical hysterectomy in stage IB cervical carcinoma. Obstet Gynecol. 1987; 69:382–385.
63. Bush RS, Jenkin RDT, Allt WEC. Definitive evidence for hypoxic cells influencing cure in cancer therapy. Br J Cancer. 1978; 37:302–306.
64. Buxton EJ, Blackledge G, Mould JJ. The role of Ifosfamide in cervical cancer. Semin Oncol. 1989; 16:60–67.
65. Byfield JE, Calabro-Jones P, Klisak I, Kulhanian F. Pharmacologic requirements for obtaining sensitization of human tumor cells in vitro to combined 5-Fluorouracil or Ftorafur and X-rays. Int J Radiat Oncol Biol Phys. 1982; 8:1923–1933.
66. Calame RJ. Recurrent carcinoma of the cervix. Am J Obstet Gynecol. 1969; 105:380–385.
67. Calkins AR, Lester SG, Stehman FB, Mc Cammon R, Hornback NB. Intraoperative radiotherapy in advanced, recurrent or metastatic malignancy. Indians Med. 1985; 78:206–208.
68. Carlson Jr JA, Freedman RS, Wallace S, Chuang VP, Wharton JT, Rutledge FN. Intra-arterial cis-platinum in the management of squamous cell carcinoma of the uterine cervix. Gynecol Oncol. 1981; 12:92–98.
69. Cary A, Free KE, Wright RG, Shield PW. Carcinoma of the cervix-recurrence in Queensland 1982–1986. Int J Gynecol Cancer. 1992; 207–214.
70. Cavins JA, Geisler HE. Treatment of advanced, unresectable, cervical carcinoma already subjected to complete irradiation therapy. Gynecol Oncol. 1978; 6:256–260.
71. Chambers SK, Chambers JT, Holm C, Peschel RE, Schwartz PE. Sequelae of lateral ovarian transposition in unirradiated cervical cancer patients. Gynecol Oncol. 1990; 39:155–159.
72. Chang HC, Lai CH, Chen MS, Chao AS, Chen LH, Soong Y-K. Preliminary results of concurrent radiotherapy and chemotherapy with cis-platinum, vincristine, and bleomycin in bulky, advanced cervical carcinoma: A pilot study. Gynecol Oncol. 1992; 44:182–188.
73. Chapman GW. Survival of advanced age females with carcinoma. Gynecol Oncol. 1992; 46:287–291.
74. Choo YC, Choy TK, Wong LC, Ma HK. Potentiation of radiotherapy by Cis-dichlorodiamine platinum (II) in advanced cervical carcinoma. Gynecol Oncol. 1986; 23:94–100.
75. Choy D, Wong LC, Sham J, Ngan HYS, Ma HK. Dose-tumor response for carcinoma of cervix: An analysis of 594 patients treated by radiotherapy. Gynecol Oncol. 1993; 49:311–317.
76. Christensen A, Lange P, Neilsen E. Surgery and radiotherapy for invasive cancer of the cervix: Surgical treatment. Acta Obstet Gynecol. 1964; 43:59–87.
77. Chung CK, Nahhas WA, Stryker JA, Curry SL, Abt AB, Mortel R. Analysis of factors contributing to treatment failures in stages IB and IIA carcinoma of the cervix. Am J Obstet Gynecol. 1980; 138:550–556.
78. Chung CK, Nahhas WA, Stryker JA, Mortel R. Treatment outcome of recurrent cervical cancer. J Surg Oncol. 1983; 24:5–10.
79. Cohen CJ, Deppe G, Yannopoulos K, Gusberg SB. Chemosensitivity testing with cis-platinum (II) diamine-dichloride. 1. A new concept in the treatment of carcinoma of the cervix. Gynecol Oncol. 1982; 13:1–9.
80. Coleman CN. Review. Hypoxia in tumors: A paradigm for the approach to biochemical and physiologic heterogeneity. J Natl Cancer Inst. 1988; 80:310–317.

81. Coleman DL, Gallup DG, Wolcott HD, Otken LB, Stock RJ. Patterns of failure of bulky-barrel carcinomas of the cervix. Am J Obstet Gynecol. 1992; 166:916–920.

82. Connor ME, Davidson SE, Stern PL, Arrand JR, West CML. Evaluation of multiple biologic parameters in cervical carcinoma: High macrophage infiltration in HPV-associated tumors. Int J Gynecol Cancer. 1993; 3:103–109.

83. Copeland LJ, Silva EG, Gershenson DM, Morris M, Young DC, Wharton JT. Superficially invasive squamous cell carcinoma of the cervix. Gynecol Oncol. 1992; 45:307–312.

84. Corti L, Tomio L, Maluta S et al. Recurring gynaecologic cancer treated with photodynamic therapy. Photochem Photobiol. 1987; 46:949–952.

85. Cox JD, Guse C, Asbell S, Rubin P, Sause WT. Tolerance of pelvic normal tissues to hyperfractionated radiation therapy: Results of protocol 83-08 of the radiation therapy oncology group. Int J Radiat Oncol Biol Phys. 1988; 15:1331–1336.

86. Crawford ER, Robinson LS, Vaught J. Carcinoma of the cervix. Results of treatment by radiation alone and by combined radiation and surgical therapy in 335 patients. Am J Obstet Gynecol. 1965; 91:480–485.

87. Cradick RN. Carcinoma of the cervical stump. Am J Obstet Gynecol. 1958; 75:565–574.

88. Creasman WT, Rutledge FN, Fletcher GH. Carcinoma of the cervix associated with pregnancy. Obstet Gynecol. 1970; 36:495–501.

89. Crissman JD, Makuch R, Budhraja H. Histopathologic grading of squamous cell carcinoma of the uterine cervix: An evaluation of 70 stage IB patients. Cancer. 1985; 55:1590–1596.

90. Crissman JD, Budhraja M, Aron BS, Gummings G. Histopathologic prognostic factors in stage II and III squamous cell carcinoma of the uterine cervix. Int J Gynecol Pathol. 1987; 6:97–103.

91. Cunningham MJ, Dunton CJ, Corn B et al. Extended-field radiation therapy in early-stage cervical carcinoma: Survival and complications. Gynecol Oncol. 1991; 43:51–54.

92. Dale RG. The use of small fraction numbers in high dose-rate gynecological afterloading: Some radiobiological considerations. Br J Radiol. 1990; 63:290–294.

93. Darne J, Soutter WP, Ginsberg R, Sharp F. Nuclear and "cytoplasmic" estrogen and progesterone receptors in squamous cell carcinoma of the cervix. Gynecol Oncol. 1990; 35:216–219.

94. Dattoli MJ, Gretz HF, Beller U. Analysis of multiple prognostic factors in patients with stage IB cervical cancer: Age as a major determination. Int J Radiat Oncol Biol Phys. 1989; 17:41–47.

95. Davidson SE, Symonds RP, Lamont D, Watson ER. Does adenocarcinoma of uterine cervix have a worse prognosis than squamous carcinoma when treated by radiotherapy? Gynecol Oncol. 1989; 33:23–26.

96. Davy M, Bentzen H, Jahren R. Simple hysterectomy in the presence of invasive cervical cancer. Acta Obstet Gynecol Scand. 1977; 56:105–108.

97. Delgado G, Coglar H, Walker P. Survival and complications in cervical cancer treated by pelvic and extended field radiation after para-aortic lymphadenectomy. Am J Roentgenol. 1978; 130:141–143.

98. Delgado G, Goldson AL, Ashayeri E, Hill LT, Petrilli ES, Hatch KD. Intraoperative radiation in the treatment of advanced cervical cancer. Obstet Gynecol. 1984; 63:246–252.

99. Delgado G, Bundy BN, Fowler WC. A prospective surgical pathological study of stage I squamous carcinoma of the cervix: A Gynecologic Oncology Group study. Gynecol Oncol. 1989; 35:314–320.

100. Delgado G, Bundy B, Zaino R, Sevin B-U, Creasman WT, Major F. Prospective surgical-pathological study of disease-free interval in patients with stage IB squamous cell carcinoma of the cervix: A gynecologic oncology group study. Gynecol Oncol. 1990; 38:352–357.

101. Deppe G, Malviya VK, Han I et al. A preliminary report of combination chemotherapy with cisplatin and mitomycin-c followed by radical hysterectomy or radiation therapy in patients with locally advanced cervical cancer. Gynecol Oncol. 1991; 42:178–181.

102. Deutsch M, Parsons JA. Radiotherapy for carcinoma of the cervix recurrent after surgery. Cancer. 1974; 34:2051–2055.

103. DeVita Jr VT. The relationship between tumor mass and resistance to chemotherapy. Cancer. 1983; 51:1209–1220.

104. DeWys WD. Studies correlating the growth rate of a tumor and its metastases and providing evidence for tumor-related system growth-retarding factors. Cancer Res. 1972; 32:374–379.

105. Dewey WC, Hopwood LE, Sapareto SA, Gerweck LE. Cellular responses to combinations of hyperthermia and radiation. Radiology. 1977; 123:463–474.

106. Dickson RJ, Late results of radium treatment of carcinoma of the cervix. Clin Radiol. 1972; 23:528–535.

107. DiSaia PJ, bundy BN, Curry SL, Schlaerth J, Thigpen JT. Pahse III study on the treatment of women with cervical cancer, stage IIB, IIIB, and IVA (confined to the pelvis and/or periaortic nodes), with radiotherapy alone versus radiotherapy plus immunotherapy with intravenous corynebacterium parvum: A gynecologic oncology group study. Gynecol Oncol. 1987; 26:386–397.

108. Dische S, Anderson PJ, Sealy R, Watson ER. Carcinoma of the cervix—anaemia, radiotherapy and hyperbaric oxygen. Br J Radiol. 1983; 56:251–255.

109. Dosoretz DE, Tepper JE, Shim DS et al. Intraoperative electron beam irradiation in gynecologic malignant disease. Appl Radiol. 1984; 13:61–63.

110. Dottino PR, Plaxe SC, Beddoe AM, Johnston C, Cohen CJ. Induction chemotherapy followed by radical surgery in cervical cancer. Gynecol Oncol. 1991; 40:7–11.

111. Downey GO, Potish RA, Adcock LL, Prem KA, Twiggs LB. Pretreatment surgical staging in cervical carcinoma: Therapeutic efficacy of pelvic lymph node resection. Am J Obstet Gynecol. 1989; 160:1055–1061.
112. Drescher CW, Hopkins MP, Roberts JA. Comparison of the pattern of metastatic spread of squamous cell cancer and adenocarcinoma of the uterine cervix. Gynecol Oncol. 1989; 33:340–343.
113. Drescher CW, Reid GC, Terada K et al. Continuous infusion of low-dose 5-fluorouracil and radiation therapy for poor-prognosis squamous cell carcinoma of the uterine cervix. Gynecol Oncol. 1992; 44:227–230.
114. Durrance FR. Radiotherapy following simple hysterectomy in patients with stage I and II carcinoma of the cervix. Am J Roentgenol Radium Ther Nucl Med. 1968; 102:165–169.
115. Durrance FY, Fletcher GH, Rutledge FN. Analysis of central recurrent disease in stage I and II squamous cell carcinomas of the cervix on intact uterus. Am J Roentgenol. 1969; 106:831–838.
116. Dyson JED, Joslin CAF, Rothwell RI. Flow cytofluorometric evidence for the differential radioresponsiveness of aneuploid and diploid cervix tumors. Radiother Oncol. 1987; 8:263–272.
117. Einhorn N, Patek E, Sjöberg B. Outcome of different treatment modalities in cervix carcinoma stage IB and IIA. Cancer. 1985; 55:949–955.
118. Ellis F. Dose, time and fractionation: a clinical hypothesis. Clin Radiol. 1969; 20:1–7.
119. Erickson KR, Truitt JS, Bush SE, Ritcher N, Pathak D, Khan KM. Interstitial implantation of gynecologic malignancies using Syed-Neblett template: Update of results, technique, and complications. Endocurie, Hypertherm Oncol. 1989; 5:99–105.
120. Evans JC, Bergsjo P. The influence of anemia on the results of radiotherapy in carcinoma of the cervix. Radiology. 1965; 81:709–716.
121. Evans Jr SR, Hilaris BS, Barber HRK. External vs. interstitial irradiation in unresectable recurrent cancer of the cervix. Cancer. 1971; 28:1284–1288.
122. Evans LS, Kersh CR, Constable WC. Concomitant 5-Fluorouracil and Mitomycin-C with radiotherapy in the primary management of advanced gynecologic malignancy. Int J Radiat Oncol Biol Phys. 1987; 13(1):129.
123. Falappa P, Trodella L, Cotroneo AR, Turriziani A. Advanced carcinoma of the cervix treated by continuous pelvic arterial infusion with cytostatic and radiation therapy. Europ J Radiol. 1982; 2:307–309.
124. Feder BH, Syed AMN, Neblett D. Treatment of extensive carcinoma of the cervix with the "Transperineal Parametrial Butterfly." A preliminary report on the revival of Waterman's approach. Int J Radiat Oncol Biol Phys. 1978; 4:735–842.
125. Fedorkow DM, Robertson DI, Duggan MA, Nation JG, McGregor SE, Stuart GCE. Invasive squamous cell carcinoma of the cervix in women less than 35 years old: Recurrent versus nonrecurrent disease. Am J Obstet Gynecol. 1988; 158:307–311.
126. Figge DC, Tamimi HK. Patterns of recurrence of carcinoma following radical hysterectomy. Am J Obstet Gynecol. 1981; 140:213–220.
127. Fiorica JV, Roberts WS, Greenberg H, Hoffman MS, LaPolal JP, Cavanagh D. Morbidity and survival patterns in patients after radical hysterectomy and postoperative adjuvant pelvic radiotherapy. Gynecol Oncol. 1990; 36:343–347.
128. Fletcher GH. Cancer of the uterine cervix: Janeway Lecture. Am J Roentgenol Radium Ther Nucl Med. 1971; 111:225–242.
129. Folkman J, Langer R, Linhardt RJ, Haudenschild C, Taylor S. Angiogenesis inhibition and tumor regression caused by heparin or a heparin fragment in the presence of cortisone. Science. 1983; 221:719–725.
130. Foon KA, Bernhardt MI, Oldham RK. Monoclonal antibody therapy: Assessment by animal tumor models. J Biol Resp Modif. 1982; 1:277–304.
131. Franchi M, La Fianza A, Babilonti L et al. Clinical value of computerized tomography (CT) in assessment of recurrent uterine cancers. Gynecol Oncol. 1989; 35:31–37.
132. Frei III E, Miller D, Clark JR, Fallon BG, Ervin TJ. Clinical and scientific considerations in preoperative (neoadjuvant) chemotherapy. In: Recent results in cancer research Berlin, Heidelberg: Springer; 1986:1–5.
133. Friedberg V, Beck T. Ergebnisse operativer Therapie des Zervixkarzinoms im Stadium II B. Geburtsh u Frauenheilk. 1989; 49:782–786.
134. Friedberg V. Ergebnisse von 108 Exenterationsoperationen bei fortgeschrittenen gynäkologischen Karzinomen. Geburtsh u Frauenheilk. 1989; 49.
135. Friedlander ML, Atkinson K, Coppleson JVM et al. The integration of chemotherapy into the management of locally advanced cervical cancer: A pilot study. Gynecol Oncol. 1984; 19:1–7.
136. Friedman M, Pearlman AW. Carcinoma of the cervix: Radiation salvage of surgial failures. Radiology. 1965; 84:801–811.
137. Fuller A, Elliott N, Kosloff C, Hoskins W, Lewis J. Determinants of increased risk for recurrence in patients undergoing radical hysterectomy for stage IB and IIA carcinoma of the cervix. Gynecol Oncol. 1989; 33:34–39.
138. Fu YS, Reagan JW. Benign and malignant epithelial lesions of the uterine cervix. In: Pathology of the uterine cervix, vagina, and vulva. Bennington JL, ed. San Francisco: WB Saunders, 1989; 225–335.
139. Fu KK, Phillips TL. High-dose-rate versus low-dose-rate intracavitary brachytherapy for carcinoma of the cervix. Int J Radiat Oncol Biol Phys. 1990; 19:791–796.
140. Gaddis Jr O, Morrow CP, Klement V, Schlaerth JB, Nalick RH. Treatment of cervical carcinoma employing a template for transperineal interstitial Ir192 brachytherapy. Int J Radiat Oncol Biol Phys. 1983; 9:819–827.

141. Gallion HN, Van Nagell JR, Donaldson GS. Combined radiation therapy and extrafascial hysterectomy in the treatment of stage IB barrel-shaped cervical cancer. Cancer. 1985; 56:262–265.

142. Gallion HH, Maruyama V, Van Nagell JR. Treatment of stage IIIB cervical cancer with Californium-252 fast-neutron brachytherapy and external photon therapy. Cancer. 1987; 59:1709–1712.

143. Garton GR, Gunderson LL, Webb MJ et al. Intraoperative radiation therapy in gynecologic cancer: The Mayo clinic experience. Gynecol Oncol. 1993; 48:328–332.

144. Garza de La J, Guadarrama R, Ramirez J, Candelario S. Cisplatin, epirubicin and cyclophosphamide + radiotherapy in stage IIB, IIIB cervix carcinoma. Proc Am Soc Clin Oncol. 1987; 6:A441.

145. Gauthier P, Gore I, Shingleton H. Identification of histopathologic risk groups in stage IB squamous cell carcinoma of the cervix. Obstet Gynecol. 1985; 66:569.

146. Giaroli A, Sananes C, Sardi JE et al. Lymph node metastases in carcinoma of the cervix uteri: Response to neoadjuvant chemotherapy and its impact on survival. Gynecol Oncol. 1990;39:34–39.

147. Girardi F, Haas J. The importance of the histologic processing of pelvic lymph nodes in the treatment of cervical cancer. Int J Gynecol Cancer. 1993; 3:12–17.

148. Goellner JR. Carcinoma of the cervix: Clinicopathologic correlation of 196 cases. Am J Clin Pathol. 1976; 66:775–785.

149. Goertz SR, Ali MM, Goplerud D. "A Controversy Reviewed"—Treatment of para-aortic disease. Int J Radiat Oncol Biol Phys. 1988; 15(1): 232–233.

150. Goldhirsch A, Greiner R, Bleher A et al. Combination of chemotherapy with methotrexate, bleomycin, and CIS-platinum and radiation therapy for locally advanced carcinoma of the cervix. Am J Clin Oncol. 1986; 9:12–14.

151. Goldie JH. Scientific basis for adjuvant and primary (neoadjuvant) chemotherapy. Seminars in Oncology. 1987; 14:1–7.

152. Goldson AL, Delgado G, Hill LT. Intraoperative radiation of the paraaortic nodes in cancer of the uterine cervix. Obstet Gynecol. 1978; 52:713–717.

153. Goldson AL. Past, present, and prospects of intraoperative radiotherapy. Seminars in Oncology. 1981; 8(1):59–64.

154. Goodman HM, Niloff JM, Buttlar CA et al. Adenocarcinoma of the cervical stump. Gynecol Oncol. 1989; 35:188–192.

155. Goodman HM, Buttlar CA, Niloff JM et al. Adenocarcinoma of the uterine cervix: Prognostic factors and patterns of recurrence. Gynecol Oncol. 1989; 33:241–247.

156. Goolsby CD, Daly JW, Skinner OD, Gibbs CE. Combination of 5-Fluorouracil and radiation as primary therapy of carcinoma of the cervix. Obstet Gynecol. 1968; 32:674–676.

157. Gorai I, Yanagibashi T, Minaguchi H. Immunological modulation of lymphocyt subpopulation in cervical cancer tissue by sizofiran and OK-432. Gynecol Oncol. 1992; 44:137–146.

158. Gordon AN, Bornstein J, Kaufmann R, Estrada RG, Adams E, Adler-Storthz K. Human papillomavirus associated with adenocarcinoma and adenosquamous carcinoma of the cervix: Analysis by in situ hybridization. Gynecol Oncol. 1989; 35:345–348.

159. Graham J, Graham R, Hirabayashi K. Recurrent cancer of the cervix uteri. Surg Gynecol Obstet. 1968; 126:799–804.

160. Green TH, Morse WJ. Management of invasive cervical cancer following inadvertent simple hysterectomy. Obstet Gynecol. 1969; 33:763–769.

161. Greer BE, Easterling TR, McLennon DA. Fetal and maternal considerations in the management of stage IB cervical cancer during pregnancy. Gynecol Oncol. 1989; 34:61–65.

162. Grigsby PW, Perez CA, Kuske RR. Adenocarcinoma of the uterine cervix: Lack of evidence for a poor prognosis. Radiother Oncol. 1988; 12:289–296.

163. Grigspy PW, Perez CA. Radiotherapy alone for medically inoperable carcinoma of the cervix: Stage IA and carcinoma in situ. Int J Radiat Oncol Biol Phys. 1991; 21:375–378.

164. Gunderson LL, Weems WS, Hebertson RM, Plenk HP. Correlation of histopathology with clinical results following radiation therapy for carcinoma of the cervix. Am J Roentgenol Radium Ther Nucl Med. 1974; 120:74–87.

165. Gunderson LL, Shipley WU, Suit HD et al. Intraoperative irradiation. A pilot study combining external beam photons with "boost" dose intraoperative electrons. Cancer. 1982; 49:2259–2266.

166. Gupta BD, Ayyagari S, Sharma SC, Negi PS, Patel F. In: Brachytherapy Mould RF, ed. The Netherlands: Nucleotron Trading BV, Leersum; 1989; 307–308.

167. Gustafsson DC, Kottmeier HL. Carcinoma of the cervix associated with pregnancy. Acta Obstet Gynecol Scand. 1962; 41:1–21.

168. Guthrie D. Treatment of carcinoma of the cervix with bromocriptine. Br J Obstet Gynecol. 1982; 89; 853–855.

169. Guttmann R. Significance of postoperative irradiation in carcinoma of the cervix: A ten year survey. Radiotherapy. 1970; 108:102–108.

170. Hacker NF, Berek JS, Lagasse LD, Charles EH, Savage EW, Moore G. Carcinoma of the cervix associated with pregnancy. Obstet Gynecol. 1982; 59:735–746.

171. Haie C, Pejovic MH, Gerbaulet A et al. Is prophylactic para-aortic irradiation worthwhile in the treatment of advanced cervical carcinoma? Results of a controlled clinical trial of the EORTC radiotherapy group. Radiother Oncol. 1988; 11:101–112.

172. Hale RJ, Buckley CH, Fox H, Wilcox FL, Tindall VR, Logue JP. The morphology and distribution of lymph node metastases in stage IB/IIA cervical carcinoma: Relationship to prognosis. Int J Gynecol Cancer. 1991; 1:233–237.

173. Hale RJ, Ryder WDJ, Wilcox FL, Buckley CH, Tindall VR. Cervical carcinoma: a hazard model in early stage disease. Int J Gynecol Cancer. 1992; 2:79–82.

174. Halpin TF, Frick II HC, Munnell EW. Critical points of failure in the therapy of cancer of the cervix: A reappraisal. Am J Obstet Gynecol. 1972; 114:755–764.
175. Hanks GE, Herring DF, Kramer S. Patterns of care outcome studies: Results of the national practice in cancer of the cervix. Cancer. 1983; 51:959–967.
176. Hasumi K, Sakamoto A, Sugano H. Microinvasive carcinoma of the uterine cervix. Cancer. 1980; 45:928–931.
177. Hatch KD, Cervical Cancer. In: Practical Gynecologic Oncology Berek JS, Hacker NF, eds. Baltimore, Hong Kong, London, Sydney: Willims + Wilkins; 1989:241–284.
178. Heaton D, Yordan E, Reddy S et al. Treatment of 29 patients with bulky squamous cell carcinoma of the cervix with simultaneous Cisplatin, 5-Fluorouracil, and Split-Course hyperfractionated radiation therapy. Gynecol Oncol. 1990; 38:323–327.
179. Hellmann K. Antimetastatic drugs: Laboratory to clinic. Clin Exp Metastasis. 1984; 2:1–4.
180. Henk JM. Does hyperbaric oxygen have a future in radiation therapy? Int J Radiat Oncol Biol Phys. 1981; 7:1125–1128.
181. Henriksen E. Dispersion of cervix cancer. Radiology 1950; 54:812–815.
182. Hensche UK. Afterloading applicator for radiation therapy of carcinoma of the uterus. Radiology. 1960; 74:834.
183. Himmelmann A, Willén R, Iosif S, Prien-Larsen J, Ranstam J, Astedt B. Prospective histopathologic malignancy grading to indicate the degree of postoperative treatment in early cervical carcinomas. Gynecol Oncol. 1992; 46:37–41.
184. Hintz BL, Kagan AR, Chan P. Radiation tolerance of the vaginal mucosa. Int J Radiat Oncol Biol Phys. 1980; 6:711–716.
185. Hiraoka O, Nakai T, Shimizu C. Modified pelvic vascular bed isolation chemotherapy: Theoretical basis, surgical procedure, and two clinical case reports. Gynecol Oncol. 1980; 9:135–152.
186. Hirst DG. Oxygen delivery to tumors. Int J Radiat Oncol Biol Phys. 1986; 12:1271–1277.
187. Hirst DG. Anemia: A problem or an opportunity in radiotherapy? Int J Radiat Oncol Biol Phys. 1986; 12:2009–2017.
188. Hoffman MS, Roberts WS, Bryson SCP, Kavanagh Jr JJ, Cavanagh D, Lyman GH. Treatment of recurrent and metastatic cervical cancer with cis-platin, doxorubicin, and cyclophosphamide. Gynecol Oncol. 1988; 29:32–36.
189. Hoffman MS, Kavanagh JJ, Roberts WS et al. A phase II evaluation of cisplatin, bleomycin, and mitomycin-c in patients with recurrent squamous cell carcinoma of the cervix. Gynecol Oncol. 1991; 40:144–146.
190. Hopkins MP, Peters WA, Anderson W, Morley GW. Invasive cervical cancer treated initially by standard hysterectomy. Gynecol Oncol. 1990; 36:7–12.
191. Hopkins MP, Morley GW. Stage I B squamous cell cancer of the cervix: Clinicopathologic features related to survival. Am J Obstet Gynecol. 1991; 164:1520–1529.
192. Horiot JC, Nabid A, Chaplain G. Clinical experience with multiple daily fractionation in the radiotherapy of head and neck cancer. Cancer Bulletin. 1982; 34:230.
193. Horiot JC, Pigneux J, Pourquier H. Radiotherapy alone in carcinoma of the intact uterine cervix according to GH Fletcher Guidelines: A French Cooperative study of 1383 cases. Int J Radiat Oncol Biol Phys. 1988; 14:605–611.
194. Hoskins WJ, Ford JH, Lutz MH, Averette HE. Radical hysterectomy and pelvic lymphadenectomy for the management of early invasive cancer of the cervix. Gynecol Oncol. 1976; 4:278–290.
195. Hoskin PJ, Blake PR. Cis-platin, methotrexate and bleomycin (PMB) for carcinoma of the cervix: The influence of presentation and previous treatment upon response. Int J Gynecol Cancer. 1991; 1:75–80.
196. Howard GCW, Sathiaseelan V, King GA, Dixon AK, Anderson A, Bleehen NM. Regional hyperthermia for extensive pelvic tumors using an annular phased array applicator: a feasibility study. Br J Rad. 1986; 59; 1195–1201.
197. Höckel M, Kutzner J, Bauer H, Friedberg V. Eine neue experimentelle Methode zur Behandlung von Beckenwandrezidiven gynäkologischer Malignome. Geburtsh u Frauenheilk. 1989; 49:981–986.
198. Höckel M, Knapstein PG, Kutzner J. A novel combined operative and radiotherapeutic treatment approach for recurrent gynecology malignant lesions infiltrating the pelvic wall. Surg Gynecol Obstet. 1991; 173:297–302.
199. Höckel M, Schlenger K, Knoop C, Vaupel P. Oxygenation of carcinomas of the uterine cervix: Evaluation by computerized O_2 tension measurements. Cancer Res. 1991; 51:6098–6102.
200. Höckel M, Knapstein PG. The combined operative and radiotherapeutic treatment (CORT) of recurrent tumors infiltrating the pelvic wall: First experience with 18 patients. Gynecol Oncol. 1992; 46:20–28.
201. Höckel M, Vorndran B, Schlenger K, Baussmann E, Knapstein PG. Tumor oxygenation: A new predictive parameter in locally advanced cancer of the uterine cervix. Gynecol Oncol. 1993; 51:141–149.
202. Höckel M, Knapstein PG, Hohenfellner R, Rösler HP, Kutzner J. Die kombinierte operative and radiotherapeutische Behandlung (CORT) von Beckenwandrezidiven: Erfahrungsbericht nach 3 Jahren. Geburtsh u Frauenheilk. 1993; 53:169–176.
203. Höckel M, Knoop C, Schlenger K et al. Intratumoral pO2 predicts survival in advanced cancer of the uterine cervix. Radiother Oncol. 1993; 26:45–50.
204. Höckel M, Müller T. A new template assembly for transperineal interstitial irradiation. Radiother Oncol. 1994; 31:262–264.
205. Höckel M, Schlenger K, Doctrow S, Kissel T, Vaupel P. Therapeutic Angiogenesis. Arch Surg. 1993; 128:423–429.

206. Hreshchyshyn MM. Hydroxyurea with irradiation for cervical carcinoma—preliminary report. Cancer Chemotherapy Rept. 1968; 52:601–602.

207. Hreshchyshyn MM, Aron BS, Boronow RC, Franklin III EW, Shingleton HM, Blessing JA. Hydroxyurea or placebo combined with irradiation to treat stages III B and IV cervical cancer confined to the pelvis. Int J Radiat Oncol Biol Phys. 1979; 5:317–322.

208. Hsu CT, Yu MH, Lee CYG, Jong HL, Yeh MY. Ectopic production of prolactin in uterine cervical carcinoma. Gynecol Oncol. 1992; 44:166–171.

209. Hunter RE, Longscope C, Keough P. Steroid hormone receptors in carcinoma of the cervix. Cancer. 1987; 60:392.

210. Hurt WG, Silverberg SG, Frable WJ. Adenocarcinoma of the cervix. Histopathologic and clinical features. Am J Obstet Gynecol. 1977; 129:304–315.

211. Ilijas M. Proposal of a modified (FIGO 1985) classification of stages I and II cancer of the uterine cervix. Gynecol Oncol. 1992; 47:210–215.

212. Inoue T. Prognostic significance of the depth of invasion, and cell types. A study of 628 cases with stage IB, IIA and IIB cervical carcinoma. Cancer. 1984; 54:3035–3042.

213. Inoue T, Chihara T, Morita K. The prognostic significance of the size of the largest nodes in metastatic carcinoma from the uterine cervix. Gynecol Oncol. 1984; 19:187–193.

214. Issels RD, Wadepohl M, Tiling K, Müller M, Sauer H, Wilmanns W. Regional hyperthermia combined with systemic chemotherapy in advanced abdominal and pelvic tumors: First results of a pilot study employing an annular phased array applicator. In: Recent Results in Cancer Research Berlin, Heidelberg: Springer; 1988:236–243.

215. Itoh N, Sawairi M, Hanabayashi T, Mori H, Yamawaki Y, Tamaya T. Neoadjuvant intraarterial infusion chemotherapy with a combination of mitomycin-c, vincristine, and cisplatin for locally advanced cervical cancer: A preliminary report. Gynecol Oncol. 1992; 47:391–394.

216. Iwasaka T, Yokoyama M, Oh-Uchida M et al. Detection of human papillomavirus genome and analysis of expression of c-myc and ha-ras oncogenes in invasive cervical carcinomas. Gynecol Oncol. 1992; 46:298–303.

217. Jacobs AJ, Perez CA, Camel HM, Kao MS. Complications in patients receiving both irradiation and radical hysterectomy for carcinoma of the uterine cervix. Gynecol Oncol. 1985; 27:412–419.

218. Jain RK. Delivery of novel therapeutic agents in tumors: Physiological barriers and strategies. J Natl Cancer Inst. 1989; 81:570–576.

219. Jakobsen A, Bichel P, Ahrons S, Nyland M, Knudsen J. Is radical hysterectomy always necessary in early cervical cancer? Gynecol Oncol. 1990; 39:80–81.

220. Jampolis S, Andras EJ, Fletcher GH. Analysis of sites and causes of failures of irradiation in invasive squamous cell carcinoma of the intact uterine cervix. Radiol. 1975; 115:681–685.

221. Jarrell MA, Heintz N, Howard P et al. Squamous cell carcinoma of the cervix: HPV 16 and DNA ploidy as predictors of survival. Gynecol Oncol. 1992; 46:361–366.

222. Ji HX, Syrjänen S, Klemi P, Chang F, Tosi P, Syrjänen K. Prognostic significance of human papillomavirus (HPV) type and nuclear DNA content in invasive cervical cancer. Int J Gynecol Cancer. 1991; 1:59–67.

223. Jobson V, Homesley H, Muss H. Chemotherapy of advanced squamous carcinoma of the cervix: A phase I–II study of high-dose cisplatin and cyclophosphamide. Am J Clin Oncol. 1984; 7:341–345.

224. Jobsen JJ, Leer JWH, Cleton FJ, Hermans J. Treatment of locoregional recurrence of carcinoma of the cervix by radiotherapy after primary surgery. Gynecol Oncol. 1989; 33:368–371.

225. John M, Cooke JK, Flam M, Padmanabhan A, Mowry PA. Preliminary results of concomitant radiotherapy and chemotherapy in advanced cervical carcinoma. Gynecol Oncol. 1987; 28:101–110.

226. John B, Scarbrough EC, Nguyen PD, Antich PP. A diverging gynecological template for radioactive interstitial/intracavitary implants of the cervix. Int J Radiat Oncol Biol Phys. 1988; 15:461–465.

227. John M, Flam M, Sikic B et al. Preliminary results of concurrent radiotherapy and chemotherapy in advanced cervical carcinoma: A phase I–II prospective intergroup NCOG-RTOG study. Gynecol Oncol. 1990; 37:1–5.

228. Jones Jr TK, Levitt SH, King ER. Retreatment of persistent and recurrent carcinoma of the cervix with irradiation. Radiology. 1970; 95:167–174.

229. Kalra J, Cortes E, Chen S et al. Effective multimodality treatment for advanced epidermoid carcinoma of the female genital tract. J Clin Oncol. 1985; 3:917–924.

239. Kapp DS, Fischer D, Gutierrez E. Pretreatment prognostic factors in carcinoma of the uterine cervix: A multivariate analysis of the effects of age, stage, histology and blood counts on survival. Int J Radiat Oncol Biol Phys. 1983; 9:445–455.

231. Kapp DS, Lawrence R. Temperature elevation during brachytherapy for carcinoma of the uterine cervix: Adverse effect on survival and enhancement of distant metastasis. Int J Radiat Oncol Biol Phys. 1984; 10:2281–2292.

232. Kapp DS, Cox RS, Fessenden P et al. Parameters predictive for complications of combined hyperthermia (HT) and radiation therapy (XRT). Radiat Oncol Biol Phys. 1988; 15(1):122.

233. Kataoka M, Kuwamura M, Nishiyama Y, Hamada K, Hamamoto K, Matsu-Ura S. Results of the combination of external-beam and high-dose-rate intracavitary irradiation for patients with cervical carcinoma. Gynecol Oncol. 1992; 44:48–52.

234. Kato T, Nemoto R, Mori H, Takahashi M, Tamakawa Y, Harada M. Arterial chemoembolization with microencapsulated anticancer drug. An approach to selective cancer chemotherapy with sustained effects. JAMA 1981; 245:1123–1127.

235. Kavanagh Jr JJ. Regional chemotherapeutic approaches to the management of pelvic malignancies. Cancer Bulletin, 1984; 36:52–55.

236. Keettel WC, Van Voorhis LW, Latourette HB. Management of recurrent carcinoma of the cervix. Am J Obstet Gynecol. 1968; 102:671–679.

237. Kenter GG, Cornelisse CJ, Aartsen EJ et al. DNA ploidy level as prognostic factor in low stage carcinoma of the uterine cervix. Gynecol Oncol. 1990; 39:181–185.

238. Kersh CR, Constable WC, Spaulding CA, Hahn SS, Andersen WA, Taylor PT. A phase I–II trial of multimodality management of bulky gynecologic malignancy. Combined chemoradiosensitization and radiotherapy. Cancer. 1990; 66:30–34.

239. Ketcham AS, Hoye RC, Taylor PT, Deckers PJ. Radical hysterectomy and lymphadenectomy for carcinoma of the uterine cervix. Cancer. 1971; 28:1271–1277.

240. Keys H, Blessing J et al. Hydroxyurea and radiation for stages III B and IVA cervix cancer: Analysis of recurrence patterns and radiation factors. Int J Radiat Oncol Biol Phys. 1980; 6:1429.

241. Kim DS, Moon H, Hwang YY, Cho SH. Preoperative adjuvant chemotherapy in the treatment of cervical cancer stage IB, II A and II B with bulky tumor. Gynecol Oncol. 1988; 29:321–332.

242. Kim RY, Black NC, Salter MM. Lurleen B. Wallace cervical-uterine applicator. Intracavitary treatment of cancer of the uterine cervix. Alabama J Med Sci. 1988; 25:288–290.

243. Kim D, Moon H, Kim K, Hwang Y, Cho S, Kim S. Two-year survival: Preoperative adjuvant chemotherapy in the treatment of cervical cancer stages IB and II with bulky tumor. Gynecol Oncol. 1989; 33:225–230.

244. Kim RY, Trotti A, Wu CJ. Radiation alone in the treatment of cancer of the uterine cervix: Analysis of pelvic failure and dose response relationship. Int J Radiat Oncol Biol Phys. 1989; 17:973–978.

245. Kim JW, Sung HR, Kim DK, Song CH. Estrogen and progesterone receptor assay in carcinoma of the cervix with monoclonal antibodies. Gynecol Oncol. 1992; 47:306–310.

246. King LA, Tase T, Twiggs LB. Prognostic significance of the presence of human papillomavirus DNA in patients with invasive carcinoma of the cervix. Cancer. 1989; 63:897–900.

247. Kinney WK, Alvarez RD, Reid GC et al. Value of adjuvant whole-pelvis irradiation after Wertheim hysterectomy for early-stage squamous carcinoma of the cervix with pelvic nodal metastasis: A matched-control study. Gynecol Oncol. 1989; 34:258–262.

248. Kline JC, Schultz AE, Vermund H, Peckham BM. High dose radiotherapy for carcinoma of the cervix: Method and results. Am J Obstet Gynceol. 1969; 104:479–484.

249. Knapstein PG, Friedberg V, Sevin BU. Reconstructive surgery in gynecology. Stuttgart: Thieme; 1990.

250. Knee R, Field RS, Peters LJ. Concomitant boost radiotherapy for advanced squamous cell carcinoma of the head and neck. Radiother Oncol. 1985; 4:1.

251. Kolstad P. Follow-up study of 232 patients with stage I A1 and 411 patients with stage I A2 squamous cell carcinoma of the cervix (microinvasive carcinoma). Gynecol Oncol. 1989; 33:265–272.

252. Koren G, Weiner L, Lishner M, Zemelickes D, Finegan J. Cancer in pregnancy: Identification of unanswered questions on maternal and fetal risks. Obstet Gynecol Surv. 1991; 45:509–514.

253. Kottmeier HL, Gray MJ. Rectal and bladder injuries in relation to radiation stage dosage in carcinoma of the uterine cervix. Am J Obstet Gynecol. 1961; 82:74–82.

254. Kottmeier HL. Complications following radiation therapy in carcinoma of the cervix and their treatment. Am J Obstet Gynecol. 1964; 88:854–866.

255. Kottmeier HL. Annual report on the results of treatment in carcinoma of the uterus, vagina and ovary. Int Fed Gynecol Obstet. 1973; 15.

256. Kovalic JJ, Grigsby PW, Perez CA, Lockett MA. Cervical stump carcinoma. Int J Radiat Oncol Biol Phys. 1991; 20:933–938.

257. Kramer C, Deschel RE, Goldberg N. Radiation treatment of FIGO stage IVA carcinoma of the cervix. Gynecol Oncol. 1989; 32:323–326.

258. Krebs HB, Helmkamp F, Sevin BU, Poliakoff SR, Nadji M, Averette HE. Recurrent cancer of the cervix following radical hysterectomy and pelvic node dissection. Obstet Gynecol. 1982; 59:422–427.

259. Krishnan L, Cytacki EP, Wolf C et al. Dosimetric analysis in brachytherapy of carcinoma of the cervix. Int J Radiat Oncol Biol Phys. 1990; 18:965–970.

260. Kumar L, Bhargava VL. Chemotherapy in recurrent and advanced cervical cancer. Gynecol Oncol. 1991; 40:107–111.

261. Kumar PP, Good RR, Jones EO, Bartone FF, Scott JC. Retreatment of recurrent pelvic tumors with Iodine-125. Radiat Med 1989; 7:150–159.

262. Kuske RR, Perez CA, Grigsby PW et al. Phase I/II study of definitive radiotherapy and chemotherapy (cisplatin and 5-fluorouracil) for advanced or recurrent gynecologic malignancies. Am J Clin Oncol (CCT). 1989; 12:467–473.

263. Kyriakos M, Kempson RL, Perez CA. Carcinoma of the cervix in young women. Obstet Gynecol. 1971; 38:930–944.

264. Lam K, Astrahan M, Langholz B et al. Interstitial thermoradiotherapy for recurrent or persistent tumors. Int J Hyperthermia. 1988; 4:259–266.

265. Lanciano RM, Won M, Coja RJ. Pretreatment and treatment factors associated with improved outcome in squamous cell carcinoma of the uterine cervix: A final report of 1973 and 1978 Patterns of Care Studies. Int J Radiat Oncol Biol Phys. 1990; 126.

266. LaPolla JP, Schlaerth JB, Gaddis O, Morrow CP. The influence of surgical staging on the evaluation and treatment of patients with cervical carcinoma. Gynecol Oncol. 1986; 24:194–206.

267. LaPolla JP, Roberts WS, Greenberg H et al. Treatment of advanced gynecologic malignancies with intraarterial chemotherapy and accelerated fractionation radiation therapy: A preliminary report. Gynecol Oncol. 1990; 37:55–59.

268. Larson DM, Stringer CA, Copeland LJ. Stage IB cervical carcinoma treated with radical hysterectomy and pelvic lymphadenectomy: Role of adjuvant radiotherapy. Obstet Gynecol. 1987; 69:378–381.

269. Larson DM, Copeland LJ, Stringer CA, Gershenson DM, Malone JM, Edwards CL. Recurrent cervical carcinoma after radical hysterectomy. Gynecol Oncol. 1988; 30:381–387.

270. Lee RB, Neglia W, Park RC. Cervical carcinoma in pregnancy. Obstet Gynecol. 1981; 58:584–589.

271. Lee YN, Wang KL, Lin MH et al. Radical hysterectomy with pelvic lymph node dissection for treatment of cervical cancer: A clinical review of 954 cases. Gynecol Oncol. 1989; 32:135–142.

272. Lehtovirta P, Viinikka L, Ylikorkala O. Comparison between squamous cell carcinoma-associated antigen and CA-125 in patients with carcinoma of the cervix: Gynecol Oncol. 1990; 37:276–278.

273. Leibel S, Bauer M, Wasserman T et al. Radiotherapy with or without misonidazole for patients with stage IIIB or stage IVA squamous cell carcinoma of the uterine cervix: Preliminary report of a Radiation Therapy Oncology Group randomized trial. Int J Radiat Oncol Biol Phys. 1987; 13(4): 541–549.

274. Lele SB, Piver MS, Mang TS, Dougherty TJ, Tomczak MK. Photodynamic therapy in gynecologic malignancies. Gynecol Oncol. 1989; 34:350–352.

275. Lewandowski GS, Copeland LJ. A potential role for intensive chemotherapy in the treatment of small cell neuroendocrine tumors of the cervix. Gynecol Oncol. 1993; 48:127–131.

276. Lifshitz S, Railsback LD, Buchsbaum HJ. Intra-arterial pelvic infusion chemotherapy in advanced gynecologic cancer. Obstet Gynecol. 1978; 52:476–480.

277. Ling CC, Spiro IJ, Kubiatowicz DO et al. Measurement of dose distribution around Fletcher-Suit-Delcos colpostats using a Therados radiation field analyzer (RFA-3). Med Phys. 1984; 11:326–330.

278. Lipsztein R, Kredentser D, Dottino P et al. Combined chemotherapy and radiation therapy for advanced carcinoma of the cervix. Am J Clin Oncol (CCT). 1987; 10:527–530.

279. Liu W, Meigs JV, Radical hysterectomy and pelvic lymphadenectomy: A review of 473 cases including 244 for primary invasive carcinoma of the cervix. Am J Obstet Gynecol. 1955; 69:1–32.

280. Liversage WE. A general formula for equating protracted and acute regimes of radiation. Br J Radiol. 1969; 42:432–440.

281. Lockhart III WL, McKemie III CR, Wright S, Peacocke N, Pantazis C, Ades EW. An immunochemotherapy protocol for enhanced tumoricidal activity: In vivo treatment with IL-2 prior to chemotherapy. J Clin Lab Immunol. 1987; 24: 101–103.

282. Logue JP, Hale RJ, Wilox FL, Hunter RD, Buckley CH, Tindall VR. Carcinoma of the cervix: An analysis of prognostic factors, treatment and patterns of failure following Wertheim's hysterectomy. Int J Gynecol Cancer. 1992; 2:323–327.

283. Look KY, Rocereto TF. Relapse patterns in FIGO stage IB carcinoma of the cervix. Gynecol Oncol. 1990; 38:114–120.

284. Lopez MJ, Kraybill WG, Fuchs GJ, Johnston WD, Sala JM, Bricker EM. Transvaginal parametrial needle biopsy for detection of postirradiation recurrent cancer of the cervix. Cancer. 1988; 61:275–278.

285. Lotocki RJ, Krepart GV, Paraskevas M, Vadas G, Heywood M, Fung Kee Fung M. Glassy cell carcinoma of the cervix: A bimodal treatment strategy. Gynecol Oncol. 1992; 44:254–259.

286. Lovecchio JL, Averette HE, Donato D, Bell J. 5-year survival of patients with periaortic nodal metastases in clinical stage IB and IIA cervical carcinoma. Gynecol Oncol. 1989; 34:43–45.

287. Lovett RD, Kuske RR, Perez CA et al. Preliminary evaluation of toxicity and tumor response to radiotherapy with cis-platinum and 5-fluorouracil for advanced or recurrent gynecologic malignancies. Int J Radiat Oncol Biol Phys. 1987; 13(1): 129–130.

288. Lucraft HH. Radiotherapy following primary surgery for carcinoma of the uterine cervix. Clin Radiol. 1981; 32:347–353.

289. Ludgate SM, Crandon AJ, Hudson CN, Walker O, Langlands AO, Synchronous 5-fluorouracil, mitomycin-C, and radiation therapy in the treatment of locally advanced carcinoma of the cervix. Int J Radiat Oncol Biol Phys. 1988; 15:893–899.

290. Lutz MH, Underwood PB, Razier JC, Putney FW. Genital malignancy in pregnancy. Am J Obstet Gynecol. 1977; 129:536–542.

291. Magrina JF. Types of pelvic exenterations: A reappraisal. Gynecol Oncol. 1990; 37:363–366.

292. Malfetano JH, Keys H. Aggressive multimodality treatment for cervical cancer with paraaortic lymph node metastases. Gynecol Oncol. 1991; 42:44–47.

293. Malviya VK, Han I, Deppe G et al. High-dose-rate afterloading brachytherapy, external radiation therapy, and combination chemotherapy in poor-prognosis cancer of the cervix. Gynecol Oncol. 1991; 42:233–238.

294. Mandelblatt J, Richart R, Thomas L et al. Is human papillomavirus associated with cervical neoplasia in the elderly? Gynecol Oncol. 1992; 46:6–12.

295. Manetta A, Podczaski ES, Larson JE, De Geest K, Mortel R. Scalene lymph node biopsy in the preoperative evaluation of patients with current cervical cancer. Gynecol Oncol. 1989; 33:332–334.

296. Maor MH, Gillespie B, Peters LJ et al. Neutron therapy in cervical cancer: results of a phase II RTOG study. Int J Radiat Oncol Biol Phys. 1986; 12(1):99–110.

297. Maor MH, Gillespie BW, Peters LJ. Neutron therapy in cervical cancer: Results of a phase III RTOG study. Int J Radiat Oncol Biol Phys. 1988; 14:883–891.

298. Marcial VA, Blanco MS, De Leon E. Persistent tumor cells in the vaginal smear during the first year after radiation therapy of carcinoma of the uterine cervix. Prognostic significance. Am J Roentgenol. 1968; 102:170–175.

299. Marcial VA, Amato D, Marks RD. Split-course versus continuous pelvis irradiation in carcinoma of the uterine cervix: A prospective randomized clinical trial of the Radiation Therapy Oncology Group. Int J Radiat Oncol Biol Phys. 1983; 9:431–436.

300. Marcial LV, Marcial VA, Krall JM, Lanciano RM, Coia LR, Hanks GE. Comparison of 1 vs 2 or more intra-cavitary brachytherapy applications in the management of carcinoma of the cervix, with irradiation alone. Int J Radiat Oncol Biol Phys. 1991; 20:81–85.

301. Marcial VA, Marcial LV. Radiation therapy of cervical cancer. Cancer. 1993; 71:1438–1445.

302. Martinez A, Cox RS, Edmundson GK. A multiple-site perineal applicator (MUPIT) for treatment of prostatic, anorectal and gynecologic malignancies. Int J Radiat Oncol Biol Phys. 1984; 10:297–305.

303. Maruyama Y, Van Nagell JR, Yoneda J et al. Feasibility study of californium-252 for the therapy of stage IV cervical cancer. Cancer. 1988; 61:2448–2452.

304. Maruyama Y, Van Nagell JR, Yoneda J et al. Efficacy of brachytherapy with Californium-252 neutrons versus Cesium-137 photons for eradication of bulky localized cervical cancer: Single-Institution Study. J Natl Cancer Inst. 1988; 80:501–506.

305. Masterson JG. The role of surgery in the treatment of early carcinoma of the cervix. Clin Obstet Gynecol. 1967; 10:922–939.

306. Milas L, Hirata H, Hunter N, Peters LJ. Effect of radiation-induced injury of tumor bed stroma on metastatic spread of murine sarcomas and carcinomas. Cancer Res. 1988; 2166–2120.

307. Miller B, Dockter M, El Torky M, Photopulos G. Small cell carcinoma of the cervix: A clinical and flow-cytometric study. Gynecol Oncol. 1991; 42:27–33.

308. Miller BE, Copeland LJ, Hamberger AD et al. Carcinoma of the cervical stump. Gynecol Oncol. 1984; 18:100–108.

309. Million RR, Rutledge F, Fletcher GH. Stage IV carcinoma of the cervix with bladder invasion. Am J Obstet Gynecol. 1972; 133:239–246.

310. Mitani Y, Yukinari S, Jimi S, Iwasaki H. Carcinomatous infiltration into the uterine body in carcinoma of the uterine cervix. Am J Obstet Gynecol. 1964; 89:984–989.

311. Mohan R, Ding IY, Toraskar J, Chui C, Anderson LL, Nori D. Computation of radiation dose distributions for shielded cervical applicators. Int J Radiat Oncol Biol Phys. 1985; 11:823–830.

312. Montana GS, Fowler WC, Varia MA. Carcinoma of the cervix stage III: Results of radiation therapy. Cancer. 1986; 57:148–154.

313. Morales P, Hussey DH, Maor MH, Hamberger AD, Fletcher GH, Wharton JT. Preliminary report of the M.D. Anderson Hospital randomized trial of neutron and photon irradiation for locally advanced carcinoma of the uterine cervix. Int J Radiat Oncol Biol Phys. 1981; 7:1533–1540.

314. Morley GW, Seski JC. Radical pelvic surgery versus radiation therapy for stage I carcinoma of the cervix (exclusive of microinvasion). Am J Obstet Gynecol. 1976; 126:785–798.

315. Morris M, Gershenson DM, Eifel P, Silva EG, Mitchell MF, Burke TW, Warton JT. Treatment of small cell carcinoma of the cervix with cisplatin, doxorubicin, and etoposide. Gynecol Oncol. 1992; 47:62–65.

316. Morrow CP, DiSaia PJ, Mangan CF, Lagasse LD. Continuous pelvic arterial infusion with bleomycin for squamous carcinoma of the cervix recurrent after irradiation therapy. Cancer Treat Rep. 1977; 61:1403–1405.

317. Morrow CP. Is pelvic radiation beneficial in the postoperative management of stage IB squamous cell carcinoma of the cervix with pelvic node metastasis treated by radical hysterectomy and pelvic lymphadenectomy? Gynecol Oncol. 1980; 10:105–110.

318. Munnell EW, Bonney Jr WA. Critical points of failure in the therapy of cancer of the cervix. A study of 250 recurrences. Am J Obstet Gynecol. 1961; 81:521–534.

319. Murdoch JB, Grimshaw RN, Morgan PR, Monaghan JM. The impact of loop diathermy on management of early invasive cervical cancer. Int J Gynecol Cancer. 1992; 2:129–133.

320. Murphy WT, Schmitz A. The results of re-irradiation in cancer of the cervix. Radiology. 1956; 67:378–385.

321. Muss HB, Jobson VW, Homesley HD, Welander C, Ferree C. Neoadjuvant therapy for advanced squamous cell carcinoma of the cervix: Cisplatin followed by radiation therapy—A pilot study of the gynecologic oncology group. Gynecol Oncol. 1987; 26:35–40.

322. Nahhas WA, Sharkey FE, Whitney CW. The prognostic significance of vascular channel involvement and deep stromal penetration in early cervical carcinoma. Am J Clin Oncol. 1983; 6:259–264.

323. Nelson Jr JH, Macasaet MA, Lu T et al. The incidence and significance of para-aortic lymph node metastases in late invasive carcinoma of the cervix. Am J Obstet Gynecol. 1974; 118:749–756.

324. Nelson III AJ, Fletcher GH, Wharton JT. Indications for adjunctive conservative extrafascial hysterectomy in selected cases of carcinoma of the uterine cervix. Amer J Obstet Gynecol. 1975; 123:91–99.

325. Nelson Jr JH, Boyce J, Macasaet M et al. Incidence, significance, and follow-up of para-aortic lymph node metastases in late invasive carcinoma of the cervix. Am J Obstet Gynecol. 1977; 128:336–340.

326. Nevin J, Soeters R, Dehaeck K, Bloch B, Van Wyk L. Advanced cervical carcinoma associated with pregnancy. Int J Gynecol Cancer. 1993; 3:57–63.

327. Newton M. Radical hysterectomy or radiotherapy for stage I cervical cancer. Am J Obstet Gynecol. 1975; 123:535–542.

328. Ngan HYS, Chan SYW, Wong LC, Choy DTK, Ma HK. Serum squamous cell carcinoma antigen in the monitoring of radiotherapy treatment response in carcinoma of the cervix. Gynecol Oncol. 1990; 37:260–263.

329. Nguyen PD, Berchmans J, Munoz AK, Yazigi R, Graham M, Franklin P. Mitomycin-c/5FU and radiation therapy for locally advanced uterine cervical cancer. Gynecol Oncol. 1991; 43:220–225.

330. Nisker JA, Shubat M. Stage IB cervical carcinoma and pregnancy: Report of 49 cases. Am J Obstet Gynecol. 1983; 145:203–206.

331. Noguchi H, Shiozawa I, Kitahara T. Uterine body invasion of carcinoma of the uterine cervix as seen from surgical specimens. Gynecol Oncol. 1988; 30:173–182.

332. Nori D, Hilaris BS, Kim HS et al. Interstitial irradiation in recurrent gynecological cancer. Int J Radiat Oncol Biol Phys. 1981; 7:1513–1517.

333. Oberfield RA. Volume 86: Intra-arterial infusion in tumors of the pelvis. In: Recent Results in Cancer Research. Berlin: Springer; 1983:15–25.

334. Orr Jr JW, Kerr-Wilson RH, Bodiford C et al. Nutritional status of patients with untreated cervical cancer. Am J Obstet Gynecol. 1985; 151:625–635.

335. O'Quinn AG, Barranco SC, Costanzi JJ. Tumor cell kinetics-directed chemotherapy for advanced squamous carcinoma of the cervix. Gynecol Oncol. 1984; 18:135–144.

336. O'Reilly SE, Swenerton KD, Manji M, Acker B, Benedet JL, Elit L. Concomitant cisplatin (DDP) and radiotherapy (RT) in advanced cervical squamous cell carcinoma (SCC). Proc Am Soc Clin Oncol. 1986; 5:115.

337. Panici PB, Scambia G, Baiocchi G et al. Neoadjuvant chemotherapy and radical surgery in locally advanced cervical cancer. Cancer. 1991; 67:372–374.

338. Panici PB, Greggi S, Scambia G et al. High-dose cisplatin and bleomycin neoadjuvant chemotherapy plus radical surgery in locally advanced cervical carcinoma: A preliminary report. Gynecol Oncol. 1991; 41:212–216.

339. Paravasiliou C, Yiogarakis D, Pappas J, Keramopoulos A. Treatment of cervical carcinoma by total hysterectomy and postoperative irradiation. Int J Radiat Oncol Biol Phys. 1980; 6:871–874.

340. Parker Jr RL, Welander CE, Homesley HD, Jobson VW, Kawamoto EH. Use of the human tumor stem cell assay to study chemotherapy sensitivity in cancer of the cervix. Obstet Gynecol. 1984; 64:412–416.

341. Park RC, Patow WE, Rogers RR, Zimmerman EA. Treatment for stage I carcinoma of the cervix. Obstet Gynecol. 1973; 117–122.

342. Park TK, Choi DH, Kom SN et al. Role of induction chemotherapy in invasive cervical cancer. Gynecol Oncol. 1991; 41:107–112.

343. Parsons JT, Thar TL, Bova FJ, Million RR. An evaluation of split-course irradiation for pelvic malinancies. Int J Radiat Oncol Biol Phys. 1980; 6:175–181.

344. Patsner B, Sedlacek TV, Lovecchio JL. Para-aortic node sampling in small (3-cm or less) stage IB invasive cervical cancer. Gynecol Oncol. 1992; 44:53–54.

345. Patton Jr TJ, Kavanagh JJ, Delclos L et al. Five-year survival in patients given intra-arterial chemotherapy prior to radiotherapy for advanced squamous carcinoma of the cervix and vagina. Gynecol Oncol. 1991; 42:54–59.

346. Paunier JP, Delclos L, Fletcher GH. Causes, time of death, and sites of failure in squamous cell carcinoma of the uterine cervix on intact uterus. Radiology. 1967; 88:555–562.

347. Pearcey RG, Maclean GD. A phase I/II study combining radical radiotherapy with concurrent cisplatin in the treatment of advanced squamous cell carcinoma of the cervix. Int J Gynecol Cancer. 1992; 2:215–219.

348. Perez CA, Camel HM, Kao MS, Askin F. Randomized study of preoperative radiation and surgery of irradiation alone in the treatment of stage IB and IIA carcinoma of the uterine cervix: Preliminary analysis of failures and complications. Cancer. 1980; 45:2759–2768.

349. Perez CA, Breaux S, Madoc-Jones H. Radiation therapy alone in the treatment of carcinoma of the uterine cervix. I. Analysis of tumor recurrence. Cancer. 1983; 51:1393–1402.

350. Perez CA, Breaux S, Bedwinek JM. Radiation therapy alone in treatment of the uterine cervix. II. Analysis of complications. Cancer. 1984; 54:235–246.

351. Perez CA, Kao MS. Radiation therapy alone or combined with surgery in the treatment of barrel-shaped carcinoma of the uterine cervix (stages IB, IIA, IIB). Int J Radiat Oncol Biol Phys. 1985; 11:1903–1904.

352. Perez CA, Camel HM, Walz BJ. Radiation therapy alone in the treatment of carcinoma of the uterine cervix. A 20 year experience. Gynecol Oncol. 1986; 23:127–140.

353. Perez CA, Camel HM, Koa MS, Askin F. Randomized study of preoperative radiation and surgery or irradiation alone in the treatment of stage IB and IIA carcinoma of the uterine cervix. Final report. Gynecol Oncol. 1987; 27:129–140.

354. Perez CA, Brady LW. Uterine cervix. In: Principles and practice of radiation oncology. Philadelphia: JB Lippincott; 1992; 1143–1202.

355. Perez CA, Kurman RJ, Stehman FB, Thigpen JT. Uterine Cervix. In: Hoskins WJ, Perez CA, Young RC, eds. Gynecologic Oncology. Philadelphia: JB Lippincott; 1992:591–662.

356. Perkins PL, Chu AM, Jose B. Posthysterectomy megavoltage irradiation in the treatment of cervical carcinoma. Gynecol Oncol. 1984; 17:340–348.

357. Petersen LK, Mamsen A, Jakobsen A. Carcinoma of the cervical stump. Gynecol Oncol. 1992; 46:199–202.

358. Pettersson F. Annual report on the results of treatment in gynecological cancer. Stockholm: Panorama Press AB; 1988.

359. Petrovich Z, Lam K, Astrahan M, Luxton G, Langholz B. Interstitial radiotherapy combined with interstitial hyperthermia in the management of recurrent tumors. In: Recent Results in Cancer Research. Berlin: Springer; 1988; 136–140.

360. Pfeiffer D, Stellwag B, Pfeiffer A, Bolringhaus P, Meser W, Scheidel P. Clinical implications of the epidermal growth factor receptor in the squamous cell carcinoma of the uterine cervix. Gynecol Oncol. 1989; 33:151–156.

361. Phillips RA, Tolmach LJ. Repair of potentially lethal damage in irradiated HeLa cells. Radiat Res. 1966; 19:413.

362. Phillips TL, Fu KK. Quantification of combined radiation therapy and chemotherapy effects on critical normal tissues. Cancer. 1976; 37:1186–1200.

363. Phillips TL, Wasserman TH, Johnson RJ, Levin VA, VanRaalte G. Final report on the Untied States phase I clinical trial of the hypoxic cell radiosensitizer, Misonidazole (Ro-07-0582, NSC Nr.2610337). Cancer. 1981; 48:1697–1704.

364. Photopulos GJ, Shirley Jr REL, Ansbacher R. Evaluation of conventional diagnostic tests for detection of recurrent carcinoma of the cervix. Am J Obstet Gynecol. 1977; 129; 533–535.

365. Photopulos GJ, Zwaag RV, Miller B, Bielskis W, Veerling PJ. Vaginal radiation brachytherapy to reduce central recurrence after radical hysterectomy for cervical carcinoma. Gynecol Oncol. 1990; 38:187–190.

366. Pierquin B, Marinello G, Mege JP, Crook J. Intracavitary irradiation of carcinomas of the uterus and cervix: The Creteil method. Int J Radiat Oncol Biol Phys. 1988; 15:1465–1473.

367. Pillai MR, Balaram P, Chidambaram S, Padmanabhan TK, Nair MK. Development of an immunological staging system to prognosticate disease course in malignant cervical neoplasia. Gynecol Oncol. 1990; 37:200–205.

368. Pilleron JP, Durand JC, Hamelin JP. Prognostic value of node metastasis in cancer of the uterine cervix. Am J Obstet Gynecol. 1974; 119:458.

369. Pinto JM, Jussa Walla DJ, Shetty PA. Pre-radiation chemotherapy in carcinoma cervix. A preliminary report. Ind J Cancer. 1980; 17:179–180.

370. Piver MS, Rutledge F, Smith JP. Five classes of extended hysterectomy for women with cervical cancer. Obstet Gynecol. 1974; 44:265–272.

371. Piver MS, Barlow JJ, Vongtama V, Webster J. Hydroxyurea and radiation therapy in advanced cervical cancer. Am J Obstet Gynecol. 1974; 120:969–972.

372. Piver MS, Chung WS. Prognostic significance of cervical lesion size and pelvic node metastases in cervical carcinoma. Obstet Gynecol. 1975; 46:507–510.

373. Piver MS, Barlow JJ, Vongtama V, Blumenson L. Hydroxyurea as a radiation sensitizer in women with carcinoma of the uterine cervix. Am J Obstet Gynecol. 1977; 129; 379.

374. Piver MS, Barlow JJ, Krishnamsetty R. Five-year survival (with no evidence of disease) in patients with biopsy-confirmed aortic node metastasis from cervical carcinoma. Am J Obstet Gynecol. 1981; 139:575–578.

375. Piver MS, Barlow JJ, Vongtama V, Blumenson L. Hydroxyurea: a radiation potentiator in carcinoma of the uterine cervix. A randomized double-blind study. Am J Obstet Gynecol. 1983; 147:803–808.

376. Piver MS, Barlow JJ, Lele SB, Maniccia M. Weekly cis-Diaminedichloroplatinum II as induction chemotherapy in recurrent carcinoma of the cervix. Gynecol Oncol. 1984; 18:313–319.

377. Piver MS, Krishnamsetty R, Emrich L. Survival of non-surgically staged patients with negative lymphangiogram stage IIB carcinoma of the cervix treated by pelvic radiation plus hydroxyurea. Am J Obstet Gynecol. 1985; 151:1006–1008.

378. Piver MS, Lele SB, Malfetano JH. Cis-diaminedichloroplatinum II-based combination chemotherapy for the control of extensive paraaortic lymph node metastases in cervical cancer. Gynecol Oncol. 1987; 26:71–76.

379. Piver MS, Marchetti DL, Patton T. Radical hysterectomy and pelvic lymphadenectomy versus radiation therapy for small (≥ 3 cm) stage IB cervical carcinoma. Am J Clin Oncol. 1988; 11:21–24.

380. Podczaski ES, Palumbo C, Manetta A. Assessment of pretreatment laparotomy in patients with cervical carcinoma prior to radiotherapy. Gynecol Oncol. 1989; 33:71–75.

381. Potish R, Adcock L, Jones T Jr et al. The morbidity and utility of periaortic radiotherapy in cervical carcinoma. Gynecol Oncol. 1983; 15:1–9.

382. Potish RA, Twiggs LB, Okagaki T, Prem KA, Adcock LL. Therapeutic implications of the natural history of advanced cervical cancer as defined by pretreatment surgical staging. Cancer. 1985; 56:956–960.

383. Potish RA, Twiggs LB, Adcock LL, Savage JE, Prem KA, Levitt SH, Effect of cis-platinum on tolerance to radiation therapy in advanced cervical cancer. Am J Clin Oncol 1986; 9:387–391.

384. Potter ME, Hatch KD, Potter MY, Shingleton HM, Baker VV. Factors affecting the response of recurrent squamous cell carcinoma of the cervix to cisplatin. Cancer. 1989; 63:1283–1286.

385. Potter ME, Alvarez RD, Gay FL, Shingleton HM, Soong SJ, Hatch KD. Optimal therapy for pelvic recurrence after radical hysterectomy for early-stage cervical cancer. Gynecol Oncol. 1990; 37:74–77.

386. Pourquier H, Dubois JB, Deland R. Cancer of the uterine cervix: Dosimetric guidelines for prevention of late rectal and rectosigmoid complications are a result of radiotherapeutic treatment. Int J Radiat Oncol Biol Phys. 1982; 8:1887–1895.

387. Prasasvinichai S, Glassburn JR, Brady LW, Lewis GC. Treatment of recurrent carcinoma of the cervix. Int J Radiat Oncol Biol Phys 1978; 4:957–961.

388. Prempree T, Scott RM. Treatment of stage IIIB carcinoma of the cervix. Cancer. 1978; 42:1105–1113.

389. Prempree T, Kwon T, VillaSanta U, Scott RM. Management of late second or late recurrent squamous cell carcinoma of the cervix uteri after successful initial radiation treatment. Int J Radiat Oncol Biol Phys. 1974; 5:2053–2057.

390. Prempree T, Patanaphan V, Sewchand W, Scott RM. Parametrial implants in the treatment of stage IIIB carcinoma of the cervix. Cancer. 1980; 46:1485–1491.

391. Prempree T. Parametrial implant in stage IIIB cancer of the cervix. III. A five-year study. Cancer. 1983; 52:748–750.

392. Prempree T, Pantanaphan V, Sewchand W. The influence of patient's age and tumor grade on the prognostic of carcinoma of the cervix. Cancer. 1983; 51:1764–1771.

393. Prempree T, Amornmarn R, Villasanta U, Kwon T, Scott RM. Retreatment of very late recurrent invasive squamous cell carcinoma of the cervix with irradiation. II. Criteria for patients' selection to achieve the success. Cancer. 1984; 54:1950–1955.

394. Pringle J, Rawlings G, Sturgeon J, Fine S, Black B. Concurrent radiation, mitomycin-C and 5-fluorouracil in poor prognosis carcinoma of cervix: preliminary results of a phase I–II study. Int J Radiat Oncol Biol Phys. 1984; 10:1785–1790.

395. Puthawala AA, Syed AMN, Fleming PA, Disaia PJ. Re-irradiation with interstitial implant for recurrent pelvic malignancies. Cancer. 1982; 50:2810–2814.

396. Puthawala AA, Syed AMN, Sheikh K, Rafie S, McNamara CS. Interstitial hyperthermia for recurrent malignancies. Endocurie, Hypertherm Oncol. 1985; 1:125–131.

397. Rafla S, Parikh K, Tchelebi M, Youssef E, Selim H, Bishay S. Recurrent tumors of the head and neck, pelvis, and chest wall: Treatment with hyperthermia and brachytherapy. Radiology. 1989; 172:845–850.

398. Raju KS, Bates TD, Taylor RW. Primary adenocarcinoma of the cervix: Treatment and results. Br J Obstet Gynaecol. 1987; 94:1212–1217.

399. Raju KS, Kjorstad KE, Abeler V. Prognostic factors in the treatment of stage IB adenocarcinoma of the cervix. Int J Gynecol Cancer. 1991; 1:69–74.

400. Ramm K, Vergote IB, Kaern J, Tropé CG. Bleomycin-ifosfamide-cis-platinum (BIP) in pelvic recurrence of previously irradiated cervical carcinoma: A second look. Gynecol Oncol. 1992; 46:203–207.

401. Randall ME, Barrett RJ. Interstitial irradiation in the management of recurrent carcinoma of the cervix. After previous radiation therapy. NCMJ. 1988; 49:306–308.

402. Randall ME, Constable WC, Hahn SS. Results of radiotherapeutic management of carcinoma of the cervix with emphasis on the influence of histologic classification. Cancer. 1988; 62:48–53.

403. Randall ME, Evans L, Greven KM, McCinniff AJ, Doline RM. Interstitial reirradiation for recurrent gynecologic malignancies: Results and analysis of prognostic factors. Gynecol Oncol. 1993; 48:29–31.

404. Rando RF, Sedlacek TV, Hunt J. Verrucous carcinoma of the vulva associated with an unusual type 6 human papillomavirus. Obstet Gynecol. 1986; 67:705–755.

405. Reagan JW, Fu YS. Histologic types and prognosis of cancers of the uterine cervix. Int J Radiat Oncol Biol Phys. 1979; 5:1015–1020.

406. Remy JC, Di Maio T, Fruchter RG et al. Adjunctive radiation after hysterectomy in stage IB squamous cell carcinoma of the cervix. Gynecol Oncol. 1990; 38:161–165.

407. Rettenmaier MA, Berman ML, DiSaia PJ, Burns RG, Berns MW. Photoradiation therapy of gynecologic malignancies. Gynecol Oncol. 1984; 17:200–206.

408. Rettenmaier MA, Moran MF, Ramsinghani NF et al. Treatment of advanced and recurrent squamous carcinoma of the uterine cervix with constant intraarterial infusion of cisplatin. Cancer. 1988; 61:1301–1303.

409. Rettenmaier MA, Casanova DM, Micha JP. Radical hysterectomy and tailored postoperative radiation therapy in the management of bulky stage IB cervical cancer. Cancer. 1989; 63:2220–2223.

410. Rice GC, Hoy C, Schimke RT. Transient hypoxia enhances the frequency of dihydrofolate reductase gene amplification in chinese hamster ovary cells. Proc Natl Acad Sci USA. 1986; 83:5978–5982.

411. Riou D, Faver M, Jeannel D, Bourhis J, Le Doussal V, Orth G. Association between poor prognosis in early-stage invasive cervical carcinomas and nondetection of HPV DNA. Lancet. 1990; 335:1171–1174.

412. Roberts WS, Kavanagh JJ, Greenberg H et al. Concomitant radiation therapy and chemotherapy in the treatment of advanced squamous carcinoma of the lower female genital tract. Gynecol Oncol. 1989; 34:183–186.

413. Roberts WS, Hoffman MS, Kavanagh J et al. Further experience with radiation therapy and concomitant intravenous chemotherapy in advanced carcinoma of the lower female genital tract. Gynecol Oncol. 1991; 43:233–236.

414. Roh HD, Boucher Y, Kalnicki S, Buchsbaum R, Bloomer WD, Jain RK. Interstitial hypertension in carcinoma of the uterine cervix in patients: Possible correlation with tumor oxygenation and radiation response. Cancer Res. 1991; 51:6695–6698.

415. Rotman M, John M, Boyce J. Prognostic factors in cervical carcinoma: Implications in staging and management. Cancer. 1981; 48:560–567.

416. Rotman M, John M, Choi K, Marcial V, Hornback N, Martz K. Prophylactic irradiation of the para-aortic lymph node chain in carcinoma of the cervix. A radiation therapy oncology group study update. Int J Radiat Oncol Biol Phys. 1986; 12:94.

417. Rotman M, Choi K, Guze C, Marcial V, Hornback N, John M. Prophylactic irradiation of the para-aortic lymph node chain in stage IIB and bulky stage IB carcinoma of the cervix, initial treatment results of RTOG 7920. Int J Rad Oncol Biol Phys. 1990; 19:513–521.

418. Rotman M, Aziz H. Techniques in the radiation treatment of carcinoma of the uterine cervix. Int J Radiat Oncol Biol Phys. 1991; 20: 173–175.

419. Rotmensch J, Senekjian EK, Ghodratollah J, Herbst AL. Evaluation of bolus cis-Platinum and continuous 5-Fluorouracil infusion for metastatic and recurrent squamous cell carcinoma of the cervix. Gynecol Oncol. 198; 29: 76–81.

420. Rubin P, Keys H, Salazar O. New designs for radiation oncology research in clinical trials. Seminars in Oncology. 1981; 8: 453–472.

421. Rubin P. The Franz Buschke Lecture: Late effects of chemotherapy and radiation therapy: A new hypothesis. Int J Radiat Oncol Biol Phys. 1984; 10: 5–34.

422. Rubin SC, Brookland R, Mikuta JJ, Mangan C, Sutton G, Danoff B. Para-aortic nodal metastases in early cervical carcinoma: Long-term survival following extended-field radiotherapy. Gynecol Oncol. 1984; 18: 213–217.

423. Ruch RM, Pitcock JA, Ruch WAJ. Microinvasive carcinoma of the cervix. Am J Obstet Gynecol. 1976; 125: 87–92.

424. Runowicz CD, Wadler S, Rodriguez-Rodriguez L, et al. Concomitant cisplatin and radiotherapy in locally advanced cervical carcinoma. Gynecol Oncol. 1989; 34: 395–401.

425. Rustin GJS, Newlands ES, Southcott BM, Singer A. Cisplatin, vincristine, methotrexate and bleomycin (POMB) as initial or palliative chemotherapy for carcinoma of the cervix. Br J Obstet Gynaecol. 1987; 94: 1205–1211.

426. Rutgers DH, van der Linden PM, van Peperzeel HA. DNA-flow cytometry of squamous cell carcinomas from the human uterine cervix: The identification of prognostically different subgroups. Radiother Oncol. 1986; 7: 249–258.

427. Rutledge FN, Gutierrez AG, Fletcher GH. Management of stage I and II adenocarcinomas of the uterine cervix on intact uterus. Am J Roentgenol. 1968; 102: 161–164.

428. Rutledge FN, Galakatos AE, Wharton JT, Smith JP. Adenocarcinoma of the uterine cervix. Am J Obstet Gynecol. 1975; 122: 236–245.

429. Rutledge FN, Wharton JT, Fletcher GH. Clinical studies with adjunctive surgery and irradiation therapy in the treatment of carcinoma of the cervix. Cancer. 1976; 38: 596–602.

430. Rutledge FN, Mitchell MF, Munsell M, Bass S, McGuffee V, Atkinson EN. Youth as a prognostic factor in carcinoma of the cervix: A matched analysis. Gynecol Oncol. 1992; 44: 123–130.

431. Saigo PE, Cain JM, Kim WS. Prognostic factors in adenocarcinoma of the uterine cervix. Cancer. 1986; 57: 1584–1593.

432. Sala JM, De Leon AD. Treatment of carcinoma of the cervical stump. Radiology. 1963; 81: 300–306.

433. Sapozink MD, Gibbs Jr FA, Gates KS, Stewart JR. Regional hyperthermia in the treatment of clinically advanced, deep seated malignancy: Results of a pilot study employing an annular array applicator. Int J Radiat Oncol Biol Phys. 1984; 10: 775–786.

434. Sardi J. Early results of a randomized trial with neoadjuvant chemotherapy in squamous carcinoma cervix uteri. In: IGCS, 3rd biennial meeting. Cairns, Australia; 1991.

435. Sardi J, Sananes C, Giaroli A et al. Results of a prospective randomized trial with neoadjuvant chemotherapy in stage IB, bulky, squamous carcinoma of the cervix. Gynecol Oncol. 1993; 49: 156–165.

436. Saunders N, Landon CR. Management problems associated with carcinoma of the cervix diagnosed in the second trimester of pregnancy. Gynecol Oncol. 1988; 30: 120–122.

437. Schmidt HC, Tscholakoff D, Hricak H, Higgins CB. MR image contrast and relaxation times of solid tumors in the chest, abdomen, and pelvis. J Comput Assist Tomogr. 1985; 9: 738–748.

438. Schoeppel SL, Weeks KJ, Lichter AS et al. Clinical application of a CT compatible version of the Fletcher System intracavitary applicator. Int J Radiat Oncol Biol Phys. 1988; 15(1): 140.

439. Schreiner P, Siracka E, Siracky J, Manka I. The effect of anemia on the radiotherapy results of the uterine cervix cancer. Neoplasma. 1975; 22: 655–660.

440. Seegenschmiedt MH, Brady LW, Sauer R. Interstitial thermoradiotherapy: Review on technical and clinical aspects. Am J Clin Oncol (CCT). 1990; 13: 352–363.

441. Senekjian EK, Hubby M, Bell DA. Clear cell adenocarcinoma (CCA) of the vagina and cervix in association with pregnancy. Gynecol Oncol. 1986; 24: 207–219.

442. Sersa G, Willingham V, Milas L. Anti-tumor effects of tumor necrosis factor alone or combined with radiotherapy. Int J Cancer 1988; 42: 129–134.

443. Sevin B-U, Nadji M, Averette HE, Hilsenbeck S, Smith D, Lampe B. Microinvasive carcinoma of the cervix. Cancer. 1992; 70: 2121–2128.

443a. Sevin B-U, Nadji M, Greening SE, Ng APB, Nordquist SRB, Girtanner RE, Averette HE. Fine needle aspiration cytology in gynecologic oncology: early detection of occult persistent or recurrent cancer after radiation therapy. Gynecol Oncol. 1980; 9: 351–360.

444. Sewchand W, Prempree T, Patanaphan V, Bautro N, Sott RM. Radium implant to the parametrium in the treatment of stage IIIB carcinoma of the cervix: Analysis of dosimetry. Int J Radiat Oncol Biol Phys. 1980; 6: 927–934.

445. Shafik A. Anal submucosal injection: A new route for drug administration in pelvic malignancies. IV. Submucosal anal injection in the treatment of cancer of uterine cervix—Preliminary study. Am J Obstet Gynecol. 1989; 161: 69–72.

446. Shield PW, Wright RG, Free K, Daunter B. The accuracy of cervicovaginal cytology in the detection of recurrent cervical carcinoma following radiotherapy. Gynecol Oncol. 1991; 41: 223–229.

447. Shigematsu Y, Nishiyama K, Masaki N et al. Treatment of carcinoma of the uterine cervix by remotely controlled afterloading intracavitary

radiotherapy with high-dose rate: A comparative study with a low-dose rate system. Int J Radiat Oncol Biol Phys. 1983; 9:351–356.

448. Shimm DS, Kittelson JM, Oleson JR, Aristizabal SA, Cetas TC. Interstitial thermoradiotherapy: Thermal dosimetry, clinical results, and complications. Int J Radiat Oncol Biol Phys. 1988; 15(1):124.

449. Shingleton HM, Orr JW. In: Cancer of the cervix. Diagnosis and Treatment Shingleton HM, Orr JW, eds. New York: Churchill Livingston; 1987.

450. Shu-Mo C, Xiang-E W, Qi W. High dose-rate afterloading in the treatment of cervical cancer of the uterus. Int J Radiat Oncol Biol Phys. 1989; 16:335–338.

451. Sidhu GS, Koss LG, Barber HRK. Relation of histologic factors to the response of stage I epidermoid carcinoma of the cervix to surgical treatment. Obstet Gynecol. 1970; 35:329.

452. Simon NL, Gore H, Shingleton HM. Study of superficially invasive carcinoma of the cervix. Obstet Gynecol. 1986; 68:19–24.

453. Sinclair WK. The combined effect of hydroxyurea and X-rays on chinese hamster cells in vitro. Cancer Res. 1968; 28:198.

454. Sivanesaratnam V, Jayalakshmi P, Loo C. Surgical management of early invasive cancer of the cervix associated with pregnancy. Gynecol Oncol. 1993; 48:68–75.

455. Smith HO, Stringer CA, Kavanagh JJ, Gershenson DM, Edwards CL, Wharton JT. Treatment of advanced or recurrent squamous cell carcinoma of the uterine cervix with mitomycin-c, bleomycin, and cisplatin chemotherapy. Gynecol Oncol. 1993; 48:11–15.

456. Soerensen FB, Bichel P, Jakobsen A. DNA level and stereologic estimates of nuclear volume in squamous cell carcinomas of the uterine cervix. Cancer 1992; 69:187–199.

457. Soisson AP, Soper JT, Clarke-Pearson DL, Berchuck A, Montana G, Creasman WT. Adjuvant radiotherapy following radical hysterectomy for patients with stage IB and IIA cervical cancer. Gynecol Oncol. 1990; 37:390–395.

458. Sommers GM, Grigsby PW, Perez CA et al. Outcome of recurrent cervical carcinoma following definitive irradiation. Gynecol Oncol. 1989; 35:150–155.

459. Stanhope CR, Smith JP, Wharton JT. The effect of age on survival. Gynecol Oncol. 1980; 10:188–193.

460. Steel GG, Peckham MJ. Exploitable mechanisms in combined radiotherapy-chemotherapy: The concept of additivity. Int J Radiat Oncol Biol Phys. 1979; 5:85–91.

461. Stehman FB, Bundy BN, Keys H, Currie JL, Mortel R, Creasman WT. A randomized trial of hydroxyurea versus misonidazole adjunct to radiation therapy in carcinoma of the cervix. A preliminary report of a Gynecologic Oncology Group Study. Am J Obstet Gynecol. 1988; 159:87–94.

462. Stehman FB, Bundy BN, DiSaia PH. Carcinoma of the cervix treated with irradiation therapy. I. A multi-variate analysis of prognostic variables in the Gynecologic Oncology Group. Cancer. 1991; 67:2776–2785.

463. Stendahl U, Willén H, Willén R. Invasive squamous cell carcinoma of the uterine cervix. I. Definition of parameters in a histopathologic malignancy grading system. Acta Radiol Oncol. 1980; 19:467–480.

464. Stendahl U, Eklund G, Willen H, Willen R. Invasive squamous cell carcinoma of the uterine cervix. III. A malignancy grading system for indication of prognosis after radiation therapy. Acta Radiol Oncol. 1981; 20:231–243.

465. Stendahl U, Eklund G, Willen R. Prognosis of invasive squamous cell carcinoma of the uterine cervix: A comparative study of the predictive values of clinical staging IB-III and a histopathologic malignancy grading system. Int J Gynecol Pathol. 1983; 2:42–54.

466. Strang P, Eklund GM, Stendahl U, Frankendal B. S-phase rate as a predictor of early recurrences in carcinoma of the uterine cervix. Anticancer Res. 1987; 7:807–810.

467. Sugimura M, Kobayashi H, Kanayama N, Terao T. Clinical significance of urokinase-type plasminogen activator (uPA) in invasive cervical cancer of the uterus. Gynecol Oncol. 1992; 46:330–336.

468. Suit HD, Moore EB, Fletcher GH, Worsnop R. Modification of Fletcher ovoid system for afterloading, using standard-sized radium tubes (milligram and microgram). Radiology. 1963; 81:126–131.

469. Suit HD, Westgate SJ. Impact of improved local control on survival. Int J Radiat Oncol Biol Phys. 1986; 12:453–458.

470. Surwit EA, Manning MR, Aristizabal SA, Oleson JR, Cetas TC. Interstitial thermoradiotherapy in recurrent gynecologic malignancies. Gynecol Oncol. 1983; 15:95–102.

471. Swan DS, Roddick JW. A clinical-pathological correlation of cell type classification for cervical cancer. Am J Obstet Gynecol. 1973; 116:666–670.

472. Swenerton KD, Evers JA, White GW, David A. Intermittent pelvic infusion with vincristine, bleomycin, and mitomycin C for advanced recurrent carcinoma of the cervix. Cancer Treat Rep. 1979; 63:1379–1381.

473. Syed AMN, Puthawala AA, Neblett D et al. Transperineal interstitial-intracavitary "Syed-Neblett" applicator in the treatment of carcinoma of the uterine cervix. Endocurie, Hypertherm Oncol. 1986; 2:1–13.

474. Symmonds RE. Morbidity and complications of radical hysterectomy with pelvic lymph node dissection. Am J Obstet Gynecol. 1966; 94:663–678.

475. Tanaka Y, Sawada S, Murata T. Relationship between lymph node metastases and prognosis in patients irradiated postoperatively for carcinoma of the uterine cervix. Acta Radiol Oncol. 1984; 23:455–459.

476. Tannock I. Response of aerobic and hypoxic cells in a solid tumor to adriamycin and cyclophosphamide and interaction of the drugs with radiation. Cancer Res. 1982; 42:4921–4926.

477. Tattersall MHN, Ramirez C, Coppleson M. A randomized trial comparing platinum-based chemo-

therapy followed by radiotherapy vs. radiotherapy alone in patients with locally advanced cervical cancer. Int J Gynecol Cancer. 1992; 2:244–251.

478. Teicher BA, Holden SA, Al-Achi A, Herman TS. Classification of antineoplastic treatments by their differential toxicity toward putative oxygenated and hypoxic tumor subpopulations in vivo in the FSaIIC murine fibrosarcoma. Cancer Res. 1990; 50:3339–3344.

479. Thipgen T, Vance RB, Balducci L, Blessing J. Chemotherapy in the management of advanced or recurrent cervical and endometrial carcinoma. Cancer. 1981; 48:658–665.

480. Thipgen T, Vance R, Lambuth B et al. Chemotherapy for advanced or recurrent gynecologic cancer. Cancer. 1987; 60:2104–2116.

481. Thomas G, Dembo A, Beale F et al. Concurrent radiation, mitomycin C and 5-fluorouracil in poor prognosis carcinoma of the cervix. Preliminary results of a Phase I–II study. Int J Radiat Oncol Biol Phys. 1984; 10:1785–1790.

482. Thomas G, Dembo AJ. Is there a role for adjuvant pelvic radiotherapy after radical hysterectomy in early stage cervical cancer? Int J Gynecol Cancer. 1991; 1:1–8.

483. Thomas G, Dembo AJ, Myhr T, Black B, Pringle JF, Rawlings G. Long-term results of concurrent radiation and chemotherapy for carcinoma of the cervix recurrent after surgery. Int J Gynecol Cancer. 1993; 3:193–198.

484. Thompson JD, Capota TA, Franklin EW, Dale E. The surgical management of invasive cancer of the cervix in pregnancy. Am J Obstet Gynecol. 1975; 21:853–863.

485. Tinga DJ, Timmer PR, Bouma J, Aalders JG. Prognostic significance of single versus multiple lymph node metastases in cervical carcinoma stage IB. Gynecol Oncol. 1990; 39:175–180.

486. Tinga DJ, Bouma J, Aalders JG. Patients with squamous cell versus adeno(squamous) carcinoma of the cervix, what factors determine the prognosis? Int J Gynecol Cancer. 1992; 2:83–91.

487. Trauth BC, Klas C, Peters AMJ et al. Monoclonal antibody-mediated tumor regression by induction of apoptosis. Science. 1989; 245:301–304.

488. Trott KR. Radiation–chemotherapy interactions. Int J Radiat Oncol Biol Phys. 1986; 12:1409–1413.

489. Tsukamoto N, Kaku T, Matsukuma K. The problem of stage IA (FIGO, carcinoma of the uterine cervix. Gynecol Oncol. 1985; 34:1–6.

490. Twiggs LB, Potish RA, McIntyre S, Adcock LL, Savage JE, Prem KA. Concurrent weekly cis-platinum and radiotherapy in advanced cervical cancer: a preliminary dose escalating toxicity study. Gynecol Oncol. 1986; 24(2):143–148.

491. Underwood PB, Wilson WC, Kreutner A. Radical hysterectomy: A critical review of 22 years' experience. Am J Obstet Gynecol. 1979; 134:889–898.

492. Van Bommel P, Van Lindert A, Kock H, Leers W, Neijt J. A review of prognostic factors in early-stage carcinoma of the cervix (FIGO IB and IIA) and implications for treatment strategy. Eur J Obstet Gynecol Reprod Biol. 1987; 26:69–84.

493. Van Bommel PFJ, Van den Brule AJC, Helmerhorst TJM et al. HPV DNA presence and HPV genotypes as prognostic factors in low-stage squamous cell cervical cancer. Gynecol Oncol. 1993; 48:333–337.

494. Van Dam PA, Watson JV, Lowe DG, Shepherd JH. Flow cytometric DNA analysis in gynecologic oncology. Int J Gynecol Cancer. 1992; 2:57–65.

495. Van Herik M, Fricke RE. The results of radiation therapy for recurrent cancer of the cervix uteri. Am J Roentgenol. 1955; 73:437–441.

496. Van Herik M. Fever as a complication of radiation therapy for carcinoma of the cervix. Am J Roentgenol Radium Ther Nucl Med. 1965; 43:104–109.

497. Van Herik M, Decker DG, Lee RA, Symmonds RE. Late recurrence in carcinoma of the cervix. Am J Obstet Gynecol. 1970; 108:1183–1186.

498. Van Nagell JR, Roddick JW, Lowin DM. The staging of cervical cancer: Inevitable discrepancies between clinical staging and pathologic findings. Am J Obstet Gynecol. 1971; 110:973–978.

499. Van Nagell JR, Donaldason ES, Wood EG. Small cell cancer of the uterine cervix. Cancer. 1977; 40:2253.

500. Van Nagell JR, Donaldason ES, Parker JC. The prognostic significance of cell type and lesion size in patients with cervical cancer treated by radical surgery. Gynecol Oncol. 1977; 5:152.

501. Van Nagell JR, Donaldason ES, Wood EG. The significance of vascular invasion and lymphocytic infiltration in invasive cervical cancer. Cancer. 1978; 41:228–234.

502. Van Nagell Jr JR, Rayburn W, Donaldson ES et al. Therapeutic implications of patterns of recurrence in cancer of the uterine cervix. Cancer. 1979; 44:2354–2361.

503. Van Nagell JR, Greenwell N, Powell DF. Microinvasive carcinoma of the cervix. Am J Obstet Gynecol. 1983; 145:981–991.

504. Vaquer S, Jordá J, López de La Osa E, Alvarez de Los Heros J, López-García N, Alvarez de Mon M. Clinical implications of natural killer (NK) cytotoxicity in patients with squamous cell carcinoma of the uterine cervix. Gynecol Oncol. 1990; 35:90–92.

505. Vaupel P. Pathophysiological mechanisms of hyperthermia in cancer therapy. In: Biological Basis of Oncologic Thermotherapy Gautherie, M, ed. Heidelberg: Springer; 1990:73–134.

506. Vennin P, Hecquet B, Poissonnier B et al. Comparative study of intravenous and intraarterial cis-Platinum on intratumoral platinum concentration in carcinoma of the cervix. Gynecol Oncol. 1989; 32:180–183.

507. Vermorken JB, Mangioni C, Van den Burg MEL, Pecorelli S, Rotmensz N, Dalesio O. EORTC-GCCG phase II trials in disseminated cancer of the uterine cervix. Gin Med Repr. 1985; 10:125–131.

508. Vermorken JB, Landoni F, Pecorelli S et al. Phase II study of vindesine in disseminated squamous cell carcinoma of the uterine cervix: An EORTC gynecological cancer cooperative group study. Int J Gynecol Cancer. 1991; 1:248–252.

509. Vermorken JB. The role of chemotherapy in squamous cell carcinoma of the uterine cervix: A review. Int J Gynecol Cancer. 1993; 3:129–142.

510. Vigario G, Kurohara SS, George FW. Association of hemoglobin levels before and during radiotherapy with prognosis in uterine cervix cancer. Radiology. 1973; 106:649–652.

511. Volterrani F, Tana S, Lozza L et al. Sequential chemotherapy-radiotherapy in the treatment of advanced cervical carcinoma. The Cervix & l.f.g.t. 1990; 8:217–222.

512. Waggener RG, Lange J, Feldmeier J, Eagan P, Martin S. 3-D Gynecological implant dosimetry using an asymmetric Cs-137 source dose rate table. Int J Radiat Oncol Biol Phys. 1988; 15(1):245.

513. Walker J, Bloss JD, Liao SY, Berman M, Berden S, Wilczynski SP. Human papillomavirus genotypes as a prognostic indicator in carcinoma of the uterine cervix. Obstet Gynecol. 1989; 74:781–785.

514. Wang CC. Altered fractionation radiation therapy for gynecologic cancers. Cancer. 1987; 60:2064–2067.

515. Ward BG, Forbes IJ, Cowled PA, McEvoy MM, Cox LW. The treatment of vaginal recurrences of gynecologic malignancy with phototherapy following hematoporphyrin derivative pretreatment. Am J Obstet Gynecol. 1982; 142:356.

516. Wasserman TH, Carter SK. The integration of chemotherapy into combined modality treatment of solid tumors. VIII. Cervical cancer. Cancer Treat Rep. 1977; 4:25–46.

517. Wasserman TH, Stetz J, Philips TL. Radiation therapy oncology group clinical trials with misonidazole. Cancer. 1981; 47:2382–2390.

518. Way S. Microinvasive carcinoma of the cervix. Acta Cytol. 1964; 8:14.

519. Webb MJ, Symmonds RE. Wertheim hysterectomy: A reappraisal. Obstet Gynecol. 1979; 54:140–145.

520. Webb MJ, Symmonds RE. Site or recurrence of cervical cancer after radical hysterectomy. Am J Obstet Gynecol. 1980; 138:813–817.

521. Weeks KJ, Schoeppel SL, Dennett C. Dose measurements and calculations for a CT compatible version of the Fletcher System. Int J Radiat Oncol Biol Phys. 188. 1988; 15(1):188.

522. Welander CE, Homesley HD, Barrett RJ. Combined interferon alfa and doxorubicin in the treatment of advanced cervical cancer. Am J Obstet Gynecol. 1991; 165:284–291.

523. Wentz WB, Reagan JW. Survival in cervical cancer with respect to cell type. Cancer 1959; 12:384–388.

524. West CML, Davidson SE, Hendry JH, Hunter RD. Prediction of cervical carcinoma response to radiotherapy. Lancet 1991; 338:818.

525. Wharton JT, Jones III HW, Day Jr TG, Rutledge FN, Fletcher GH. Preirradiation celiotomy and extended field irradiation for invasive carcinoma of the cervix. Obstet Gynecol. 1977; 49:333–338.

526. Wheelock JB, Krebs HB, Goplerud DR. Bleomycin, Vincristine, and Mitomycin C (BOM) as second-line treatment after failure of cis-platinum-based combination chemotherapy for recurrent cervical cancer. Gynecol Oncol. 1990; 37:21–23.

527. WHO handbook for reporting results of cancer treatment. World Health Organization Geneva. 1979.

528. Williamson JF, Lulu B. Theoretical calculation of those distributions about shielded gynecological colpostats. Int J Radiat Oncol Biol Phys. 1988; 15(1): 244.

529. Willis G. Jennings B, Ball RY, New NE, Gibson I. Analysis of ras point mutations and human papillomavirus 16 and 18 in cervical carcinomata and their metastases. Gynecol Oncol. 1993; 49:359–364.

530. Wimbusch PR, Fletcher GH. Radiation therapy of carcinoma of the cervical stump. Radiology. 1969; 93:655–658.

531. Withers HR. Biological basis of High-LET radiotherapy. Radiology. 1973; 108:131–137.

532. Withers HR. Neutron radiobiology and clinical consequences. Strahlentherapie. 1985a; 161:739–745.

533. Withers HR. Biologic basis for altered fractionation schemes. Cancer. 1985b; 55:2086–2095.

534. Wolff JP, Lacour J, Chassagne D, Berend M. Cancer of the cervical stump: A study of 173 patients. Obstet Gynecol. 1972; 39:100–106.

535. Wong LC, Choo YC, Choy D, Sham JST, Ma HK. Long-term follow-up of potentiation of radiotherapy by cis-platinum in advanced cervical cancer. Gynecol Oncol. 1989; 35:159–163.

536. Wong RC, DeCosse JJ. Cytoreductive surgery. Surg Gynecol Obstet. 1990; 170:276–281.

537. Woods D, Bechtel W, Charnsangavej C et al. Gluteal artery occlusion: Intra-arterial chemotherapy of pelvic neoplasms. Radiology. 1985; 155:341–343.

538. Yabuki Y, Asamoto A, Hoshiba T, Nishimoto H, Kitamura S. Dissection of the cardinal ligament in radical hysterectomy for cervical cancer emphasis on the lateral ligament. Am J Obstet Gynecol. 1991; 164:7–14.

539. Yordan EL, Jurado M, Kiel K et al. Intra-operative radiation therapy in the treatment of pelvic malignancies: A preliminary report. Bailliere's Clinical Obstet Gynecol. 1988; 2:1023–1034.

540. Yuhas JM, Pazmino NH. Inhibition of subcutaneously growing Line 1 carcinomas due to metastatic spread. Cancer Res. 1974; 34:2005–2010.

541. Zanetta GM, Katzmann JA, Keeney GL, Kinney WK, Cha SS, Podratz KC. Flow-cytometric DNA analysis of stages IB and IIA cervical carcinoma. Gynecol Oncol. 1992; 46:13–19.

6 Malignancies of the Ovary and Fallopian Tube

J. T. Soper

Ovarian and Tubal Carcinoma

Ovarian carcinoma has the highest death : case ratio of all gynecological malignancies. It is the fourth leading cause of cancer-related death for women in the United States. Between 1983 and 1993, the annual incidence in the United States rose from 18 200 to 22 000, with annual mortality increasing from 11 500 to 13 500.[14] The increases in incidence and mortality most likely reflect the aging of the population in general, but these figures serve to emphasize the magnitude of the problem caused by this disease.

Epithelial ovarian carcinoma accounts for the majority of primary ovarian malignancies. Many epidemiological associations have been defined that impart an increased risk for the development of these lesions. These include a personal history of prior breast or colon cancer, infertility, nulliparity, a high-fat diet, and perineal talc use.[13] Unfortunately, these factors result in only small increases (2–4 fold) in the relative risk for the development of ovarian cancer. Although a family history of ovarian cancer increases the risk of developing ovarian cancer, the majority of epithelial ovarian malignancies develop in women who lack a high-risk family history.

Less than 10% of women with ovarian cancer have a family history of a single relative with this cancer. Kerlikowske and associates[97] reviewed the available case control studies in the literature. Their estimation of the odds ratio for ovarian cancer in women with a family history of ovarian cancer in one first or second degree relative was 3 : 1. Although this increased to 4–6 : 1 in women with two or three relatives (one first degree and/or one or more second degree relative), the magnitude of the risk imparted by a simple family history of ovarian cancer is too small to justify prophylactic oophorectomy as a routine procedure in these individuals. Ovarian cancer risk is also increased in women with a family history of breast and colon malignancies and comprises a portion of the Lynch II syndrome.[13] However, these individuals have an increased risk of malignancy at multiple sites, thus potentially lessening the impact of prophylactic intervention. A more complex pedigree with multiple family members affected with ovarian cancer or peritoneal carcinomatosis may increase the odds ratio to as high as 39 : 1; with a lifetime risk of approximately 50%.[85] The isolation and cloning of the BRCA genes may allow for the identification of women who are at extreme risk in these families. In these patients, prophylactic oophorectomy may reduce the risk of developing ovarian cancer, but this type of pedigree is observed in less than 1–2% of patients with ovarian cancer. Therefore, intervention (even in these high-risk patients) is unlikely to have a major impact on the overall incidence and mortality of ovarian cancer.

Unfortunately, epithelial ovarian carcinoma usually presents with few specific symptoms. The majority of women have advanced-stage disease at the time of diagnosis. For this reason, screening strategies using tumor markers and ultrasound imaging are undergoing evaluation, particularly in high-risk women with a family history of ovarian cancer. Although promising, these strategies have not been proven effective or cost-effective in the early detection of asymptomatic ovarian cancer.

The management of epithelial ovarian carcinoma has evolved over the past 50 years from management with minimal surgery and limited adjunctive therapy to aggressive surgery and increasingly complex adjunctive therapies. Initial experience with alkylating agents suggested responses in a substantial proportion of patients with advanced disease and yielded significant improvements in short-term survival when compared with placebo results.[21, 206] Further identification of active agents, particularly platin compounds and use of combination chemotherapy regimens, have resulted in improved response rates and short-term survival.[225] Aggressive surgical management has also resulted in an overall improvement in short-term survival of women with advanced-stage disease.[35] Despite refinements in adjunctive therapies and surgical management, however, the overall long-term survival of women with epithelial ovarian carcinoma has remained relatively stagnant over the past three decades. Ten-year progression-free survival for women with stage III and IV ovarian cancer, treated with platin-based chemotherapy, has remained less than 10%.[78, 223]

Nonepithelial malignant neoplasms of the ovary account for only about 10% of primary ovarian malignancies. Advances in the chemotherapy regimens used for malignant germ cell tumors of the testes have resulted in significantly improved survival for women with germ cell tumors of the ovaries, but these account for a minority of the cases of ovarian cancer. Stromal malignancies of the ovaries are also relatively rare, but often present unique diagnostic and management challenges.

Tubal cancer, a rare malignancy of the female genital tract, has many clinical features in common with ovarian cancer. Because the pathology, presentation, and management of tubal carcinoma is similar to epithelial ovarian carcinoma, the management of tubal carcinomas will be discussed parallel to ovarian carcinoma.

Primary Disease

▓ Pathology

A functional classification and relative distribution for the pathology of primary ovarian malignancies is displayed in Table **1**. Detailed descriptions of the pathology of each lesion are given elsewhere;[108, 192] functional differences will be emphasized.

Epithelial Ovarian Tumors

Epithelial malignancies of the ovary recapitulate epithelia of the normal müllerian tract. Serous, mucinous, endometrioid, clear cell, and Brenner tumors have both benign and malignant counterparts.[108, 192] Benign epithelial tumors typically occur in younger women, with malignant tumors occurring most often in the postmenopausal age group. Each malignant histological subtype is divided into lesions of low malignant potential (LMP) and invasive carcinomas (Table **1**). Recognition of LMP lesions is extremely important because these tumors have a markedly different biology than frankly invasive carcinomas, usually producing tumors with indolent growth and metastases that rarely result in death of the pa-

Table **1**   Histological classification of ovarian cancer

Common Epithelial:

Serous
    Borderline malignancy (low malignant potential)
    Malignant

Mucinous
    Borderline malignancy (low malignant potential)
    Malignant

Endometrioid
    Borderline malignancy (low malignant potential)
    Malignant
    Mixed müllerian tumor

Clear-cell
    Borderline malignancy (low malignant potential)
    Malignant

Brenner
    Proliferative/borderline malignancy
    Malignant

Mixed (specify subtypes)

Undifferentiated

Mixed müllerian tumor (carcinosarcoma)

Malignant Germ Cell Tumors:

Dysgerminoma

Endodermal sinus tumor (yolk sac tumor)

Embryonal carcinoma

Polyembryoma

Choriocarcinoma (nongestational)

Teratoma
    Immature
    Carcinoid
    Malignant degeneration of epithelial
      elements

Mixed (specify types)

Mixed Germ Cell/Stromal (Gonadoblastoma)

Sex Cord/Stromal Tumors:

Granulosa cell tumors

Thecoma-fibroma tumors

Sertoli-stromal cell tumors, androblastomas,
    Sertoli-Leydig cell tumors

Sex cord tumors with annular tubules

Gynandroblastoma

Steroid (lipid) cell tumors

Unclassified

tient. The histological features used to diagnose LMP tumors include cellular stratification and piling up, mitotic activity, and often impressive nuclear atypia. The distinction between LMP and very well-differentiated invasive carcinoma must usually be made on the basis of identification of a pushing interface into adjacent tissue versus destructive stromal invasion.[108, 192] Histological grading of the frankly invasive carcinomas provides a general indication of the aggressiveness of tumor biology. Stage for stage, the histological subtypes are of less importance in predicting tumor behavior than the degree of histological grade. Mixed müllerian tumors (carcinosarcomas) are also probably derived from malignant differentiation of epithelial elements (Table **1**,[108])

Germ Cell Tumors

Although 15–20% of all ovarian neoplasms are of germ cell origin, most of these tumors are benign mature teratomas (dermoid cysts) of the ovaries. Malignant germ cell tumors comprise only about 5% of ovarian malignancies.[192] Germ cell tumors are derived from the primordial germ cells of the ovary and can arise anywhere along the path of embryonic migration of the germ cells from the caudal yolk sac of the dorsal mesentery before they are incorporated into the sex cords of the developing gonads.[204] Because malignant germ cell tumors of testicular origin are much more common than those of ovarian origin,[14] most of the advances in the management of ovarian germ cell malignancies have resulted from the results of treatment of testicular tumors.

Major histological subtypes of germ cell malignancies of the ovaries include dysgerminoma, immature teratoma, endodermal sinus tumor, and mixed germ cell tumors (Table **1**). Embryonal carcinoma, primary ovarian choriocarcinoma, and polyembryoma are rare entities. Gonadoblastomas are mixed germ cell/stromal cell tumors (Table **1**) that have a premalignant potential and may develop into dysgerminoma in women with gonadal dysgenesis.

Dysgerminomas are the most common malignant germ cell malignancy of the ovary, comprising about 40% of cases.[114, 192] Histologically analogous to testicular seminoma, dysgerminomas are derived from germ cells that have not differentiated to form embryonic or extraembryonic structures. Unlike other germ cell malignancies, 10–15% of dysgerminomas are bi-

lateral.[192, 233] The median age at diagnosis is 20 years. Similar to other germ cell malignancies of the ovary, dysgerminomas usually grow rapidly, presenting most frequently as lower abdominal pain and mass. Due to rapid growth, a substantial proportion present with acute symptoms of rupture. A small proportion of dysgerminomas arise in gonadoblastomas of women with gonadal dysgenesis and who harbor a Y chromosome.[218] Lesions that are comprised predominantly of dysgerminoma but contain areas of a more aggressive germ cell tumor are classified as a mixed germ cell tumor.[192] Multinucleate giant cells that secrete hCG can develop in pure dysgerminomas, leading to elevations of serum hCG in a few patients, but pure dysgerminomas do not produce alpha-fetoprotein (AFP). Therefore, patients thought to have pure dysgerminoma, but who have circulating levels of AFP should be treated as if they have a mixed germ cell tumor rather than a pure dysgerminoma.

Although benign (mature) teratomas comprise almost 15% of all ovarian neoplasms, immature teratomas account for fewer than 1% of all ovarian malignancies.[192] Immature teratomas are the second most common germ cell malignancy of the ovary, containing tissue elements of embryonic origin.[114, 192] More than 50% of immature teratomas of the ovary are diagnosed in females between 10 and 20 years of age. Bilaterality is extremely uncommon in immature teratoma; the most frequent neoplasm in the contralateral ovary is mature teratoma (dermoid cyst). Immature teratomas are classified histologically on the basis of the degree of differentiation and quantity of immature neural tissue. Grading ranges from grade 1 lesions, which have well-differentiated cells (except in rare foci of immature tissue) to grade 3 lesions, in which large portions of the tumor exhibit atypical embryonal cells with frequent mitotic activity.[159, 192] In a study by Norris et al., prognosis varied directly in proportion to grade in the prechemotherapy era, with 82% survival in patients with grade 1, 63% in grade 2, and only 30% in those with grade 3 lesions.[159] Therefore, surgery alone is considered adequate therapy for patients with stage I, grade 1 immature teratomas, but all other patients with immature teratomas are treated with additional therapy. Peritoneal implants with completely mature histology (grade 0) do not affect prognosis and are often found during restaging laparotomy after combination chemotherapy.[57]

Endodermal sinus tumors are the next most frequent histological subtype, comprising approximately 20% of malignant germ cell tumors of the ovary.[112, 192] They are thought to be derived from extraembryonal germ cells that differentiate into the yolk sac. Histologically, these lesions are characterized by papillary projections, which contain a single blood vessel and are covered with a peripheral lining of malignant epithelioid cells (Schiller–Duval bodies). The median age at diagnosis is 19 years. These tumors frequently present with extremely rapid growth and have the potential for rapid intra-abdominal spread. Serum AFP levels are most often elevated in patients with this tumor and serve as sensitive tumor markers for diagnosis and during therapy.[228] In contrast to dysgerminomas, where survival among patients with stage I lesions was favorable, survival of less than 15% was recorded for patients with stage I endodermal sinus tumors in the prechemotherapy era.[40, 112]

Embryonal carcinomas are extremely malignant and rare germ cell neoplasms, which represent less than 5% of all ovarian germ cell malignancies.[113, 192] They are usually poorly differentiated and may be confused histologically with endodermal sinus tumors or choriocarcinoma, although these tumors lack Schiller–Duval bodies and clear dimorphic differentiation into sycytio- and cytotrophoblastic elements. Because they are derived from primitive germ cells, both hCG and AFP can be secreted by these tumors and are useful as tumor markers for monitoring during therapy in individual cases.

Pure nongestational choriocarcinoma of the ovary is an extremely rare malignancy.[56, 192] Differential diagnosis should include metastasis from a uterine or tubal primary gestational choriocarcinoma and gestational choriocarcinoma derived from a primary ovarian pregnancy. In the majority of cases of nongestational ovarian choriocarcinoma, other malignant germ cell elements comprise a portion of the tumor. Largely because of the reluctance to diagnose nongestational choriocarcinoma in women of reproductive age, the majority of cases of pure ovarian choriocarcinoma have been reported in children. Because these tumors secrete hCG, prepubertal children may present with isosexual precocious puberty. Unlike gestational choriocarcinoma, primary ovarian choriocarcinoma is not exquisitely sensitive to simple single-agent chemotherapeutic regimens.

Polyembryoma is an extremely rare germ cell tumor that has been reported in only a handful of patients.[192] Histologically, it is characterized by multiple embryonal bodies and represents parthenogenesis from germ cells.

Mixed germ cell tumors contain at least two malignant germ cell elements.[113, 192] In one series, the components in decreasing order of frequency were dysgerminoma (80%), endodermal sinus tumor (70%) immature teratoma (53%), choriocarcinoma (20%), and embryonal carcinoma (16%), with the most common mixture consisting of dysgerminoma and endodermal sinus tumor.[113] The mixed tumors can secrete either hCG, AFP, neither tumor marker, or both, depending upon the histological types comprising the individual tumor. The behavior of mixed tumors depends largely upon the most malignant element of the individual lesion. Size of the primary tumor <10 cm and tumors with < one-third comprised of endodermal sinus tumor, choriocarcinoma, or grade 3 immature teratoma have a favorable prognosis compared to lesions that are large or contain a large proportion of unfavorable histological subtypes.[113]

Stromal Tumors

Tumors derived from the sex cords and stroma represent about 6% of ovarian tumors and are the most common hormonally active ovarian neoplasms.[192, 259] Although many histological types of stromal tumors exist (Table **1**), the two most important categores comprise the granulosa-theca and Sertoli-Leydig cell tumors. Fibromas, rare benign tumors, and sarcomas account for the remainder of tumors derived from the ovarian stroma.

Tumors of the granulosa-theca cell elements most frequently present in peri- and postmenopausal women. If any granulosa cell elements are present, the neoplasm is classified as a granulosa cell tumor and is considered to have a low malignant potential.[192, 260] Pure theca cell tumors are often hard to distinguish histologically from fibromas and are almost always benign, unless there is sarcomatous degeneration with high mitotic activity and anaplasia.[260] Granulosa cell tumors can elaborate any of the sex steroid hormones, but estrogen production is the most frequent and patients often present with tender or swollen breasts and irregular uterine bleeding. Endometrial adenocarcinoma develops in association with approximately 10% of patients with granulosa cell tumors and up to 50% develop associated endometrial adenomatous hyperplasia.[52, 54] The majority of patients present with stage IA, or less frequently stage IC, disease. Rupture occurs preoperatively in approximately 14% of granulosa cell tumors. Prognosis is stongly determined by the stage of disease at presentation, with survival of >85% of patients with stage I lesions, compared to very poor survival in patients with stage III disease. Granulosa cell tumors may recur more than 5–10 years after primary surgery, but the majority of recurrences develop within the first 3 years of original diagnosis.[52, 54, 220, 260]

Fewer than 5% of granulosa cell tumors present before puberty; three-quarters of these patients present with isosexual precocious puberty caused by estrogen production from the tumor.[116] Almost all of prepubertal patients with granulosa cell tumors, and a substantial proportion of those who develop these lesions before the age of 30 years, have juvenile granulosa cell tumors,[260] Histologically, juvenile granulosa cell tumors may be extremely anaplastic, with high mitotic activity. They tend to have a clinical course similar to the more bland adult granulosa cell tumors. Outcome is largely dependent upon stage.

Sertoli-Leydig cell tumors are rare tumors comprised of cells that resemble Sertoli cells, Leydig cells, and indifferent stromal cells of the testes.[192] Bilaterality is rare. Altough almost half of Sertoli-Leydig cell tumors secrete androgens and produce signs of virilization, others produce estrogen, progesterone, or are hormonally inactive.[181, 261] The median age of onset is 25 years, with less than 5% occurring in prepubertal girls. Outcome is related to the stage of disease and histological differentiation. The majority of patients present with stage IA disease and survivals of 92–100% have been reported for these patients regardless of histological grade.

Ovarian fibromas represent approximately 4% of all ovarian neoplasms and are almost always benign.[259] Approximately 40% of patients with ovarian fibromas >10 cm in diameter will have acellular ascites, but only about 1% of ovarian fibromas present with ascites and hydrothorax (Meigs syndrome).[188] The ascites will resolve with removal of the ovarian fibroma. Other rare stromal and sex cord tumors of the ovary are encountered. Unless there is sarcomatous degeneration, the majority behave clinically in a manner similar to theca cell tumors and should be considered to have a very low malignant potential.

Tubal Malignancies

Almost all primary tubal malignancies of the fallopian tube are epithelial carcinomas. Most often these have a serous histology, although other histological types have been reported.[193] By convention, epithelial malignancies that involve both the ovary and the tube are not considered of tubal origin unless there is a clear transition between normal and malignant tubal epithelium, the dominant mass involves the tube, and ovarian involvement is limited to surface or angiolymphatic metastases. Other stromal tumors and sarcomas rarely develop from the fallopian tube.

▪ Surgery of Primary Disease

Development and Routes of Spread

Epithelial ovarian carcinoma is presumed to be derived from elements of the ovarian surface (germinal) epithelium. It is hypothesized that early growth begins within epithelial inclusion cysts buried within the substance of the ovary.[126] Initially this produces cyst formation. Transformation into a benign epithelial neoplasm may precede the development of malignant transformation, although this remains unproven. Several major routes of spread can occur after malignant transformation and stromal invasion:

1. Capsular penetration and adherence with the potential for direct invasion of adjacent organs, such as the peritoneum of the broad ligament, fallopian tube, or serosa of the bowel.

2. Exfoliation of cells from capsular excrescences into peritoneal fluid with peritoneal surface metastases. The shed cells initially follow the normal circulation of fluid through the peritoneal cacity, in the direction of colonic peristalsis up the right pericolic gutter, to the right diaphragm, and down the left pericolic gutter into the pelvis. All peritoneal surfaces are at risk for implantation metastases, including the omentum, diaphragm, and serosa and mesentery of the bowel. Implants involving the diaphragm may penetrate through

the diaphragmatic lymphatics or defects in the diaphragm, producing pleural seeding and malignant pleural effusion.

3. Two major lymphatic chains can be involved as primary sites for the lymphatic metastases of ovarian cancer. In contrast to the testes, the ovaries are intrapelvic organs that have alternative routes of lymphatic drainage. The para-aortic chain can become involved by metastasis via the lymphatic channels that accompany the infundibulopelvic ligament directly to the para-aortic and precaval lymph nodes in the region of the renal vessels. Lymph channels in the broad ligament and parametrium pass laterally to the external iliac, hypogastric, and obturator pelvic lymph nodes, resulting in frequent involvement of the pelvic nodes. Rarely, ovarian carcinomas can metastasize directly to the groin nodes via lymphatic channels in the round ligaments.

4. Hematogenous spread occurs very rarely in the absence of intra-abdominal and/or lymphatic spread. Parenchymal liver, pulmonary, bony, or central nervous system metastasis occurs in less than 5–10% of cases at diagnosis.

Early peritoneal and lymphatic metastases of epithelial ovarian carcinoma are usually clinically occult. Because no anatomic barrier exists between the pelvis and upper abdomen or retroperitoneal lymph nodes after the ovarian capsule is invaded, the diagnosis of ovarian carcinoma confined to the ovaries or pelvis can only be made after the existence of metastatic disease has been excluded through a meticulous and comprehensive surgical staging laparotomy.

Germ cell and stromal malignancies of the ovary have similar potential patterns of metastatic spread. However, because germ cell malignancies are exquisitely sensitive to chemotherapy, meticulous staging laparotomy to define early disease is of relatively less importance than for other histological types of ovarian malignancies.

Tubal carcinomas metastasize along the same routes of spread as epithelial ovarian carcinomas, with predominantly intraperitoneal and lymphatic dissemination. Because the fallopian tube has a thin muscular wall that is richly permeated with lymphatic channels, lymphatic metastasis may occur more frequently than in ovarian malignancies. Although there is less information regarding distribution of spread in tubal car-

Table **2**   FIGO Surgical Staging for Ovarian Carcinoma

Stage I:		Growth limited to the ovary(ies)
	IA:	Growth limited to *one* ovary. No ascites, no external excrescences, capsule intact
	IB:	Growth limited to *both* ovaries. No ascites, no external excrescences, capsule intact
	IC:	Tumor extent either stage IA or IB but with *malignant* ascites or positive peritoneal washings, capsular excrescences, or tumor rupture
Stage II:		Pelvic metastasis/extension of tumor
	IIA:	Metastasis/extension to the uterus and/or tubes
	IIB:	Metastasis/extension to other pelvic tissues
	IIC:	Tumor extent either stage IIA or IIB but with *malignant* ascites or positive peritoneal washings, capsular excrescences, or tumor rupture
Stage III:		Tumor metastasis outside the pelvis to involve peritoneal surfaces or retroperitoneal/inguinal lymph nodes
	IIIA:	Tumor grossly confined to the pelvis but with histologically proven metastasis to peritoneal surfaces
	IIIB:	Grossly apparent peritoneal metastasis, < 2 cm in largest diameter
	IIIC:	Grossly apparent peritoneal metastasis, > 2 cm in largest diameter, and/or positive retroperitoneal or inguinal lymph nodes
Stage IV:		Distant or hepatic parenchymal metastasis

Note: For ascites to result in classification of stage IC or IIC, cytology must contain malignant cells.
Note: Metastasis to the serosa of the liver without parenchymal involvement is classified as stage III disease.
Modified from: International Federation of Obstetrics and Gynecology: FIGO revised staging for ovarian cancer. Am J Obstet Gynecol. 1989; 156:263–264.

cinoma than for ovarian carcinoma, at least one-third of patients will have para-aortic metastasis.[229]

Staging

The revised (1986) International Federation of Obstetrics and Gynecology (FIGO) staging system for ovarian cancer (Table **2**) is based on the natural history and patterns of spread for epithelial ovarian carcinoma.[90] The stage is assigned on the basis of surgical laparotomy. Although lymph node dissection may not be required to assign stage in patients with bulky upper abdominal disease (stage III C), it is critical that metastases to the para-aortic and pelvic nodes are identified before assigning patients to lower stages. Although an official FIGO staging system for tubal cancer has not been developed, it is recommended that a modification of the ovarian cancer staging system be used to classify disease spread in this disease.[173]

Presentation and Preoperative Evaluation of Ovarian and Tubal Cancer

Screening for Epithelial Ovarian Cancer

Several prospective studies are investigating the utility of using transvaginal ultrasound and/or serum tumor markers (predominantly serum CA 125) for screening asymptomatic women for ovarian carcinoma. The available technology, however, is unlikely to have sufficient sensitivity and specificity to have a favorable impact on the survival of patients in the general population. The optimal sequence of studies (ultrasound first or second), combinations of tumor markers, and interval between screenings have not yet been determined.[13] Although participation of patients in carefully conducted screening trials is encouraged, the indiscriminate use of office ultrasound and serum CA 125 values for this purpose should be discouraged.

Presenting Signs and Symptoms

The majority of patients with epithelial ovarian carcinomas present in the early postmenopausal years with a vague and nonspecific history of discomfort, abdominal bloating, and a variety of gastrointestinal symptoms. Patients with early ovarian carcinomas may even have these symp-toms.[216] Patients are often seen by several physicians without receiving a specific diagnosis until a pelvic mass is discovered on abdominal computed tomography (CT) scan or the patient develops ascites. Almost all gynecologic oncologists have experienced patient referrals from general surgeons who made the diagnosis of abdominal carcinomatosis at the time of cholecystectomy or umbilical hernia repair. Although it is unfortunate that these patients were subjected to their surgical procedure before the diagnosis was suspected by pelvic examination, it is unlikely that their survival was adversely affected by the procedure. Unfortunately, given the unproven efficacy of screening for any patient population, serendipitous identification of a pelvic mass is the best means for early detection of ovarian cancer.

Germ cell malignancies of the ovaries tend to grow rapidly, frequently producing abdominal pain and abdominopelvic mass in girls or young women. Because these tumors have the potential to outgrow the blood supply to the central tumor, spontaneous hemorrhage or rupture with symptoms of an acute abdomen are observed in about 10 % of patients. In this setting, the correct diagnosis is often not considered until the tumor is discovered at the time of an emergent laparotomy. Production of hCG by mixed or pure ovarian choriocarcinomas can result in isosexual precocious puberty in prepubertal girls.

Stromal cell tumors often present with symptoms related to hormone production. It should be emphasized that even though granulosa cell tumors are classically thought to produce estrogen and Sertoli-Leydig cell tumors testosterone, any steroid hormone can be secreted by an individual stromal tumor. The tumor can also be hormonally inactive. In girls or women with estrogen-secreting tumors, isosexual pseudo-precocious puberty, menstrual irregularities, postmenopausal bleeding, adenomatous hyperplasia, and endometrial cancer are frequently observed. Patients with androgen-secreting tumors present with symptoms ranging from those of slight androgen excess to florid virilization, depending on the hormone and level of production. Other symptoms of stromal cell tumors are nonspecific, except that a small subset of granulosa cell tumors rupture spontaneously and present with acute hemoperitoneum.

The typical diagnostic triad associated with fallopian tubal cancer is noted in only about 15 %

of patients, but consists of a watery vaginal discharge (*hydrops tubae profluens*), pelvic pain, and a pelvic mass.[193] Vaginal discharge or abnormal bleeding is noted in more than half of patients with tubal cancer. Otherwise, the clinical presentation of these patients is similar to patients with ovarian cancer.

Diagnostic Evaluation

The most important clinical sign that should prompt a further evaluation aimed at excluding ovarian carcinoma is the finding of a pelvic mass on physical examination. In premonopausal women with unilateral, small, cystic masses, observation for a limited interval is preferred to allow funtional cysts of the ovary time to regress. Essentially all other patients who have significant pelvic masses with other clinical features, including those of reproductive age who have persistence of a clinically benign mass, should undergo operative evaluation and surgical removal of the mass. A few postmenopausal women with trivial (< 0.5–1 cm diameter) simple cysts defined by ultrasound and associated with no pelvic fluid and with normal CA 125 values can be serially monitored. However, even though the risk of malignancy in small (< 3–5 cm) simple cysts is extremely low, current practice dictates surgical removal in a postmenopausal woman unless the patient is entered onto a research protocol.

The majority of diagnostic tests used for the evaluation of women with an adnexal mass should be used to segregate patients into four groups: those patients unlikely to have a gynecological cause of a pelvic mass, those likely to have benign functional cysts of the ovary, those likely to have benign neoplasms, and those likely to have ovarian cancer. Patients who have bowel symptoms or occult fecal blood should undergo an evaluation of the lower gastrointestinal tract with a barium enema or colonoscopy to exclude colonic or other gastrointestinal pathology, such as diverticulitis, other inflammatory bowel disease, or colonic carcinoma. Likewise, patients upper with gastrointestinal symptoms should undergo endoscopy or upper GI series to exclude upper gastrointestinal tract involvement. Other patients are unlikely to benefit from these evaluations.

Extensive further diagnostic testing to discriminate between benign and malignant adnexal masses may not be useful if the patient will be explored in a setting where patients with malignancy can undergo comprehensive surgical staging and definitive debulking. However, characterization of the mass as probably benign or malignant is advisable to decide whether the patient should be referred to an institution where comprehensive gynecologic oncology services are available. Furthermore, the only adnexal masses that should be approached in a freestanding day surgery unit are those that are clearly benign by noninvasive tests.

Transvaginal or abdominal ultrasound and CA-125 values can provide complimentary information about the nature of pelvic masses. In premenopausal patients, unilateral and mostly cystic adnexal masses up to approximately 8 cm in diameter are most likely to be functional cysts, and less than 2 % are malignant.[63, 65, 130, 145]

Although there are sparse data characterizing the ultrasound and flow characteristics of corpora hemorrhagicum and corpora luteum, an occasional premenopausal patient will present with a 4–8 cm mixed solid-cystic mass that has ominous flow characteristics on Doppler-flow analysis. In our experience, these are most often functional cysts of the ovaries that will resolve with observation, provided there are no internal papillations on ultrasound or other findings on clinical examination that are suspicious for malignancy. Patients with presumed functional cysts of the ovaries should be reevaluated within 6–8 weeks. Moderate-dose oral contraceptives may be used to suppress ovulation and avoid detection of a second functional cyst,[217] but probably do not hasten regression of functional cysts. Cysts that persist or enlarge should be presumed neoplastic and be removed surgically. If the cyst has decreased in size at the initial follow-up evaluation but is still present, a follow-up examination in another 4–6 weeks is warranted to ensure complete regression of the cyst.

Cysts > 8 cm in women of reprodutive age should be surgically evaluated unless the patient is receiving ovulation induction agents. With the introduction of low-dose oral contraceptives that do not always inhibit ovulation, women who develop cysts while on low-dose oral contraceptives should be observed while taking a higher-dose (> 35 mcg estrogen) oral contraceptive.

Unfortunately, many studies that compare ultrasound characteristics of pelvic masses to final diagnosis are limited by their failure to separate findings in premenopausal and postmenopausal women. Furthermore, older studies used transabdominal ultrasound, while more recent series have used transvaginal ultrasound, where the transducer provides more detail for visualization of the ovaries. However, ultrasound characteristics of size, septations, intracystic papillations, and pulsatility index provide useful information about the likelihood of malignancy.

Even in premenopausal women, larger adnexal masses are more likely to be malignant than smaller masses. Between 20% and 57% of premenopausal patients with masses > 10 cm, and up to 64% of postmenopausal patients with large masses have malignant disease.[65, 76, 187] The risk of malignancy in purely unilocular cysts without any solid areas is less than 1%.[65, 151, 187] However, Granberg et al.[65] reported that the risk of malignancy increased from 8% in patients with multilocular tumors that lacked a solid component to 70% in those with multilocular tumors that had solid regions within the lesion. Requard and associates[176] observed that 28 (87.5%) of 32 tumors with septae thicker than 1–3 mm in diameter were malignant, although others did not find that thin septae by themselves were reassuring.[145]

Intracystic papillations are associated with a high risk of malignancy. Granberg et al.[65] found that 73 (93%) of 79 masses with this characteristic were malignant. It should be emphasized that the entire cyst wall should be evaluated for papillations. In some patients with large masses, transvaginal and abdominal ultrasounds must be combined to give a complete assessment of the cyst wall.

The Doppler effect, caused by focusing an ultrasound signal on blood moving in a vessel, has been used in an attempt to detect the characteristically high flow of blood in the vessels of an ovarian malignancy. Both systolic and diastolic flow can be calculated using the Doppler wave form and used to calculate various indices or ratios. Weiner et al.[248] found that a pulsatility index (systolic flow–diastolic flow/mean flow) of <1 was characteristic of ovarian malignancies. In their experience, the sensitivity (94%) and specificity (97%) for correctly predicting malignancy or benignancy of the calculated pulsatility index was superior to both the ultrasonic features and the CA 125 level. Other small series have confirmed their findings, but the number of premenopausal patients studied to date has been small.[16, 110, 115]

The CA 125 antigen has been measured in the sera of women with active ovarian carcinoma. It has been found to correlate with the response of disease to therapy. Several studies have documented that elevations of CA 125 above threshold, usually 35 or 65 µ/ml are strongly predictive of malignancy in patients with pelvic masses, particularly in postmenopausal women.[132, 212, 239] Elevated levels have a sensitivity of approximately 85–95% and a specificity in a similar range in this age group. In premenopausal women with adnexal masses, CA 125 levels are of limited value because of the frequent diagnoses of inflammatory masses, endometriosis, and leiomyomata, which can falsely elevate serum CA 125 levels. Both Jacobs et al.[93] and Finkler et al.[53] reported that the use of CA 125 in conjuction with ultrasound for the evaluation of women with pelvic masses improved the accuracy for prediction of malignancy above the accuracy for either test alone. Neither of these studies evaluated Doppler-flow characteristics of the masses; it remains to be seen whether a combination of Doppler flow studies and CA 125 values will enhance diagnostic accuracy.

In prepubertal and premenopausal women with a pelvic mass, the incidence of ovarian germ cell and stromal tumors is relatively increased compared to epithelial malignancies. Specific tumor markers (AFP and hCG) should be obtained preoperatively in these patients in addition to CA 125 level. Because of the rapid clearance of AFP or hCG when a stage I malignancy is resected, elevated markers might be missed if the studies are performed only during the postoperative period.

Abdominopelvic CT scans or upper GI contrast studies might diagnose or exclude occult pancreatic or hepatobiliary malignancy in a patient presenting with malignant ascites in the absence of a distinct pelvic mass, but otherwise will rarely obviate the need for a surgical exploration. Elevated carcinoembryonic antigen (CEA) levels may be present in patients with either mucinous ovarian carcinomas or gastrointestinal malignancies.

The use of primary surgical debulking lessens the value of primary CT imaging for assigning stage of disease. The CT scan is most useful as a postoperative baseline study to determine if patients with bulky residual have disease that can be followed with noninvasive studies. Nelson et al.,[156] (however), recently reported that findings

Table 3 Discrimination between benign and malignant adnexal masses using clinical, ultrasound, and CA-125 characteristics

	Benign	Malignant
Clinical		
Age	20–50 years +++	< 20, > 50 years +++
Laterality	Unilateral ++	Bilateral ++
Size	< 8 cm +++	> 8 cm ++
Nodularity	–	+++
Ultrasound		
Simple cyst	++++	–
Multilocular	Thin septae ++	Thick septae or solid component +++
Papillary excrescences	–	++++
Ascites	–	++++
Doppler color flow	Low flow, High pulsatility +++	High flow, Low pulsatility +++
CA 125		
< 50 years	< 35 u/ml +	> 35 u/ml +
> 50 years	< 35 u/ml +++	> 35 u/ml +++
		> 65 u/ml ++++

Grading of correlation: not associated –, strength of positive associated indicated by number of +.

on CT could be used to predict the potential for optimal primary cytoreductive surgery with a sensitivity of 92.3% and specificity of 79.3%. Although the use of neoadjuvant chemotherapy followed by interval debulking is not standard management for patients with ovarian cancer, their study creates the possibility of using noninvasive imaging to make decisions regarding the feasibility of primary debulking, and for selecting patients who are unlikely to be optimally debulked to receive experimental regimens before attempting surgery. However, it should be noted that 6 (33%) of 18 patients having unfavorable characteristics for optimal debulking could be successfully cytoreduced.

A summary of the clinical, ultrasound, and CA 125 characteristics that are useful in discriminating between benign and malignant pelvic masses is given in Table **3**.

Surgery for Early Disease

Studies performed in the past 25 years have helped to define the extent of surgery needed to define stage in epithelial ovarian carcinomas. Although similar routes of spread are involved in germ cell, stromal, and tubal malignancies, the efficacy of comprehensive staging laparotomy in patients who have apparent early stage disease with these lesions has not been established. Until these lesions have been adequately studied, however, it is recommended that comprehensive staging laparotomies be performed to define extent of disease in all patients. While precise surgical staging is important, the main therapeutic effect of primary surgery in early disease is the removal of all or most of the gross tumor burden, to prepare the patient for postoperative adjuvant therapy.

Comprehensive Staging Laparotomy

The majority of women who are explored for ovarian carcinoma undergo initial surgery by general obstetrician–gynecologists or general surgeons. McGowan et al.[140] evaluated the completeness of surgical staging in 291 women with ovarian carcinoma of all stages and found that 46% had incomplete documentation of stage at their initial laparotomy. Thirty-five percent and 52% of those explored by general surgeons and obstetrician–gynecologists, respectively, had complete documentation of stage, compared to 97% of patients who were initially explored by gynecologic oncologists. Trimbos et al.[237] evaluated completeness of surgical staging in women thought to have early ovarian carcinoma. Only 15% of patients explored in community hospitals had a complete comprehensive staging laparotomy, including only 5% explored by an obstetrician–gynecologist and 38% explored by an obstetrician–gynecologist, assisted by a vascular surgeon. Omissions resulting in incomplete staging were divided almost equally between procedures associated with an increased risk or difficulty, such as lymphadenectomy, and very

Table 4 Distribution of positive findings in restaged patients with apparent stage I and II epithelial ovarian cancer

Site	Frequency (%)
Peritoneal cytology	20
Diaphragm	7.5
Omentum	7
Abdominal peritoneum	10
Pelvic peritoneum	10
Pelvic lymph nodes	9
Para-aortic lymph nodes	12

Compiled from: Buchsbaum, 1989; Young, 1983; Soper, 1992; Soper, 1994.

simple procedures, such as performing omental biopsy or obtaining peritoneal washings for cytology, which reflected a lack of knowledge of the anatomic sites at risk for metastasis.

Other investigators have reexplored women who were presumed to have early epithelial ovarian carcinoma but underwent an incomplete initial staging procedure. When these patients were subjected to a pretherapy comprehensive restaging laparotomy, 22–30% were upstaged, with 20–23% having occult stage III disease.[19, 215, 257] In the study by Young et al.,[257] the stage was increased in 18% of patients with presumed stage I disease and in 44% of those with presumed stage II disease. The distribution of positive findings in studies of staging laparotomy in patients with apparent early ovarian cancer (Table 4) emphasizes the need to assess both the peritoneal cavity and retroperitoneal lymph nodes meticulously in patients with apparent early stage disease. In our experience, the majority of the patients were upstaged on the basis of biopsies that reveal histological evidence of clinically occult disease rather then obvious metastatic disease that had been overlooked at the primary surgery.[215]

A significant proportion of patients with LMP epithelial lesions also have their stage of disease increased through comprehensive staging laparotomy. Recent studies have suggested that between 12.5–29% of patients with apparent early stage LMP epithelial lesions are upstaged on the basis of histopathological findings.[120, 138, 178, 208] It should be emphasized that the identification of occcult metastatic involvement by LMP lesions

may not indicate a worsened prognosis or aid in the selection of therapy for individual patients. However, a diagnosis of epithelial LMP by frozen section is unreliable. Up to 30% of lesions thought to be LMP lesions are found to be invasive epithelial ovarian carcinomas when the entire ovarian specimen is histologically analyzed.[178] In this situation, the surgeon should always presume that the patient may have an invasive epithelial lesion and perform a comprehensive staging laparotomy if a frozen section diagnosis of an epithelial LMP lesion is obtained.

The components of a comprehensive staging laparotomy for women with apparent early ovarian carcinoma are detailed in Table 5. Less than 25% of patients referred for management of early disease have an incision that is adequate for evaluation of the upper abdomen and diaphragms.[215, 258] In most cases, adequate incision consists of a generous midline incision extending above the umbilicus. In the event that a patient with an unanticipated ovarian carcinoma is diagnosed at the time of exploration through a Pfannenstiel incision, the inferior epigastric vessels can be sacrificed and the incision con-

Table 5 Comprehensive staging laparotomy for early epithelial ovarian carcinoma

Midline abdominal incision

Peritoneal washings for cytology[a]
  Ascites
  Pelvis
  Bilateral pericolic gutters
  Diaphragm

Total abdominal hysterectomy/bilateral salpingo-oophorectomy[b]

Omentectomy

Meticulous peritoneal exploration
  Biopsies of adhesions/suspicious lesions
  Random biopsies of normal peritoneum in pelvis and upper abdomen

Diaphragm biopsies or scraping for cytology

Bilateral selective pelvic and para-aortic lymphadenectomy

[a] May pool specimens and submit together for cytopathology.
[b] May retain uterus and/or contralateral ovary in highly selected patients who desire to retain child-bearing capacity.

verted into a Maylard incision. This usually allows adequate exposure to complete a comprehensive staging laparotomy. Alternatively, a second midline incision can be made to allow visualization of the upper abdominal contents. A complete and thorough peritoneal exploration should be performed initially, with biopsy of any suspicious peritoneal lesions.

Ascites or peritoneal washings should be obtained from the pelvis, gutters, and diaphragms, and submitted for cytology. The critical factor is whether the peritoneal washings have malignant cytology, rather than the relative distribution of positive cytology. Therefore, the washings can be pooled and submitted as a single specimen to spare expense. Ascites associated with early ovarian carcinoma have malignant cytology in less than 50% of cases.[19] In contrast, specimens from more than 20% of patients with no clinical evidence of ascites will have malignant cytology.[19, 169, 213, 257] Specimens for cytology should therefore be obtained in all patients with apparent early ovarian cancer.

In most patients with early epithelial ovarian carcinoma, stromal tumors, and tubal carcinomas, bilateral salpingo-oophorectomy and hysterectomy should be performed, along with complete removal of all pelvic disease. The infundibulopelvic ligament(s) and broad ligament(s) should be resected widely on the affected side(s) to ensure complete removal of ovarian tissue. Patients of reproductive age with epithelial lesions of low malignant potential, well-differentiated apparent stage IA epithelial carcinomas, unilateral stromal tumors, and virtually all patients with germ cell tumors can be conservatively managed with unilateral salpingo-oophorectomy, as will be discussed subsequently.

A complete peritoneal exploration should be performed with manual and visual inspection of the diaphragms, bowel serosa and mesentery, pericolic gutters, and pelvis. Biopsies should be taken from any suspicious lesions or adhesions. A sample of the diaphragm should be taken for cytology and/or multiple biopsies should be submitted for histology even if it appears normal. In addition, random biopies are obtained from normal-appearing pelvic side walls, bladder serosa, cul-de-sac, pericolic gutters, anterior parietal peritoneum, bowel serosa, and mesentery (Table 5). Multiple specimens from single anatomic sites are pooled and submitted as single specimens for histopathology. These random biopsies detect occult peritoneal metastases in approximately 5–10% of patients at each site.[19, 169, 215, 257]

Partial omentectomy should remove at least the majority of the infracolic omentum. Our practice is to divide the omentum into ten pieces, which are submitted as a single specimen to the pathology department. Because the gross assessment of the omentum has poor sensitivity for detecting small metastases,[19] this potentially increases the yield for detection of occult metastases. We have had anecdotal cases in which only one of ten omental specimens had microscopic foci of disease.

Bilateral selective pelvic and para-aortic lymphadenectomy should be performed if there is no gross evidence of extrapelvic metastases. Selective pelvic lympadenectomy consists of removing the entire lymphatic fat pad from the anterior and medial surfaces of the external iliac vessels, the hypogastric artery, and all nodes from the obturator fossa. Lymphatic tissue lateral to or between the external iliac vessels is not removed unless suspicious nodes are encountered. The lymph nodes anterior and lateral to the common iliac arteries and aorta are removed to the level of the renal vessels, exposing the vena cava on the right side and extending above the level of the inferior mesenteric artery on the left side. The insertion of the right and left ovarian veins into the vena cava and left renal vein, respectively, should be identified. Between 5–20% of patients with apparent stage I or II ovarian epithelial carcinoma have metastases to the retroperitoneal nodes.[19, 169, 215, 257] The sensitivity of clinical assessment for nodal metastases of ovarian carcinoma is less than 50%,[215] therefore, biopsy of only suspicious nodes is not an adequate substitution for selective pelvic and para-aortic lympadenectomy.

Laparoscopic staging of early ovarian carcinoma is currently not the standard of care. Although cases have been reported of patients who have undergone primary laparoscopic management[177] or laparoscopic restaging that included pelvic and para-aortic lymph node sampling,[37] laparoscopic staging of early ovarian carcinoma should be considered an investigational procedure until it has been critically evaluated and compared to the standard open procedure. The loss of tactile appreciation for small metastases and the compromised ability to completely run

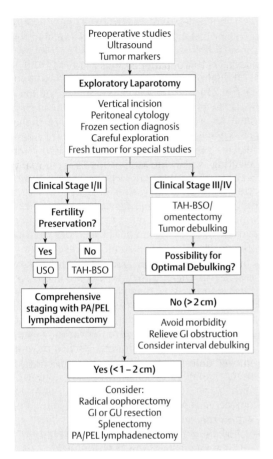

Fig. 1 Primary Surgery for Ovarian Malignancies

TAH-BSO = total abdominal hysterectomy with bilateral salpingo-oophorectomy; USO = unilateral salpingo-oophorectomy; PEL = pelvic; PA = para-aortic; GI = gastrointestinal; GU = genitourinary

ensure that women with suspected ovarian carcinoma are explored in a setting in which a comprehensive staging laparotomy can be performed at the time of the initial surgery. The general surgical management of the patient with ovarian malignancies is summarized in Figure **1**.

Conservative Surgery for Early Disease

Epithelial lesions of LMP and early ovarian invasive carcinomas occasionally develop in women of reproductive age who desire preservation of reproductive function. Malignant germ cell tumors frequently involve girls and nulliparous young women. Stromal tumors are infrequently encountered in this age group, but occasionally patients with granulosa and Sertoli-Leydig cell tumors will be of reproductive age. In women who wish to preserve childbearing potential, conservative surgery is acceptable under certain conditions (Table **6**). If an unsuspected apparent stage I A lesion is encountered in a young woman whose wishes are not known, it is advisable to

Table **6**   Criteria for conservative surgery in ovarian carcinoma

Reproductive age

Patient wishes to conserve reproductive capacity
(or is undecided)

Unilateral salpingo-oophorectomy
Comprehensive staging laparotomy
Normal contralateral ovary[a]

Epithelial carcinomas
    Low malignant potential—stage I
                              stage II (no residual)
    Invasive carcinoma—stage I A, grade 1–2

Germ cell tumors—all stages[b]

Stromal cell tumors—stage I A[c]

Close follow-up mandatory

Removal of contralateral ovary in epithelial carcinomas when child-bearing complete

---

[a] May retain noninvolved uterus for future in-vitro fertilization with donor oocytes if both ovaries involved.
[b] Karyotype if fertility not proven; may retain ovary with small superficial metastases.
[c] Endometrial biopsy if granulosa cell tumor.

the bowel in an efficient manner may outweigh the advantages of superior visibility of the diaphragm and reduced convalescence provided by the laparoscopic approach.

The importance of a comprehensive staging laparotomy in the initial management of early epithelial ovarian carcinoma cannot be overemphasized. If a patient has not been adequately evaluated at the primary surgical procedure, there is a substantial risk of occult advanced-stage disease. Should the patient undergo a potentially morbid restaging procedure or receive potentially toxic therapy for presumed advanced disease? It is the responsibility of the physician to perform only conservative surgery combined with comprehensive staging laparotomy at the initial procedure. After all pathology reports have returned, a careful discussion should be held with the patient so that a true informed consent can be obtained prior to definitive management. In young and healthy patients, a second operation can be performed safely at a later date, to complete total abdominal salpingo-oophorectomy. These organs, however, can never be replaced.

Several studies have documented compromised survival among patients treated with unilateral salpingo-oophorectomy for apparent stage I invasive epithelial ovarian carcinoma. For example, Parker et al.[165] reported that survival in their women with stage I disease decreased from approximately 80% after total abdominal hysterectomy with bilateral salpingo-oophorectomy to less than 50% after unilateral salpingo-oophorectomy. The majority of their patients, however, had staging procedures that would be considered suboptimal by contemporary standards. Williams and Dockerty[252] reported the status of contralateral ovaries in 65 women thought to have stage IA epithelial ovarian cancer. Among their patients, 31% had contralateral ovarian neoplasms and almost half of these were malignant. Of their 51 patients with grossly "normal" contralateral ovaries, 8% had contralateral malignancies ranging in size from 1–3 cm in diameter. Serous and endometrioid lesions had a 20% incidence of bilateral malignancy, compared to only 4% in mucinous lesions.

In contrast, Williams et al.[253] reviewed their experience with 29 patients thought to have stage I ovarian epithelial carcinoma who were treated with unilateral salpingo-oophorectomy only. Among 19 patients with grade 1 or 2 lesions who did not have features of rupture, excrescences, or adherence, only one developed a contralateral „recurrence" more than 10 years after primary surgery. There were at least 12 pregnancies in seven of these patients. They reported six recurrences and five deaths in ten women whose lesions had ruptured, capsular excresences, or adherence. Others have reported similar favorable survival among women who have stage IA well-differentiated ovarian carcinoma treated with unilateral salpingo-oophorectomy or with total abdominal hysterectomy and bilateral salpingo-oophorectomy and surgical staging alone.[68, 238, 258]

The development of effective chemotherapy for epithelial ovarian carcinoma has created the possibility of using conservative surgery followed by cisplatin chemotherapy for young women with higher risk epithelial ovarian carcinoma confined to one ovary, who have stage IA, grade 2 or 3 lesions or stage IC disease. In a small series reported by Colombo et al.,[37] 38 (50%) of 76 patients younger than age 40 with invasive epithelial ovarian carcinomas were treated with unilateral salpingo-oophorectomy. Nineteen (87%) of 22 patients with epithelial carcinomas attempting pregnancy after chemotherapy and unilateral salpingo-oophorectomy were able to conceive, resulting in one spontaneous abortion and 24 liveborn children. The authors did not provide any information about clinical characteristics, survival, or chemotherapeutic regimens used in their patients. Another potential fertility-sparing option in women with stage IB (bilateral ovarian involvement) disease includes retention of the uterus, treatment with chemotherapy, and impregnation using in vitro fertilization with donor oocytes. Until additional studies provide survival data and fertility results, conservative surgery followed by chemotherapy in high-risk epithelial ovarian carcinoma should only be considered in patients who have undergone comprehensive surgial staging and have been informed of the risks and benefits of this approach. A second look laparotomy is recommended after completion of chemotherapy in women with high-risk stage I/II ovarian carcinoma who have been managed with conservative surgery followed by chemotherapy.

Many authors have reported favorable outcomes for selected patients with apparent stage IA LMP epithelial lesions who have had only the affected ovary removed. Recurrence rates after unilateral salpingo-oophorectomy (averaging approximately 5%) have been reported in several series,[15, 29, 72, 103] with rare deaths caused by disease.

Furthermore, favorable outcome after cystectomy was observed in women with stage I serous LMP lesions reported by Lim-Tan et al.[123] In their series of 35 women who were initially managed with cystectomy, tumor persisted or recurred in only two ovaries and recurred in the contralateral ovary or in both retained ovaries in one patient each, for a total failure rate of 12%. Positive surgical margins or multifocal disease requiring multiple cystectomies were always associated with persistence or recurrence. Overall survival was 100% with a median follow-up of 6.5 years after initial surgery. Out of sixteen patients treated conservatively, eight had subsequent pregnancies. However, 19 of their patients underwent additional surgery after cystectomy, which suggests that the excellent outcome does not reflect the effect of ovarian cystectomy alone. Furthermore, Chambers and associates[29] reported recurrences after cystectomy in a patient with an LMP lesion who eventually developed an invasive serous carcinoma. Therefore, cystectomy should be reserved only for the unusual women with a LMP lesion who has had prior oophorectomy, in an attempt to preserve the possibility of childbearing. Despite the favorable results when retention of childbearing potential is desired, complete removal of the reproductive organs must be considered standard therapy for women with stage I LMP lesions and epithelial carcinomas who have completed childbearing.

Germ cell tumors of the ovary usually develop in girls or young women of childbearing age. Although dysgerminomas have approximately a 10% incidence of bilaterality, other histological types of germ cell malignancies are almost always unilateral, with rare surface metastases to the contralateral ovary. The preferred management in these patients is usually removal of the affected ovary, which does not compromise survival for patients with stage I germ cell malignancies.[40] Because of the high cure rate of chemotherapy, the contralateral ovary can be retained even in women with advanced germ cell malignancies.

Young girls with germ cell tumors associated with gonadoblastoma, and those who have not established menstrual or reproductive function, should be tested with peripheral lymphocyte karyotype to exclude 46, XY gonadal dysgenesis. In individuals with this karyotype, the contralateral gonad should be removed after puberty because of a high risk for developing a second malignant tumor in the contralateral gonad.[218] Even if both gonads have been removed, the uterus can be retained so that the patient can have the option for in vitro fertilization with donor oocytes and pregnancy in the future.

Unilateral salpingo-oophorectomy is also appropriate management for apparent stage I A granulosa cell tumors occurring in young women because these lesions are bilateral in only approximately 2% of patients.[10] If the uterus is retained, a dilatation and curettage should be performed to exclude the frequent coexistent endometrial adenocarcinoma or hyperplasa.[52, 54] Because malignant behavior of other stromal tumors is unusual, young women with unilateral, smooth, and encapsulated stromal tumors who have no evidence of distant metastasis can also be treated with conservative surgery.

Because these young patients undergo one or more major operative procedures, pelvic adhesions comprise a major potential cause of future infertility. The routine practice of performing a wedge biopsy of normal-appearing ovary is discouraged because of the low yield for this procedure, particularly in patients with germ cell malignancies, and risk of significant adhesive disease.[22, 98] The surgeon should use a meticulous surgical technique and avoid manipulation of the contralateral ovary unless there is clinical evidence of involvement with tumor.

The long-term effects of chemotherapy on ovarian function are poorly understood. Temporary loss of ovulation and amenorrhea are common after combination chemotherapy but permanent ovarian dysfunction or ovarian failure is uncommon.[23] Longer duration or greater cumulative doses of chemotherapy,[32, 221] alkylating agents,[245] and older age [157, 245] have an unfavorable impact on ovarian function after chemotherapy. Gershenson et al.[60] reported that 27 (68%) of 40 patients who retained a normal contralateral ovary and uterus, and who were successfully treated for germ cell malignancies of the ovary with combination chemotherapy, resumed menstruation. Twelve (75%) of their 16 patients who attempted pregnancy had 22 normal infants and one elective abortion after chemotherapy.[60] Others have reported sucessful pregnancies after multiagent chemotherapy for ovarian germ cell malignancies.[190] In treating patients who have undergone conservative surgery for early epithelial ovarian carcinoma, chemotherapy with single agent cisplatin is recommended to avoid exposure to an alkylator.

There are no good data to support the preservation of ovarian function through ovulation suppression (by administration of oral contraceptive or gonadotropin-releasing hormone analogues, e.g., Lupron). However, most patients of reproductive age require effective contraception, and oral contraceptives prevent symptoms from transient ovarian failure produced by chemotherapy.

Primary Surgery for Advanced Disease

The importance of comprehensive surgical staging laparotomy to detect occult advanced disease in patients with apparent early epithelial ovarian carcinoma has been previously emphasized. At the time of surgical exploration, however, epithelial ovarian carcinoma is often found to be widely metastatic throughout the abdominal peritoneal cavity. Under these circumstances, assignment of surgical stage is relatively straightforward. Patients with small upper abdominal metastases, <2 cm in diameter (stage III B), should undergo selective pelvic and para-aortic lymphadenectomy to exclude stage III C disease. Likewise, we usually perform lymphadenectomy in patients who have all gross evidence of metastatic disease resected because the majority of these patients will have no clinical evidence of disease upon completion of primary chemotherapy. Under these circumstances, lymph node sampling does not have to be performed at second-look laparotomy if lymph nodes were negative at primary surgery.

In patients with disseminated intra-abdominal tumors, the surgeon is not required to conduct a meticulous search for occult disease but rather is faced with management decisions regarding the optimal initial surgical procedures for the individual patient. In contrast to patients with peritoneal carcinomatosis from other solid tumors, such as colonic or pancreatic carcinomas, where lack of effective chemotherapy results in futility of surgical debulking, studies over the past 20 years have tended to support the concept of primary surgical debulking for patients with epithelial ovarian carcinoma.[35] The first steps, therefore, in the exploration of a patient with carcinomatosis from a presumed ovarian primary should focus on assessing the potential for optimal or complete surgical debulking and should be used to exclude the possibility of a gastrointestinal or pancreatic primary site of malignancy (Fig. **1**).

Primary Cytoreductive Surgery—Rationale

There are several hypothetical reasons to consider surgical debulking of chemotherapy-sensitive neoplasms.[83] Because the majority of chemotherapeutic agents produce cell kill using first-order kinetics, or elimination of a fixed and usually logarithmic proportion of surviving tumor cells with each cycle of chemotherapy[62], surgical reduction of tumor volume by a factor of several logs may reduce the number of cycles of chemotherapy required to produce a clinically or pathologically complete remission. The initial proliferation of cancer cells is exponential but eventually slows as the individual tumors outgrow blood supply and enter the plateau phase of the Gompertzian growth curve. Cells in the central portion of larger tumors tend to be in the nonproliferating phase of the growth cycle. Removal of these resting cells results in a larger proportion of actively proliferating cells comprising the total population of malignant cells, thus potentially increasing the likelihood of response to chemotherapy. Furthermore, resection of bulky masses often removes poorly vascularized tumors that have a compromised blood supply. These tumors result in impaired delivery of chemotherapeutic agents in effective concentrations to the central tumor. Removal of "older" implants of tumor might also remove clones of cells that have had a chance to develop spontaneous drug resistance.[62] Finally, removal of bulky peritoneal implants might palliate patients during early chemotherapy by allowing normalization of bowel function and nutritional uptake.

The concept of primary surgical debulking of advanced epithelial ovarian carcinoma was initially established in the 1960s, when Munnell[152] introduced the term "maximum surgical effort" and reported improved survival in patients who had a "complete operation" before treatment with radiotherapy. Griffiths[67] subsequently reported that the survival of patients with stage II and III ovarian carcinoma treated with postoperative alkylating agents significantly correlated with the amount of postoperative residual tumor, even when controlling for the size of initial extrapelvic disease.

Retrospective studies conducted over the last decade have confirmed the favorable prognostic effect of small disease residuum in women with advanced disease treated with platin-containing regimens (Table **7**). In all studies, patients who were "optimally" debulked at primary surgery had a higher incidence of complete response and negative second-look laparotomies, an improved progression-free survival, and improved overall survival compared to patients with bulky residual disease. The definition of "optimal" debulking varies among different series of patients. The

Table **7** Effect of optimal primary cytoreduction on survival in patients with advanced epithelial ovarian cancer

Author, year	Median survival (months)	
	Optimal[a]	Suboptimal
Hacker, 1983	18	6
Vogl, 1983	40	16
Delgado, 1984	45	16
Pohl, 1984	45	16
Conte, 1985	25	14
Posada, 1985	30	18
Sutton, 1986	45	23
Louie, 1986	24	15
Redman, 1986	37	26
Neijt, 1987	40	21
Hainsworth, 1988	72	13
Piver, 1988	48	21
Mean	39	17

[a] Definition of "optimal" varied among these series.

amount of residual disease is probably a continuous, rather than discrete, prognostic factor with completely debulked patients having the best chance for survival. Most contemporary investigators agree that optimal tumor debulking results in the removal of all tumors > 1 cm in diameter. Using this definition, optimal surgical debulking can be accomplished in approximately 35 – 60 % of patients with advanced disease.

In addition to the maximum size of residual tumor, the distribution and number of residual lesions also have an effect on survival after primary surgery. For example, Hoskins and colleagues[81] analyzed the prognostic effect of these factors in patients with ovarian carcinoma who were initially optimally debulked and entered into a Gynecologic Oncology Group chemotherapy trial. In this study, patients with >20 residual lesions and those who required extensive debulking to achieve and optimal residual status with tumor deposits < 1 cm had inferior survival compared to those who had a limited amount of residual lesions or limited upper abdominal disease before tumor debulking. These data suggest that tumor biology, in addition to the amount of residual tumor burden, has an impact on the survival of patients with advanced ovarian carcinoma.

Despite the evidence cited above that supports the concept of primary debulking in advanced epithelial ovarian carcinoma, a randomized trial that formally tests the hypothesis that debulking improves survival has never been completed. The Gynecologic Oncology Group, in fact, attempted such a study in the late 1980s, but closed the protocol because of poor patient accrual. A recent meta-analysis was conducted of reported series of patients with advanced epithelial ovarian cancer who were treated with surgery followed by chemotherapy.[88] Optimal surgical debulking had a minimal effect on outcome in univariate analysis, but lost significance in multivariate modelling. Both univariate and multivariate analysis suggested that the use of platin-based regimens significantly improved the outcome of patients with advanced ovarian cancer, compared to nonplatin regimens. It is clear from studies conducted by the Gynecologic Oncologic Group that extensive debulking procedures that leave patients with tumors > 2 cm in diameter do not improve survival.[82] In these patients, the effect of primary surgery on survival is questionable. Despite the lack of conclusive studies supporting primary cytoreductive surgery, however, most gynecologic oncologists support the concept.

Primary Cytoreductive Surgery— Strategy and Techniques

Cytoreductive surgery in patients with advanced ovarian carcinoma provides a challenge even for the experienced surgeon. Carcinomatosis can completely distort the anatomy of the pelvis, making recognition of individual pelvic structures difficult. Upper abdominal disease may involve multiple structures, such as omentum, small and large bowel, stomach, and spleen. Although less common, bulky lymph node metastases can also be encountered. Therefore, it is imperative that the surgeon approaching debulking surgery in patients with ovarian carcinoma has both pelvic and abdominal surgical skills to perform surgery in all sites potentially affected by disease.[35]

A generous vertical incision is usually employed to facilitate exposure of both upper abdomen and pelvis (Fig. **1**). Buchwalter or Wechsler retractors, which feature adjustable-pitch retractors on a steel ring, are extremely helpful for optimizing exposure, particularly in obese patients. Ascites or peritoneal washings should be collected for cytopathology upon entering the abdomen. Frozen sections should be liberally obtained if the diagnosis of ovarian malignancy is in doubt. Before performing extensive and potentially morbid pelvic procedures in a patient with peritoneal carcinomatosis, the surgeon should examine the upper abdomen to determine whether complete or optimal debulking appears feasible. It is also desirable to rule out a pancreatic or bowel primary malignancy before subjecting the patient to an extensive surgical cytoreductive procedure. If the pancreas cannot be palpated, the lesser sac should be entered so that the pancreas can be palpated directly. This can be accomplished either by dissecting through the omentocolic ligament and entering the lesser sac above the transverse colon, or by dividing the short gastric vessels along the greater curvature and entering the space behind the stomach.

A total abdominal hysterectomy with bilateral salpingo-oophorectomy and omentectomy should be performed in the majority of patients with advanced disease, even if bulky residual disease remains. The primary site of disease can be confirmed and the most frequent site of bulky metastatic disease removed, usually with minimal morbidity. A supracervical hysterectomy may be used to limit potential morbidity, but complete hysterectomy is preferred and can be performed in the majority of cases.

Because ovarian carcinoma usually involves the pelvic peritoneum, yet leaves the retroperitoneum relatively free, even impressive pelvic masses can be resected in toto via a "radical oophorectomy" using a lateral retroperitoneal approach above the level of the pelvic brim.[87] The infundibulopelvic ligaments can thus be isolated and divided, protecting the ureters under direct visualization. Development of the retroperitoneal pararectal and paravesicle spaces allows mobilization of the ureters and division of the mid-hypogastric or proximal uterine artery similar to a radical hysterectomy, effectively mobilizing the central pelvic complex of tumor, ovaries, uterus, and sigmoid colon. Essentially the entire pelvic peritoneum, including the anterior cul-de-sac, can be stripped off and resected along with the central pelvic tumor.

Development of the presacral space allows anterior mobilization of tumors that involve the sigmoid colon. The technique of reverse hysterectomy, which uses entry into the anterior vagina and transvaginal development of the rectovaginal space, can aid in resections of tumors that obliterate the posterior cul-de-sac. After lateral mobilization of the ureters, transection of the vaginal cuff, and development of the rectovaginal space, tumors that are adherent to the sigmoid colon can be resected en bloc with a segmental rectosigmoid resection.[4] The use of surgical staplers has facilitated performance of low rectosigmoid reanastomosis in patients with pelvic malignancies, allowing the majority of these patients to avoid colostomy.[4, 8, 211]

Other bowel resections are performed in approximately 15–30% of patients undergoing primary surgical cytoreduction for advanced epithelial ovarian carcinoma.[35] These are performed to relieve partial bowel obstructions in some patients, even though optimal disease residual status is not always achieved with these procedures. Other resections, such as partial gastrectomy, splenectomy, partial resection of the diaphragm, or lymph node resections are often incorporated into the cytoreductive procedure if performance will result in no gross disease or only minimal residual tumor burden. There are uncontrolled, retrospective data suggesting that lymphadenectomy prolongs survival in patients with stage III disease,[20] but verification of this observation requires independent confirmation from a prospective trial, which is currently being conducted internationally.[199] The use of the cavitron ultrasonic surgical aspirator[47] and argon beam laser[18] can aid in the resection of tumor deposits, particularly from flat surfaces such as the diaphragm.

It is not clear whether patients with LMP epithelial lesions of the ovary benefit from radical surgery or any adjunctive therapy.[224] Although advanced-stage disease is less common in patients with LMP epithelial lesions than in patients with invasive epithelial carcinomas, approximately 20% of patients with LMP lesions have had spread beyond the ovary.[224] In collected series of women with LMP lesions, surgical debulking by itself provides long-term survival in approximately 76% of patients with stage II or III LMP lesions.[224] In addition to providing palliation and long-term survival through removal of gross tumor, complete surgical debulking can usually be performed in these women. Furthermore, extensive sampling of metastatic deposits should be performed in patients with metastatic LMP lesions to exclude the rare patient with a primary

LMP lesion in the ovary, which is associated with metastases that have an invasive histology (Fig. 1).

Patients with pseudomyxoma peritonei also do not appear to benefit from any form of adjuvant therapy; therefore aggressive surgical removal of mucoid peritoneal deposits is the mainstay of initial management for these patients. Peritoneal lavage with copious amounts of D5W is usually performed in an effort to lyse tumor cells, but the effect of this is unproven.

The role of primary surgical debulking is less clearly defined for advanced germ cell or stromal tumors of the ovary and tubal cancers. Because germ cell malignancies are extremely chemosensitive, primary debulking of these tumors is attractive. Patients with malignant germ cell tumors that are completely debulked will rarely have residual disease at second-look laparotomy after platin-based combination chemotherapy. Granulosa cell tumors often have an indolent growth pattern; therefore, primary debulking might improve disease-free survival even if chemotherapy is not effective. Tubal carcinomas behave similarly to ovarian epithelial carcinomas, responding to similar chemotherapeutic regimens. Most gynecologic oncologists will therefore perform aggressive primary cytoreductive procedures on patients with non-epithelial ovarian and epithelial tubal malignancies. Because of the tendency for germ cell and stromal malignancies to metastasize to the retroperitoneal lymph nodes, a careful pelvic and para-aortic lymph node dissection is recommended in all cases that have minimal intraperitoneal residual disease after surgical debulking.

Complications of Primary Cytoreductive Surgery

Most studies have reported that the morbidity and mortality of aggressive primary debulking procedures are acceptable.[35, 83] In one of the largest series of 472 procedures, the most frequent complications were blood loss (> 1000 mL) and urinary tract infection, occurring in 21% and 18% of patients, respectively.[35] Major morbidity occurs in approximately 5% of patients, with operative mortality in 1–3% of patients.[35] Large and/or small intestinal resections do not significantly increase the morbidity of primary debulking procedures.[9, 35] The effect of major cytoreductive surgery upon the interval between surgery and instituion of adjuvant therapy has been less well studied. In patients in whom prolonged ileus is anticipated (because of carcinomatosis or after bowel resection), it may be sensible to start total parenteral nutrition immediately after surgery, so that chemotherapy can be begun promptly.

An important issue that needs further prospective study is the impact of aggressive debulking procedures and residual disease upon patient quality of life. Blythe and Wahl[12] used very crude measures to compare quality of life in 19 patients with advanced epithelial ovarian cancer who had undergone cytoreduction to 17 who had minimal initial surgical procedures. Their patients received alkylator chemotherapy postoperatively. They studied acceptance of colostomy, performance of normal activity, consumption of a regular diet, and "enjoyment of life." The debulked patients fared better than the nondebulked patients in all areas, with 78.9% of those debulked reporting that they "enjoyed life" in contrast to only 46% of those who underwent minimal surgery. The need for more sophisticated studies in this area is obvious.

Alternative Approaches—Neoadjuvant Chemotherapy Preceding Debulking

Because a significant proportion of patients with advanced epithelial ovarian carcinoma undergo primary exploration by general obstetrician–gynecologists or general surgeons and often have minimal attempts at cytoreductive surgery ("peek and shriek"), strategy of neoadjuvant chemotherapy for 2–4 cycles, followed by a second attempt at surgical cytoreduction and further chemotherapy has been considered. Ideally, the neoadjuvant chemotherapy would improve the status of disease enough to allow optimal interval debulking and improve survival. Lawton and associates[119] reported that 75% of patients with initial suboptimal disease status after primary surgery could be optimally debulked during an interval cytoreductive procedure after receiving neoadjuvant chemotherapy. In their experience, there was decreased morbidity and decreased incidence of bowel surgery in comparison to the literature for primary cytoreductive procedures. However, the impact on survival was not analyzed.

Preliminary results of a randomized trial in 421 patients designed to assess the survival benefit of interval debulking after neoadjuvant chemotherapy were reported by van der Burg et al.[243] In their study, patients with advanced stage III epithelial ovarian carcinoma who had stable disease or were responding to three cycles of platin-based combination chemotherapy were randomized to receive either further chemotherapy or interval debulking followed by further chemotherapy. Three hundred seventeen patients were randomized. In 36% of the explored patients, lesions were < 1 cm in diameter at interval surgery and an additional 27% could be debulked to lesions < 1 cm in diameter. No unusual complications were encountered and no surgical mortality occurred. Follow-up on 278 patients indicates prolongation of progression-free and overall survival by 5 and 6 months, respectively, in the surgical arm (p = 0.001). Interval debulking was a significant prognostic factor for both progression-free and overall survival in multivariate analysis. The GOG is conducting a randomized trial (Protocol #152) of interval debulking in patients who have had an inital attempt at debulking but are left with bulky residual disease. Patients who have not progressed after three cycles of chemotherapy are randomized to interval debulking versus no interval debulking.

Neoadjuvant chemotherapy followed by interval debulking may be a logical approach to patients who have significant comorbid illnesses, very poor functional status, or those who had a minimal attempt at primary surgical cytoreduction. Results, however, are too preliminary to consider this approach the standard of care for patients with advanced epithelial ovarian carcinoma.

Postsurgical Therapy for Primary Disease

Adjuvant Therapy for Early Epithelial Ovarian Carcinoma

The decision to use adjuvant therapy in patients with stage I or II epithelial ovarian carcinoma is individualized and based on the extent of initial staging laparotomy, clinicopathological prognostic factors, medical condition or functional status of the patient, and, in a few patients, the desire to retain reproductive capacity. Many adjuvant therapeutic modalities have been used in patients with early disease, but most studies in women with stage I and II epithelial ovarian carcinoma have included inadequately staged patients and have not been randomized trials of therapy. Although long-term survival rates lower than 70% are often cited, patients who have had comprehensive staging laparotomy (used to define early stage disease) have survival ranging between 80% and 95%.[258] It should be emphasized that even though patients with high-risk early disease have a recurrence rate that is high enough to justify adjuvant therapy, no form of treatment has been proven superior to observation in any subset of these patients.

Conventional clinicopathological factors can be used to define low-risk and high-risk subsets of patients with early epithelial ovarian carcinoma.[216] Although there is clearly a difference in survival between patients with stage I and those with stage II disease, the influence of tumor substage is much less apparent and is not of statistical significance in several studies of patients with early disease.[46, 197, 226, 247, 258]

The status of the tumor capsule has been considered to reflect the prognosis of early epithelial ovarian cancer. Conventional wisdom would suggest a worse prognosis for a lesion that has breached the tumor capsule, thereby producing surface excrescences, adherence to adjacent structures, or tumor rupture. However, these factors may reflect other poor prognostic factors, and may not impart a worsened prognosis by themselves. In the large series of patients reported by Dembo et al.,[46] only tumor adherence was related to a poor prognosis in multivariate analysis. Capsular rupture and surface excrescences were of borderline prognostic significance for stage I, grade 1 lesions in univariate analysis, but lost significance in multivariate analysis.

Webb et al.[247] reported decreased survival in women with stage I ovarian cancer who had excrescences, rupture, or capsular adherence compared to patients with intact intracystic tumors, but did not analyze the effect of other prognostic factors. Purola and Nieminen[175] noted that patients with stage I disease and tumors that had been removed intact had survival of 83%, compared to survivals of 89% and 60%, respectively, for patients whose tumors were deliberately drained to facilitate removal and those whose tumors ruptured accidentally. However, they did not control for the effects of other prognostic factors.[175] More recent studies using multi-variate analysis of prognostic factors have not been able to detect independent prognostic effects for any of these factors related to the tumor capsule.[197, 226, 258]

Older studies suggested a worsened survival for patients with stage I and II ovarian cancer who presented with ascites. In the large study reported by Dembo and associates,[46] the prescence of ascites was an independent risk factor in multivariate analysis. Unfortuantely, the majority of patients in their study did not have cytological assessment of peritoneal washings. Although peritoneal cytology has a poor sensitivity for detecting histologically confirmed peritoneal metastases,[19] the identification of malignant cells in peritoneal washings is highly suggestive of occult peritoneal spread, particularly in patients who have not undergone comprehensive staging laparotomy.

Many studies have confirmed a strong prognostic effect of histological grade for patients with early epithelial ovarian carcinoma. The recent studies by Young et al.[258] and Rubin et al.[185] suggested that clear cell histology was associated with a poor prognosis, but other investigators have not observed an effect from any single histological subtype.[46, 197, 226] In contrast, the effect of differentiation on survival is striking. In series of patients with stage I disease, survival ranges from almost 100% for LMP lesions and 85–95% for grade 1 lesions, to 35–63% for grade 3 lesions.[46, 185, 197, 224, 258]

Conventional clinicopathologial factors useful for predicting prognosis in early stage disease include: stage (I versus II), histological grade, ascites or malignant peritoneal cytology, adherence to adjacent structures, and, possibly, clear cell histology. The Gynecologic Oncology Group/Ovarian Cancer Study Group has arbitrarily defined low-risk patients as those having stage I A or I B lesions with grade 1 or 2 histological differentiation.[258] Patients with grade 3 lesions and those stage I C or II disease are considered at high risk. Others have defined low-risk disease as consisting of only early stage grade 1 lesions.[238] Classification of patients using these relatively crude systems, however, does aid in the decision-making process for the consideration of adjuvant therapy for individual patients.

Observation

Several series of patients have attempted to define low-risk subsets of patients that have such a low recurrence after primary surgery, that adjunctive therapy is not indicated. Recent prospective trials, including the observation arms from three randomized trials, are presented in Table **8**. In all studies, except for the one reported by Dembo et al.,[44] "complete" surgery (consisting of total abdominal hysterectomy with bilateral salpingo-oophorectomy and omentectomy) was required for entry of patients into the study. Young et al.[258] required a comprehensive staging laparotomy for patient entry into their trial,

Table **8**   Observation after surgery for early epithelial ovarian carcinoma

Author, year	Stage(s)	Number	Surgery[a]	Survival (%)
Dembo, 1979	I A	20	Incomplete	87[b]
Hreschchyshyn, 1980	I A/I B	29	Complete	83[b]
Young, 1990	I A/B, G 1/2	38	Comprehensive	94[b]
Trimbos, 1991	I – II A, G 1	43	Complete	88
		24	Comprehensive	100
Monga, 1991	I A/B, G 1/2	40	Complete	98

[a] Extent of surgical staging.
[b] Observation arms in randomized trials.

while Trimbos et al.[238] separately analyzed a subset of patients who underwent comprehensive surgical staging.

According to these studies, women with stage I A/B, grade 1 lesions have favorable survival without adjunctive therapy. They warrant no additional treatment beyond surgery and comprehensive staging. Although stage I A/B, grade 2 lesions were included in the observation arm of the trial reported by Young and associates,[258] only five patients with grade 2 lesions were included in the observation arm, and the majority of patients studied by Monga et al.[147] had grade 1 lesions. Therefore, further study of patients with grade 2 lesions may be warranted. Furthermore, the excellent results reported by Trimbos and colleagues[238] suggest that some women with grade 1 lesions and stage I C disease with negative cytology or stage II A disease might have excellent survival without adjuvant therapy.

Early stage LMP lesions also have an excellent prognosis when treated with surgery alone, as discussed previously. It is important to perform a critical pathology review of all epithelial lesions that have a well-differentiated histology to differentiate between LMP lesions and truly invasive, but well-differentiated, carcinomas. A substantial proportion of patients entered into cooperative group studies of early invasive ovarian carcinoma have LMP lesions when pathology review is performed.[258] In addition to the lack of evidence that adjuvant chemotherapy or radiation therapy improves the outcome in patients with LMP lesions, there are many anecdotal reports of complications from therapy. For example, leukemia has resulted from alkylator chemotherapy that was given to women with LMP lesions. This should support the current recommendation not to treat these patients after appropriate surgery.

Radiation Therapy

Radiotherapy has been frequently used in the past as adjuvant therapy for patients with early ovarian carcinoma. Because there is no anatomic barrier between the pelvis and upper abdomen, there is little rationale for the use of pelvic radiation therapy. Randomized studies from both the Princess Margaret Hospital in Toronto[44] and the GOG[86] documented that there was no improvement in the survival of patients with relatively low-risk (stage I A/B) ovarian carcinoma who

were treated with whole-pelvic radiotherapy when compared to those in the no-treatment arms. Predictably, upper abdominal failures were common after pelvic radiation.

Whole-abdominal radiation therapy, initially using the moving strip technique, was shown to be superior to whole-pelvic radiation (with or without alkylator chemotherapy) in the study reported by Dembo et al.[44] Unfortunately, patients with incomplete surgical staging with gross residual disease were included in the study, and patients with disease in stages I–III were randomized without stratification for any risk factors.

Whole abdominopelvic radiation can be given safely to patients with ovarian cancer who have not received prior chemotherapy, with major bowel complications occurring in only approximately 5% of patients.[44, 102] Dembo and associates[45] demonstrated that the use of the open field technique improved the safety of abbominopelvic irradiation when compared to the moving strip technique. Although only a small proportion of patients receiving this therapy develop severe chronic bowel complications, complications in individual patients can be extremely difficult to treat with simple therapy due to the obliterative endarteritis and fibrostenosis induced by radiation of the bowel. Additionally, a significant proportion of bone marrow is included in the abdominopelvic radiation portals. This might compromise chemotherapy tolerance later, if the patient develops a recurrence of disease.

Furthermore, some treatment regimens reduce the dose delivered to the liver and kidneys, which might create relative sanctuaries for tumor implants. Another disadvantage of whole abdominopelvic radiation therapy results from the complexity required for treatment planning. It is important to secure treatment with adequate fields that include the diaphragms. Klassen and colleagues[102] reported a high proportion of failures in patients treated with adjuvant abdominopelvic radiotherapy for early ovarian cancer in a multi-institutional trial. The researchers often violated protocol in their simulation films. They failed to cover the specified whole abdominal field.

Dembo and colleagues[44] reported superior survival among their patients with high-risk stage I and stage II disease who received whole abdominopelvic radiation therapy compared to the group that received pelvic radiotherapy combined with an alkylator. Other randomized trials, however, have reported equivalent results in patients receiving abdominopelvic irradiation compared to chemotherapy.[102, 105, 207]

Intraperitoneal Radiotherapy

Intraperitoneal administration of various radiopharmaceutical agents has a long history of use as adjuvant therapy of epithelial ovarian carcinoma. Originally, radiogold was employed, but radioactive chromic phosphate (P-32) is currently the most frequently used agent. Because P-32 emits only beta particles and has a half-life of approximately 2 weeks, it can be used with much more convenience and safety than radiogold.[180] In comparison, radiogold emits both beta and gamma particles and has a half-life of approximately 3 days. Because beta particles have a relatively superficial depth of tissue penetration compared to gamma particles, patients do not experience significant marrow exposure or radiation enteritis with P-32, as they do with radiogold.[180]

On the basis of studies performed on phantoms and in dogs, intraperitoneal P-32 is adsorbed to peritoneal surfaces within 2–3 hours after administration. A therapeutic dose of radiation is delivered to the peritoneal surfaces and omentum, with minimal depth of penetration deeper than 3 mm into the tissue.[42] The dose to retroperitoneal pelvic and para-aortic lymph nodes is minimal, but P-32 is taken up by the lymphatics of the diaphragm and sequestered in the mediastinal lymph nodes.[42] Although a small amount of radioactivity is detectable in the circulation, distribution to the marrow is calculated to be minimal in humans.[180]

Instillation of P-32 is usually accomplished via an intraperitoneal catheter, put in place at the time of laparotomy.[211, 214] At least 500 mL of normal saline are instilled into the peritoneal cavity. Distribution is documented with 1 mCi 99 m technetium sulfur colloid as a tracer, and imaging is performed in anterior-posterior fields with a gamma scintillation camera. Alternatively, a peritoneogram (using water-soluble contrast medium) can be obtained. After diffuse intraperitoneal distribution is confirmed, a dose of 15 (±10%) mCi P-32 is premixed in an additional 500 mL normal saline and instilled into the peritoneal cavity. After instillation, the patient is changed repeatedly from Trendelenburg to reverse-Trendelenburg positions for 2–3 hours to enhance peritoneal distribution of the P-32. Premixing the P-32 and changing positions frequently immediately after instillation reduces the risk of focal adsorbtion of P-32 which might cause bowel damage due to a high local dose of radiation.[42, 211, 214]

Major toxicity from intraperitoneal P-32 is relatively rare. Bowel obstruction that requires surgical therapy is observed in < 5–6% of patients treated with P-32 alone.[102, 213, 214, 242, 258] An additional 6–14% develop moderately severe abdominal pain, which requires narcotic or nonsteroidal analgesics. The pain is presumably related to a low-grade chemical peritonitis.[102, 213, 214, 242, 258] The development of leukemia after P-32 treatment has only been reported in patients who also received alkylating agent chemotherapy.[180, 213] Pelvic radiotherapy should not be combined with intraperitoneal P-32. Klassen et al.[102] reported that five (11%) of 44 patients treated with this combination for early ovarian cancer developed either severe small bowel obstruction or fistulas that required surgical correction during short-term follow-up.

Although older, uncontrolled trials suggested that treatment with an intraperitoneal radiopharmaceutial agent resulted in improved survival of early ovarian carcinoma patients when compared to historical controls,[180] it should be emphasized that no randomized trial has demonstrated improved survival after adjuvant P-32 when compared to a no-treatment arm. Three randomized trials have, however, documented equivalent survival results in patients treated with P-32 compared to groups treated with a single alkylator,[258] whole abdominopelvic radiation therapy or a single alkylator combined with pelvic radiation therapy,[102] and single-agent cisplatin.[240] Based on the low toxicity and ease of administration of P-32 compared to melphalan,[258] this agent was chosen for a current GOG study (Protocol #95), which randomized patients with high-risk (stage I grade 3, stage IC or II) early ovarian cancer to P-32 versus three cycles of platin-cyclophosphamide combination chemotherapy.

In the study by Vergote et al.,[240] patients with stage I epithelial ovarian carcinoma had disease-free survival of 82% after P-32 treatment compared to 79% after cisplatin treatment. Despite equivalent survival, these authors concluded that cisplatin was the preferred treatment for early ovarian cancer, based on the 6% incidence of late bowel complications among the patients receiving P-32. Preliminary results reported from a randomized Italian cooperative group study have suggested an improved disease-free survival for patients with stage I C disease who received single-agent cisplatin compared to the group that received intraperitoneal P-32.[11] However, patients in their study who recurred after receiving P-32, often responded to chemotherapy, while those who recurred after cisplatin usually did not respond to additional therapy, resulting in no difference in the overall survival.

Chemotherapy

Ever since the demonstration of the activity of alkylating agents, and subsequently, platin compounds in the treatment of patients with advanced stage epithelial ovarian carcinoma, chemotherapy has been evaluated as adjuvant therapy in women with early stage disease. Early randomized studies by the MD Anderson Group[207] and the GOG[86] suggested that adjuvant chemotherapy with alkylating agents achieved results that were equivalent to whole abdominopelvic radiotherapy and superior to pelvic radiotherapy, respectively. In contrast, Dembo et al.[44] observed improved survival in the whole abdominopelvic radiation therapy arm compared to the pelvic radiation-chlorambucil arm of their randomized study. However, others have reported equivalent results in randomized trials of adjuvant abdominopelvic radiation compared to combined pelvic radiotherapy-alkylator.[102, 195] All of these studies suffered from the inclusion of incompletely staged patients. They often included patients of all stages from I–III, and used relatively primitive randomization techniques that sometimes resulted in imbalances of risk factors between the treatment arms.

The only randomized trials of adjuvant therapies in patients with early ovarian carcinoma (defined by comprehensive staging laparotomy) that have been reported in final form to date are the two-part GOG/Ovarian Cancer Study Group trials reported by Young et al.[258] Although these were limited by relatively small numbers of patients in some subgroups, they provided important information about adjuvant therapy of early ovarian carcinoma. In the first study (Protocol 7601), women with low-risk (stage I A/B, grade 1, 2) early stage disease were randomized to receive either no therapy or 12 months of melphalan.

There was no therapeutic benefit for therapy with the alkylator, and both groups had survival in excess of 90%. In the second trial (Protocol 7602), high-risk patients (stage I C or II, or stage I grade 3 lesions) were randomized to recieve 18 months of melphalan or intraperitoneal P-32, with nonsignificant differences in survival of 78% and 81%, respectively.[258] Because of these discouraging results and the potential risk of leukemia associated with alkylator chemotherapy,[66] single-agent alkylators are currently not recommended for patients with early ovarian cancer.

The study by Vergote and colleagues[241] randomized treatment between six courses of moderate dose (50 mg/m^2) single-agent cisplatin in one arm and compared this with 7–10 mCi of intraperitoneal P-32 in 340 patients with stage I–III disease with no gross residual disease after primary surgery. Patients with poor intraperitoneal distribution for P-32 received whole abdominopelvic radiation therapy. Patients were not staged completely and patients with LMP lesions comprised approximately 10% of each treatment arm. Overall survival was similar in both groups of patients, with disease-free survival in stage I patients of 82% and 79%, respectively, after P-32 and cisplatin. The preliminary results of two Italian intergroup randomized studies documented improved disease-free survival in women with low-risk stage I disease who received six cycles of single-agent cisplatin (50 mg/m^2) compared to no treatment, and in those with high-risk stage I disease who received cisplatin compared to P-32.[11] However, overall survival was equivalent in both trials because salvage chemotherapy was successful only in patients who had not received cisplatin.

Initial single-arm studies of patients with early ovarian carcinoma who received adjuvant platin-containing combinations purported to show excellent survival.[48, 170] However, these included incompletely staged patients and no control arms. In contrast, Rubin and associates[185] documented only a 73% disease-free survival in 62 comprehensively staged patients with high-risk stage I disease, who were treated with platin-based combination chemotherapy. Furthermore, Piver and colleagues[171] noted a disappointing disease-free survival in patients with stage II disease who received platin-combination adjuvant therapy.

Currently, the GOG is evaluating P-32 versus three cycles of cisplatin-cyclophosphamide in

Fig. **2** Integration of surgery and adjuvant therapy for early epithelial ovarian carcinoma

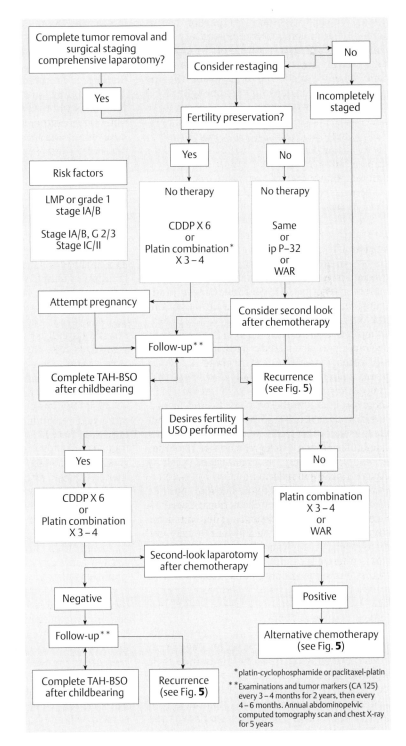

* platin-cyclophosphamide or paclitaxel-platin
** Examinations and tumor markers (CA 125) every 3–4 months for 2 years, then every 4–6 months. Annual abdominopelvic computed tomography scan and chest X-ray for 5 years

women with high-risk stage I/II epithelial ovarian carcinoma after comprehensive surgical staging (Protocol #95). The completion of the GOG and Italian studies are awaited with interest to determine whether platin-based adjuvant therapy improves the outcome for women with early epithelial ovarian carcinoma.

Current Management of Early Epithelial Ovarian Carcinoma

The suggested use of adjuvant therapy for women with early stage epithelial ovarian carcinoma is outlined in Fig. **2**. Patients with stage IA/B disease and grade 1 lesions, and all patients with stage I/II LMP lesions clearly have low-risk disease and can be observed without further therapy. Although patients with stage IA/B grade 2 lesions were included in the low-risk disease arm of the prior GOG/Ovarian Cancer Study Group trial, only five patients with lesions of this type were included in the observation arm.[258] Adjuvant therapy is reasonable in these patients. High-risk patients include patients with stage IC/II disease and those with grade 3 lesions, where survival of approximately 80% was observed after treatment of P-32 or melphalan.[258] These patients are offered participation in randomized clinical trials. In patients who are not suitable study protocol candidates, therapy is individualized and usually consists of six cycles of single-agent platin or three to four cycles of platin-cytoxan combination.

Second-look laparotomy yields positive findings in only approximtely 5% of patients with stage I/II disease who originally underwent comprehensive surgical staging and are clinically free of disease after adjuvant therapy.[186, 246] Furthermore, negative second-look laparotomy is a poor predictor of survival, particularly in patients with grade 3 or clear cell lesions.[186] Therefore, second-look laparotomy is not used in the routine management of these patients.

Therapeutic decisions are considerably more difficult in patients who underwent an incomplete staging procedure during their primary surgery. Patients who might have low-risk early stage disease are offered an immediate restaging laparotomy,[215] particularly if conservative surgery with preservation of the contralateral ovary and no further therapy is considered (Fig. **2**). Because P-32 does not provide adequate therapy for potential retroperitoneal

metastases,[213] options include abdominopelvic radiotherapy or platin-based chemotherapy. Second-look laparotomy in incompletely staged patients yields approximately 20% positive findings after chemotherapy;[185, 246] therefore a strategy using short courses of platin-based chemotherapy followed by second-look laparotomy is recommended to define patients who have occult advanced disease and require additional therapy (Fig. **2**).

Adjuvant Chemotherapy for Advanced (Stages III/IV) Epithelial Ovarian Carcinoma

It has long been recognized that patients with advanced epithelial ovarian carcinomas will almost always recur rapidly and die of disease if no further therapy is given after primary surgical therapy. This is valid even when all gross evidence of disease is surgically resected. During the earliest experience with chemotherapy of solid human tumors, epithelial ovarian cancer was recognized as a chemosensitive tumor.[194] Many single agents are active against ovarian cancer; most notable are alkylating agents, which have combined partial and complete response rates of 43 – 51%, hexamethylmelamine (42% response rate), and doxorubicin (35% response rate) in untreated patients.[235] However, response duration and overall survival of patients with advanced disease receiving these agents as monotherapy tended to be brief, and response rates with secondary therapy were low.

At approximately the same time that cisplatin was identified as an active agent in women after failure of radiotherapy or alkylator chemotherapy, combination chemotherapy was evaluated in women with advanced epithelial ovarian carcinoma. Wiltshaw and Kroner[254] and the GOG (1979) independently reported combined complete and partial response rates of approximately 30% in patients who received single-agent cisplatin as salvage chemotherapy. Young et al.[256] first reported superior activity of combination chemotherapy when compared to a single-agent alkylator. In their randomized trial, Hexa-CAF (hexamethylmelamine-cyclophosphamide-methotrexate-5-fluorouracil) significantly increased response rate (75% versus 54%), complete remissions (33% versus 16%) and longer median survival (29 months versus 17 months) compared to single-agent melphalan.

Cisplatin quickly became incorporated into combination chemotherapy regimens for advanced epithelial ovarian carcinoma. Ehrlich and associates[51] used cisplatin-doxorubicin-cyclophosphamide (PAC) in 56 patients with advanced ovarian carcinoma. They reported an overall response rate of 80% with a median survival of 33 months for complete responders. Several randomized trials reported in the early 1980s established platin-based combination therapy as the treatment of choice for patients with advanced-stage disease.[43, 154, 161, 244] However, the most efficacious platin combination has not been determined.

The Netherlands Cancer Institute randomized patients with advanced disease to cisplatin-cytoxan (CP) or a four-drug platin-based regimen (CHAP-5) that contained hexamethylmelamine. They failed to detect differences in response rates or survival.[155] Likewise, the GOG compared CP with PAC combination in 349 patients with optimally resected stage III disease (defined as residual tumors of < 2 cm at greatest diameter).[161] In this study, the dose of cyclophosphamide was increased in the CP arm. The intent was to produce a similar amount of myelosuppression as the PAC arm. The rate of pathologically determined complete response, and both progression-free interval and overall survival curves were statistically similar.

Retrospective meta-analyses of chemotherapy trials in patients with advanced ovarian carcinoma suggest that regimens with increasing dose intensity of cisplatin are associated with improved survival, while associations between increasing doses of doxorubicin and cyclophosphamide with improved survival were of only borderline significance.[121, 122] The addition of multiple agents to cisplatin combination regimens often leads to increased toxicity, with a reduction in the dose intensity of administered cisplatin in the three- and four-drug regimens. However, the maximal effect of increasing the dose intensity of cisplatin appears to occur at a dose equivalent of 25 mg/m^2/week.[121, 122] Furthermore, doses of cisplatin above 100 mg/m^2/cycle are associated with dose-limiting neurotoxicity. For these reasons, moderate-dose cyclophosphamide-cisplatin (CP) combination chemotherapy, using cisplatin doses of 50–100 mg/m^2/cycle, has been considered the standard regimen for advanced epithelial ovarian carcinoma until recently (Table **9**).

The GOG attempted to evaluate the issue of increasing the dose intensity of cisplatin by randomizing 458 patients with bulky residual (> 2 cm) advanced disease to receive totals of 400 mg/m^2 cisplatin and 4 g/m^2 cyclophosphamide over four or eight treatment cycles.[142] For patients in the higher-dose intense arm, toxicity was greater but the response rates and survival curves were identical to those for the patients in the lower-dose intensity arm. A Scottish cooperative group trial randomized 190 patients with all stages of ovarian cancer to receive cyclophosphamide 750 mg/m^2 plus cisplatin at doses of either 50 mg/m^2 or 75 mg/m^2 every 3 weeks for six cycles.[96] Patients in the dose-intense arm received 25% more total cisplatin than patients in the lower-dose arm. Survival in the dose-intense arm was significantly longer than in the lower-dose arm (125 versus 69 weeks). These results

Table **9**   Primary chemotherapeutic regimens for advanced epithelial ovarian carcinoma

Agents	Dose/cycle	Interval
Cisplatin	50–100 mg/m^2	
or		
Carboplatin	300–350 mg/m^2 (or AUC = 5–7)	q 3 wk
plus		
Cyclophosphamide	500–750 mg/m^2	
Paclitaxel	135–175 mg/m^2 [a]	
plus		
Cisplatin	75 mg/m^2 [b]	q 3 wk
or		
Carboplatin	AUC = 5	

AUC = are under the curve calculated by Calvert formula (Calvert, 1989)
[a]   Paclitaxel administered over 3–24 hours as continuous i.v. infusion; longer infusions associated with more myelosuppression.
[b]   Cisplatin is administered after paclitaxel.

must be interpreted with caution, however, due to the very heterogenous patient population studied, which included stage I or II disease in almost one-third of the study population.

Another strategy employed to increase the local dose intensity of cisplatin is the use of intraperitoneal administration of cisplatin. Intraperitoneal administration of cisplatin results in higher levels of cisplatin in the peritoneal fluid than in the peripheral circulation. The combined GOG-SWOG (GOG protocol #104) study randomized patients with small-volume residual (< 1 cm) advanced ovarian carcinoma to receive intravenous cyclophoshamide plus a fixed dose of either intravenous or intraperitoneal cisplatin. Although the study has been closed to patient accrual, no results have been presented to date.

Recent studies have evaluated the substitution of carboplatin for cisplatin in chemotherapy for epithelial ovarian carcinoma. Although the first randomized comparison of cyclophosphamide combined with cisplatin or carboplatin favored the cisplatin, equipotent doses of the platins were not used.[50] In this study, a dose of 150 mg/m^2/cycle carboplatin was compared to 60 mg/m^2/cycle cisplatin, resulting in approximately one-half the platin dose intensity in the carboplatin arm. Two subsequent mature studies compared six cycles of cyclophosphamide combined with carboplatin at doses of 300 mg/m^2/cycle versus cisplatin at doses of 50–75 mg/m^2/cycle in patients with advanced disease. These studies indicate that carboplatin can be substituted for cisplatin with no significant reduction in response rates or short-term progression-free survival.[2, 226] Although myelosuppression was more severe in the carboplatin arm, patients in the cisplatin arm of these trials had more neurotoxicity, nephrotoxicity, and emetogenic toxicity. This resulted in a slightly improved therapeutic ratio for the carboplatin regimens.

One potential disadvantage of carboplatin regimens is the loss of platin dose intensity caused by myelosuppression (most notably severe thrombocytopenia), which may delay chemotherapy or result in dose reductions when a standard dose of carboplatin is used. Dose calculations of carboplatin using renal creatinine clearance to predict a target area under the curve (AUC) of serum carboplatin levels (dose = target AUC × CrCl) can be used to individualize the carboplatin dose to the highest intensity, while avoiding dose-limiting severe thrombocyto-

penia.[25] In untreated patients, a target carboplatin AUC of approximately 5–7 can be used for initial combination therapy (Table **9**).

A recently reported cluster of three cases of acute leukemia or myelodysplasia in patients with ovarian cancer who received carboplatin-cyclophosphamide regimens is of concern.[38] Similar complications are rarely observed in patients receiving cisplatin-cyclophosphamide regimens. More experience with carboplatin regimens is required to determine whether this is a significant toxicity for carboplatin combinations. Currently, appropriate doses of carboplatin are considered to be equivalent to cisplatin in platin combination therapy (Table **9**).

Platin-paclitaxel combinations are undergoing intensive evaluation as the primary therapy for women with advanced ovarian carcinoma. When cisplatin is combined with paclitaxel, the paclitaxel must be administered first so that renal clearance of paclitaxel is not impaired. Such impairment can result in unacceptable hematological toxicity. The GOG reported preliminary results of Protocol #111, a randomized comparison of cisplatin 75 mg/m/cycle combined with either paclitaxel 135 mg/m^2/cycle administered over 24 hours or cyclophosphamide 750 mg/m^2/cycle in women with suboptimally debulked (> 1 cm) advanced ovarian carcinoma.[143] Chemotherapy was administered every 3 weeks for a total six cycles. Early results indicate a significantly higher response rate, a greater number of surgical responses, and an improved median disease-free survival for patients in the paclitaxel arm. Although these results are encouraging, the study is not mature. The magnitude of survival advantage is fairly small, with prolongation of median disease-free survival in the paclitaxel arm only by approximately 4 months. Furthermore, the paclitaxel arm had a 20% incidence of severe myelosuppression, nearly double the incidence of the cyclophosphamide arm.

A randomized study has been presented in preliminary form, which compares 24-hour versus 3-hour paclitaxel infusions in patients with previously treated ovarian cancer at two different dose levels.[227] The incidence of severe neutropenia and febrile neutropenia was much greater in the group receiving paclitaxel by the longer infusion than in the group receiving the 3-hour infusion (74% versus 17% and 12% versus 0%, respectively). There was a higher incidence of

Fig. **3** Integration of primary surgery and initial chemotherapy in advanced epithelial ovarian carcinoma

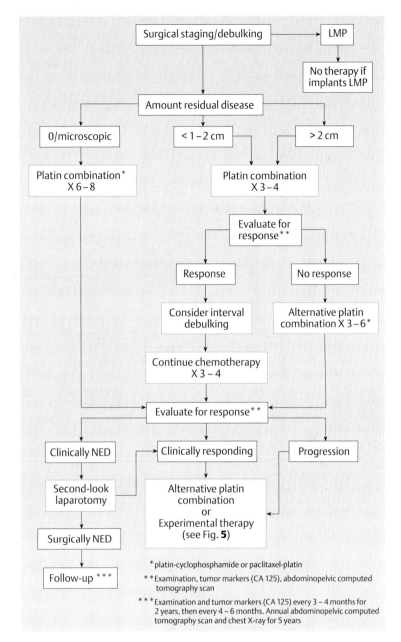

* platin-cyclophosphamide or paclitaxel-platin

* * Examination, tumor markers (CA 125), abdominopelvic computed tomography scan

* * * Examination and tumor markers (CA 125) every 3 – 4 months for 2 years, then every 4 – 6 months. Annual abdominopelvic computed tomography scan and chest X-ray for 5 years

neuropathy in patients treated with higher pacli-taxel doses. Response rates were similar for the two infusion times. These data suggest that short-infusion paclitaxel might be incorporated into primary cisplatin therapy of ovarian cancer without the high incidence of myelosuppression observed in the GOG trial. They also suggest that

carboplatin and taxol could be safely combined (in addition to the possibility of increasing the dose of paclitaxel) if a dose-intensity effect for paclitaxel is observed in ovarian cancer.

A subsequent GOG study comparing single-agent cisplatin (100 mg/m^2) and paclitaxel (200 mg/m^2) arms to cisplatin (75 mg/m^2) plus paclitaxel (135 mg/m^2) arms in patients with suboptimally debulked (> 1 cm) advanced ovarian carcinoma has completed patient accrual, but is not mature enough for analysis. Other phase I/II studies are evaluating dose-intense carboplatin-paclitaxel and cisplatin-cyclophosphamide-paclitaxel combinations in untreated patients.[100, 164] The phase I GOG trial of carboplatin-paclitaxel used a 24-hour infusion of paclitaxel.[164] Without using granulocyte-colony stimulating factor (GCSF) support, a paclitaxel dose of 135 mg/m^2 was combined with carboplatin and dosed to a target AUC of 7.5. There was no severe toxicity in the first cycle, but cumulative myelosuppression, resulting in delays in therapy, occurred after multiple cycles. Future patients will be treated using GCSF support in an attempt to accelerate the paclitaxel dose. Although these early results suggest high response rates with these regimens, hematological toxicity and cost will remain substantial concerns with paclitaxel combinations.

Suggested chemotherapy regimens for the primary therapy of patients with advanced epithelial ovarian carcinoma are outlined in Table **9**. A reasonable strategy for primary chemotherapy of advanced epithelial ovarian cancer would consist of primary therapy with a platin-cyclophosphamide or paclitaxel-cisplatin regimen following initial debulking surgery (Fig. **3**). If the patient is optimally debulked, second look-surgery should be considered after six to eight cycles of treatment, provided there is no clinical or radiographic evidence of disease progression.

In patients that are suboptimally debulked, re-evaluation should take place after three cycles of therapy. Nonresponders should receive the alternate combination (e.g., carboplatin-cyclophosphamide substituted for paclitaxel-cisplatin) or participate in clinical trials. In patients who have had evidence of disease response, interval debulking should be considered. Patients with optimal disease after interval debulking should receive further therapy with the same combination to complete six to eight cycles of therapy, while those with suboptimal residual disease should receive the alternate combination.

Adjuvant Therapy for Germ Cell Malignancies of the Ovaries

Before the development of effective chemotherapy regimens, patients with malignant germ cell tumors of the ovaries (other than dysgerminomas and grade 1 immature teratomas) frequently progressed and died rapidly after diagnosis, even when disease was thought to be confined to the ovary. With the exception of dysgerminomas, ovarian germ cell malignancies are not sensitive to radiotherapy. The sequential development of increasingly effective and less toxic regimens against germ cell malignancies of the testis, and their subsequent successful application to their rarer ovarian counterparts, is one of the success stories of modern oncology. Initial experience with vincristine-dactinomycin-cyclophosphamide (VAC) and similar combination regimens resulted in successful therapy of the

Table **10** Chemotherapy regimens for germ cell and stromal malignancies of the ovary	Regimen/Agents	Dose	Duration
	BEP		
	Bleomycin	15 U/m^2/wk	6 weeks
	Etoposide	100 mg/m^2/d × 5 days	q 21 days
	Cisplatin	20 mg/m^2/d × 5 days	
	PVB		
	Bleomycin	15 U/m^2/wk	6 weeks
	Vinblastine	0.15 mg/kg/d × 2 days	q 21 days
	Cisplatin	20 mg/m^2/d × 5 days	
	VAC		
	Vincristine	1 mg/m2 × 1	
	Dactinomycin	500 mcg/d × 5 days	q 28 days
	Cyclophosphamide	150 mg/m^2/d × 5 days	

All agents given intravenously.

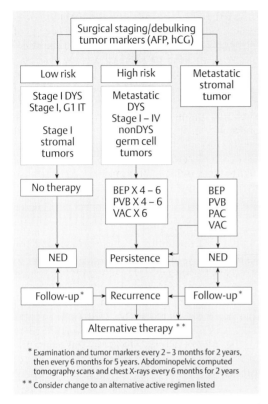

Surgical staging/debulking
tumor markers (AFP, hCG)

Low risk → Stage I DYS / Stage I, G1 IT / Stage I stromal tumors → No therapy → NED → Follow-up*

High risk → Metastatic DYS / Stage I – IV nonDYS germ cell tumors → BEP X 4 – 6 / PVB X 4 – 6 / VAC X 6 → Persistence → Recurrence

Metastatic stromal tumor → BEP / PVB / PAC / VAC → NED → Follow-up*

Alternative therapy**

* Examination and tumor markers every 2 – 3 months for 2 years, then every 6 months for 5 years. Abdominopelvic computed tomography scans and chest X-rays every 6 months for 2 years

** Consider change to an alternative active regimen listed

Fig. **4** Integration of therapy in management of ovarian germ cell and stromal tumors

majority of patients with stage I disease and substantial proportion of those with advanced-stage disease.[40] The subsequent application of cis-platin-vinblastine-bleomycin (PVB) or bleomy-cin-etoposide-cisplatin (BEP) testicular regimens to these patients resulted in cures in the majority of patients with germ cell malignancies. Relatively short but intensive treatment regimens were used.[250] Current chemotherapy regimens for germ cell malignancies are summarized in Table **10**, and overall management is summarized in Fig. **4**.

Observation

Pure dysgerminomas differ from other germ cell malignancies of the ovaries in several respects. They present as stage I lesions more often, have bilaterality in 10 – 15 % of lesions, and are much more radiosensitive than other histological subtypes.[233] In contradistinction to the other histo-logical subtypes, patients with stage I dysgermin-omas have an excellent survival after treatment with surgery alone.[233]

Published reviews of patients with dysgermi-nomas report that approximately 75 % of patients have stage I disease,[64, 107, 117, 233] however, with careful surgical staging it is expected that the true incidence of stage I disease is probably lower. Because the majority of patients with dys-germinomas are in their prime reproductive years and desire to retain child-bearing capacity, and because older strategies using adjuvant ra-diotherapy were associated with a high incidence of ovarian failure, recent trends have been to-ward management of patients with stage I A tumors with surgical resection and careful stag-ing alone.[233] The contralateral ovary should be carefully inspected and biopsied if there are any abnormalities. The primary tumor must be ade-quately sampled to exclude the possibility of a mixed germ cell tumor and to identify gonado-blastoma elements. If menstrual or reproductive function has not been established, karyotype should be performed to exclude 46, XY gonadal dysgenesis.[218]

Tumor markers should be obtained; a few pure dysgerminomas can secret hCG, but elevat-ed AFP levels suggest a mixed germ cell tumor with an occult endodermal sinus tumor element that mandates postoperative chemotherapy. Patients with elevated hCG levels should be monitored postoperatively to ensure that this tumor marker normalizes within a few weeks of surgery during follow-up. Earlier studies sug-gested that patients with tumors > 10 cm were not suitable for conservative management because of a higher recurrence rate,[107] but most contemporary clinicians will monitor patients with dysgerminoma regardless of tumor size.[233]

Patients must be closely monitored after con-servative surgical therapy, as 15 – 25 % will recur.[233] Because dysgerminomas are extremely sensitive to both chemotherapy and radio-therapy, virtually all patients with recurrent disease can be salvaged if the recurrence is diag-nosed early and treated when small-volume disease is present.

The only other germ cell tumor type with a relatively indolent biology is grade 1 immature teratoma. These lesions rarely recur after surgical resection[159] and can be monitored after conserva-tive surgery. If clinical recurrence is documented during follow-up, secondary surgical resection should be performed to document whether the recurrence continues to have grade 0–1 differentiation. If grade 0–1 elements are the only component of recurrence, it is doubtful that added chemotherapy will be of additional benefit.

Adjuvant Therapy for Early Nondysgerminomatous Germ Cell Malignancies

In the prechemotherapy experience, as many as 75% of patients with grade 3 immature teratomas and other nondysgerminomas malignancies recurred within 2 years of complete resection. Initially, protracted courses of VAC or similar regimens were used as adjuvant therapy for patients with stage I and II germ cell tumors, with apparent improved survival. In two relatively large GOG trials, the recurrence rates after adjuvant VAC chemotherapy were 28% and 24%.[205, 251] Analysis of the literature prior to 1985 revealed no apparent benefit when patients received < 6 or >6 cycles of VAC or similar combination regimens as adjuvant therapy of nondysgerminomatous germ cell malignancies.[40]

Although no randomized studies have been conducted in germ cell tumors of the ovary, the cisplatin-based combination regimens (PVB, BEP) appear to be more effective as adjuvant therapy than VAC-type regimens. In testicular germ cell tumors, the BEP regimen has at least the equivalent efficacy and reduced toxicity as the VBP regimen, producing much less neurological and gastrointestinal toxicity.[249] Bleomycin appears to be an important component of the BEP regimen. A randomized trial of BEP versus etoposide-platin in 166 patients with testicular germ cell malignancies reported 84% disease-free survival in the BEP arm compared to 69% in the etoposide-cisplatin arm.[126] Furthermore, cisplatin may be slightly better than carboplatin when treating tumors that have a potentially rapid growth pattern and where delays in retreatment caused by hematological toxicity might adversely affect outcome.[3]

Experience at the MD Anderson and preliminary data from the GOG suggest that BEP is superior to VAC-type regimens for adjuvant therapy of ovarian germ cell tumors. In the MD Anderson study, all 20 patients with early stage germ cell tumors survived free of disease after adjuvant BEP.[61] The GOG used three cycles of BEP as adjuvant therapy on women with completely resected stage I–III nondysgerminomatous malignant germ cell tumors and reported that 50 of 52 patients remained disease free during initial follow-up.[251] Both patients who failed had persistent immature teratoma at second look but remained clinically free of disease at the time of the preliminary report.

Based upon this collective experience, BEP (Table **10**) is the regimen of choice for the adjuvant therapy of completely resected ovarian germ cell malignancies. Patients with all histologies (except those with early stage dysgerminomas and grade 1 immature teratomas) should receive three to four cycles of adjuvant chemotherapy (Fig. **4**). Treatment should be initiated as soon as possible after surgery because of the rapid growth potential of these tumors and the increased difficulty when treating patients with advanced or bulky disease. Patients with elevated tumor markers (AFP or hCG) should be monitored to ensure that these markers normalize during the course of therapy, and chemotherapy should be continued for one to two cycles after normalization. Salvage chemotherapy and indications for secondary surgery are discussed in subsequent sections.

Chemotherapy for Advanced Germ Cell Malignancies

Chemotherapy of patients with advanced ovarian germ cell malignancies represents one of the true triumphs of modern chemotherapy in human solid tumors. Germ cell tumors of the ovaries rarely respond to single-agent regimens. In the 1970s, VAC and VAC-like combination regimens were applied to the treatment of these patients with significant numbers responding to chemotherapy. However, the number of long-term survivors after VAC chemotherapy was relatively small. For example, only seven (32%) of 22 patients with advanced disease who received VAC on a GOG trial were long-term survivors.[205]

Application of testicular cisplatin-combination regimens to the therapy of ovarian germ cell tumors resulted in apparent marked improvement of outcome in patients with advanced-stage disease. Small series of patients with advanced disease who received PVB were reported from Stanford, the Cross Cancer Institute, and the MD Anderson in the 1980s, resulting in an overall progression-free survival in 19 (76%) of 25 patients in these combined series.[26, 57, 230] A subsequent GOG study of patients with advanced and recurrent disease reported that 47 (53 %) of 89 patients treated with this regimen remained progression free. An additional eight patients were salvaged with second-line therapy for an overall survival of 70 %.[250] Prior radiotherapy or chemotherapy and measurable or bulky residual disease were poor prognostic factors in patients treated in this study. However, eight (27 %) of 30 patients with no prior therapy and with small volume residual disease failed PVB therapy.

Because randomized trials in patients with testicular cancer have suggested at least equivalent response rates with reduced toxicity for BEP,[249] most investigators believe that BEP is the regimen of choice for patients with advanced germ cell malignancies of the ovary. Support for the activity of the regimen includes complete responses in five of six patients with advanced nondysgerminomatous germ cell tumors that were treated with BEP at the MD Anderson.[61] Four cycles are usually administered. This is similar to the treatment strategy used for patients with advanced testicular malignancies; however, tumor marker-positive patients should be monitored closely during therapy to ensure that elevated tumor markers normalize during therapy.

Advanced dysgerminomas are also very sensitive to combination chemotherapy. Although VAC and VAC-like combinations have high response rates in this disease,[40] cisplatin-based regimens appear to have superior activity. In two GOG protocols that treated advanced germ cell tumors with PVB and BEP followed with VAC, 19 (95 %) of 20 patients with advanced dysgerminomas were alive and disease free at a median 26 months follow-up after initiation of therapy.[250] All 14 patients who underwent second-look laparotomies in these trials had negative findings. In another study, 14 patients with advanced dysgerminomas who had residual disease received BEP chemotherapy, with all patients surviving during long-term follow-up.[61] An ongoing GOG study is evaluating carboplatin-etoposide in completely resected advanced dysgerminomas.

Radiation Therapy for Dysgerminoma

In contrast to other histological subtypes of ovarian germ cell malignancies, and similar to testicular seminomas, dysgerminomas are extremely radiosensitive. In the past, adjuvant radiation

was given to many patients with stage I disease and the majority with advanced-stage disease.[233] The doses of radiation and treatment fields varied according to the extent of disease and the investigator; however, even low doses of 2500–3500 cGy were curative in some patients with incompletely resected advanced disease. Typical results were reported by DePalo and associates (1982): disease-free survival was 100 % for 13 patients with stage I disease and 61.4 % for 12 with stage III disease treated with radiotherapy. Loss of fertility following radiotherapy is a problem; therefore, chemotherapy is used in the majority of women with dysgerminomas who require postoperative treatment.

Ovarian Stromal Cell Tumors

Granulosa cell and Sertoli-Leydig cell tumors usually present in stage I upon diagnosis. Except for rare tumors with poorly differentiated histologies, these tumors should be considered lesions of low-malignant potential. Total abdominal hysterectomy with bilateral salpingo-oophorectomy and staging laparotomy should be performed in all patients who do not desire to retain fertility. Because these tumors are bilateral in less than 2 % of cases.[192] unilateral salpingo-oophorectomy and staging laparotomy should be performed for women of reproductive age who desire to retain child-bearing capacity. Endometrial adenocarcinoma is associated with approximately 5 % of granulosa tumors and adenomatous hyperplasia is present in an additional 25–50 %.[52, 54] Therefore, dilatation and curettage should be performed in all patients who are treated with conservative surgery.

Patients with advanced-stage disease should undergo debulking for palliation because there is no consistently effective chemotherapeutic regimen for these lesions. Anecdotal responses have been observed with a variety of single-agent and combination regimens, including VAC,[205] and platin-adriamycin combinations.[59, 91] The best response rates have been reported with PVB combination chemotherapy.[36, 267] Colombo et al.[36] reported six (55 %) complete and three (27 %) partial responders in their eleven patients with metastatic granulosa cell tumors. Severe hematological and nonhematological toxicity, (with two deaths caused by toxicity) was observed in their experience. Because of the reduced toxicity compared to VBP, BEP chemotherapy is currently recommended as initial therapy for patients with metastatic stromal tumors (Fig. **4**). Radiation therapy is usually reserved for palliation of pelvic recurrences.

Tubal Carcinoma

In terms of histology, pattern of spread, and behavior, tubal carcinoma is similar to epithelial ovarian carcinoma. For this reason, treatment strategies similar to those employed for ovarian cancer are used for treating patients with carcinoma of the fallopian tube. Surgical staging and debulking strategies are identical to the surgery used for ovarian cancer. It is unclear whether there is a low risk (e. g., stage IA, grade 1) subset of patients similar to the group in ovarian cancer that has a low enough risk of recurrence to be monitored without adjuvant therapy after surgery and comprehensive staging.

Chemotherapy with platin-based combination therapy in patients with residual disease produces responses in a substantial proportion of patients with tubal carcinomas.[92, 139, 166] Peters and associates[166] recorded an overall 81% response rate (with 75% complete responses) among 12 patients with advanced or recurrent tubal carcinomas who received cisplatin/doxorubicin/cyclophosphamide or cisplatin/cyclophosphamide chemotherapy, which was significantly better than response rates with nonplatin combination or single-agent therapy. Survival was significantly better in patients receiving platin-based regimens than for those receiving other forms of therapy. Furthermore, the large retrospective series analyzed by Hellstrom et al.[74] also suggested that patients who were treated with platin-based regimens had a better survival than those who received nonplatin regimens. Therefore, it is reasonable to treat patients with tubal carcinomas using epithelial ovarian cancer chemotherapy regimens.

Although pelvic radiotherapy was used to treat patients with tubal carcinomas in the past, whole abdominopelvic radiation therapy is probably more effective, given the propensity for tubal cancer to spread to the upper abdomen and lymph nodes.[75, 167, 173] Radiation therapy is not effective in treating patients with bulky residual disease (it is similarly ineffective in treating ovarian cancer), but appears to improve survival in patients with limited or microscopic residual disease. In the series reported by Hellstrom and

associates,[74] patients treated with chemotherapy had significantly improved survival compared to those treated with radiotherapy or with no adjuvant therapy (p = 0.0006). However, there are no randomized studies comparing chemotherapy to radiation in patients with optimal residual tubal cancers.

Surveillence During and After Primary Therapy

During primary chemotherapy, patients should be closely monitored for evidence of disease response and toxicity of therapy. An interval history and complete physical examination should be performed at the time of each cycle of therapy. Tolerance of prior treatment should be noted and the patient should be thoroughly questioned about symptoms referrable to toxicity of chemotherapy. Special emphasis should be placed upon the abdominal and pelvic examinations for evidence of disease response. In patients receiving cisplatin or paclitaxel, a neurological examination should be performed to screen for early signs of neuropathy. A careful pulmonary examination should be performed upon patients receiving bleomycin; fine rales or delayed expiratory phase may be the earliest signs of pulmonary fibrosis and should be evaluated by chest X-ray and pulmonary function tests. In asymptomatic patients, pulmonary function tests, with determination of carbon monoxide diffusing capacity (DL[CO]), are obtained after every other course of bleomycin.

Hematological indices and both renal and hepatic function tests should generally be evaluated prior to each course of therapy. Hematological indices are usually evaluated approximately 10 days after chemotherapy, during the anticipated nadir, to aid in the determination of dose adjustments during subsequent cycles of therapy.

Monitoring of serum tumor marker levels is helpful in the management of marker-positive patients. Serum hCG and AFP levels are extremely sensitive indicators of disease resonse in patients with germ cell tumors that secrete these markers. Among patients with epithelial ovarian carcinoma, CA 125 is the most reliable tumor marker and will be subsequently discussed in detail. Tumor markers should be obtained before primary surgery (or in the immediate postoperative interval) as a baseline and immediately prior to the first course of chemotherapy. In marker-positive patients, serial levels should be obtained before each subsequent cycle of therapy.

Bast and associates[5] first reported a correlation of serial CA 125 levels with disease response or progression in 93% of their patients with marker-positive epithelial ovarian carcinoma. Since others have then, confirmed a similar level of correlation: a fall in the CA 125 value to normal or half of its pretherapy value corresponds to clinical or surgical response, while elevations more than twice the pretherapy level indicates disease progression.[106, 240] Furthermore, the time to normalization of CA 125 values or half-life of serum CA 125 strongly corresponds to disease status at second-look laparotomy. In a study by Levin et al.,[121] 75% and 66% of patients who had normalized CA 125 levels after 3 months of therapy, had complete clinical and surgical responses. In contrast, all patients with elevated levels at this interval had persistent disease, even when CA 125 levels normalized with further therapy. Patients with CA 125 half-lives longer than 20 days have a very low chance of complete response and have shorter survival compared to those with short half-lives.[73, 89]

After completion of therapy, patients should be reevaluated with abdominopelvic CT scans, chest X-rays, serum tumor marker levels, and complete physical examinations with pelvic examination. Depending upon the type and extent of initial disease, second-look laparotomy or secondary debulking should be considered, as discussed below. Patients should be monitored at 3–4 month intervals for the first 2 years after completion of therapy, and at 6-month intervals thereafter, with examinations and tumor-marker determinations. Initially, radiographical imaging should be repeated at least every 12 months in patients with epithelial ovarian and tubal cancers. After 2 years of close follow-up, patients with germ cell malignancies have a very small incidence of recurrence, and radiographic imaging is usually not cost-effective after this interval.

Secondary Management

Currently, there is no consensus regarding the optimal secondary management for any of the categories of ovarian or tubal malignancies. Each

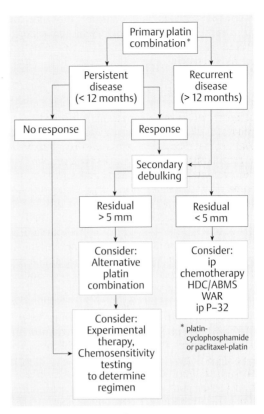

Fig. 5 Integration of surgery and salvage chemotherapy or radiotherapy in persistent or recurrent epithelial ovarian carcinoma

patient must be approached in the context of prior stage, response or lack of response to prior therapy, and functional status. While it is often easy to assume a passive and fatalistic attitude toward the patient with recurrent epithelial ovarian carcinoma, this can become a self-fulfilling prophecy; many patients will receive a temporary benefit from second-line or palliative treatment. Secondary management of epithelial ovarian carcinoma is outlined in Fig. **5**.

Secondary Surgery

Secondary surgical procedures performed on patients with ovarian carcinoma include "second-look" laparotomies for reassessment of disease status in patients with no clinical evidence of disease following primary therapy, secondary debulking procedures, and palliative procedures to relieve symptoms of bowel obstruction caused by advanced disease. The following sections will consider the role for each of these types of secondary surgery separately.

Wangenstein and associates[35] first introduced the concept of a second-look laparotomy in patients with colorectal cancers. These patients had been treated with surgery in an attempt to identify asymptomatic, occult recurrences that could be resected for cure. Rutledge and Burns[35] applied secondary reassessment surgery to patients with ovarian cancer who had completed a course of therapy and were thought to be free of disease. The term "second-look" laparotomy should be only used to describe a reassessment laparotomy, which is performed on patients who have no clinical or radiographical evidence after completion of primary therapy. In patients with disease that is not measurable by noninvasive examination or imaging techniques, a second-look laparotomy is the only means to assess response to chemotherapeutic regimens. Findings from the second-look procedure might provide information to help design further therapeutic strategies. Patients with clinically measurable disease may have other secondary surgical procedures (such as secondary debulking) utilized in their management but these procedures are not considered strictly second-look procedures.

Collected series support the validity of the concept that second-look findings provide prognostic information.[35] However, between 24–54% of patients with advaced disease, who have negative findings after platin-based chemotherapy, will eventually recur. Although it has been adopted as standard management in patients with epithelial ovarian cancer, the second-look laparotomy has been recently criticized due to lack of randomized trials or retrospective data that indiate a survival benefit for populations of patients who undergo these procedures.[55, 209] In addition, critics point to a general lack of effective second-line therapy for patients who have persistent disease at second-look procedures after completion of primary surgical debulking and platin-based chemotherapy.

However, recent retrospective studies suggest that patients with gross tumor residual that can be completely resected have improved survival.[80] Furthermore, second-line therapy is continually evolving, and past studies might not reflect response to salvage regimens and survival of patients in the future. Unfortunately, non-invasive imaging techniques and tumor marker studies often do not accurately reflect disease status in a substantial proportion of patients with advanced ovarian cancer at completion of first-line therapy. Therefore, second-look procedures will probably continue to be used to define activity of investigational protocols and to manage individual patients.

The majority of information about second-look procedures has been generated in patients with advanced epithelial ovarian carcinoma; however, the procedure has also been evaluated in patients with early epithelial ovarian carcinoma and germ cell malignancies. It is useful to briefly review the available data regarding the application of secondary evaluation of patients with ovarian and tubal maligancies to determine the current role for second-look procedures in the management of these patients.

Nonsurgical Evaluation of Residual Disease

Patients who have completed a course of primary chemotherapy after primary debulking for advanced epithelial ovarian carcinoma will have a complete clinical response in more than 50% of cases. Both computed tomography and ultrasound have been evaluated to determine efficacy for prediction of disease status after completion of primary therapy. Neither technique is sensitive enough to preclude second-look procedures. For example, collected series, which correlated radiographical findings with second-look procedures in patients clinically free of disease, reported an overall sensitivity of approximately 44% and specificity of 83% for prediction of disease status with CT scans.[35] The failure to reliably detect peritoneal implants < 2 cm in diameter, depending upon the site of involvement, is a limitation of CT.

The use of intraperitoneal contrast in conjunction with CT scanning improved the detection of small peritoneal metastases in a recent Italian study.[35] The overall sensitivity of this combined technique was 77%, with a sensitivity of 68% for prediction of peritoneal nodules < 2 cm in diameter. However, this technique failed to reliably detect implants < 5 mm in diameter. Similar to standard CT techniques, accuracy of the intraperitoneal contrast CT was highly dependent upon disease distribution, with sensitivity for prediction of disease highest for metastases involving the subphrenic and pericolic gutter areas, and lowest for implants involving the small bowel mesentery.

Despite these limitations, abdominopelvic CT is the best conventional noninvasive method for detecting residual ovarian cancer after completion of primary therapy. Patients with a positive finding on CT may be spared a major surgical procedure if fine-needle aspiration biopsy confirms persistent disease.

Recent studies have evaluated imaging with radiolabelled monoclonal antibodies directed against a tumor-associated antibody.[35] Monoclonal antibody B 72.3 was immunoconjugated with indium-111 (111 In). This monoclonal antibody reacts with TAG-72 antigens, which are expressed by most epithelial ovarian carcinomas. Immunoscintigraphy was compared with conventional CT scanning techniques in a multiinstitutional study. The immunoscintigraphy scans correctly identified persistent/recurrent ovarian cancer in 68% of patients, compared with only 44% for conventional CT techniques, including 27% of patients with negative CT scans. In contrast, CT scans were positive in only 3% of patients with negative immunoscintigraphy scans. Fifty-nine percent of patients with miliary disease and implants < 5 mm in diameter had positive immunoscintigraphy scans. Although these results are promising, they should be interpreted with caution in patients presenting after completion of primary therapy because only 30 patients who were candidates for second-look procedures were evaluated in this study. In these patients, immunoscintigraphy scan detected disease in only six of 17 patients who had persistent disease confirmed by second-look procedures.[35] Further evaluation of this technique is needed to determine its value as a substitute for second-look laparotomy.

Tumor markers have also been evaluated in patients undergoing second-look procedures. Because serum levels of CA 125 antigen are frequently elevated in patients with epithelial ovarian carcinoma, and changes in CA 125 levels correlate with response to therapy, several investigators have evaluated absolute or serial levels of CA 125 prior to second-look procedures. In the majority of studies, elevations of CA 125 reliably predict persistent disease, but 50–65% of patients with normal CA 125 values prior to second-look procedures have small volume residual disease.[35]

For example, Rubin and associates[184] compared surgicopathological findings with preoperative CA 125 levels in 96 patients evaluated with second-look laparotomy and found that while the positive predictive value of an elevated level was 100%, the predictive value of a normal CA 125 value was only 38%. They concluded that CA 125 levels were related to the amount of tumor present because patients with tumors < 1.0 cm in diameter had elevated CA 125 values in 55% of cases, compared to 80% in patients with tumors between 1 cm and 5 cm in diameter. Similar results were reported by Patsner et al. (1990) in their study of 125 women with advanced nonmucinous epithelial ovarian carcinomas. However, they were not able to correlate CA 125 levels with the amount of residual disease in their study. Based on these and other studies, CA 125 values have insufficient sensitivity to accurately identify small-volume residual disease after completion of primary chemotherapy in women with advanced epithelial ovarian carcinoma.

As previously discussed, second-look laparotomy rarely has positive findings in patients who have undergone primary comprehensive surgical staging.[186, 216, 246] Therefore, second-look laparotomy is usually reserved only for those patients with early disease who have not undergone an initial comprehensive staging laparotomy.

For many years, the second-look laparotomy was incorporated into management of patients with germ cell malignancies of the ovary. However, given the shorter natural history of germ cell malignancies, their marked sensitivity to contemporary chemotherapy, and the excellent correlation of tumor markers (hCG, AFP) with disease status in marker-positive lesions compared to epithelial ovarian carcinomas, second-look procedures have assumed a minor role in the management of these patients. In the GOG experience, eight (14%) of 56 patients who were clinically free of disease and had negative tumor markers had positive findings at second-look laparotomy, while an additional eight patients had residual immature teratoma.[250] In a series reported from MD Anderson, Gershenson et al.[57] reported that only one (2%) of 53 similar patients had positive findings. One patient developed recurrence despite a negative second-look laparotomy. An additional 13 patients had retroconversion of immature teratoma to mature glial implants; none of these patients recurred. Therefore, second-look laparotomy is usually reserved for patients with germ cell malignancies who had bulky residual disease after primary resection or who are suspected of having persistent disease after primary chemotherapy, where secondary debulking of persistent disease might be benificial prior to institution of secondary chemotherapy. Alternatively, such high-risk patients could be monitored clinically, with chemotherapy being instituted at the time of clinical recurrence of disease.

The role of second-look laparotomy in the management of stromal tumors of the ovary has not been adequately defined. Patients with stage I disease are at a relatively low risk for recurrence; therefore, second-look procedures are not advocated. Those with advanced disease and significant residual disease after primary debulking might be selected for second-look laparotomy and secondary debulking if residual disease is present after primary chemotherapy, but no data exist to support that this approach is beneficial to patients with stromal tumors.

The data supporting second-look procedures in patients with tubal cancers is equally sparse. Because of the similarity of tubal and ovarian epithelial malignancies, most gynecologic oncologists will incorporate second-look procedures into the management of patients with advanced tubal carcinoma.

Second-Look Laparotomy Procedure

Before performing second-look procedures, the surgeon should carefully review the previous operative note and pathology report to determine sites of residual disease because these represent high-yield areas that must be sampled at second-look laparotomy. Although secondary surgical assessment is usually performed by laparotomy, laparoscopy may be performed preoperatively in selected patients who are at high risk for positive findings to spare them the morbidity of laparotomy if they have diffuse and unresectable persistent disease. A recent report by Childers et al.[32] on laparoscopic para-aortic lymphadenectomy in patients with ovarian carcinoma indicates that the entire procedure could possibly be performed by laparoscopy, but prospective studies evaluating the complete laparoscopic second-look procedure have just been initiated by the GOG. Laparoscopic second-look procedures may not be feasible on a routine basis in patients who have undergone previous de-

bulking procedures because of extensive intraperitoneal adhesions that could limit the extent of intraperitoneal visualization.

The second-look laparotomy is essentially a comprehensive staging laparotomy, which is performed on a patient who has had a previous surgical procedure for ovarian cancer.[35] A midline incision is used to expose the peritoneal cavity and is extended into the epigastrium if initial exploration reveals no gross evidence of disease. Adhesions are lysed and washings are obtained from the pelvis, pericolic gutters, and diaphragms for cytological assessment. Hysterectomy and bilateral salpingo-oophorectomy should be completed if they were not performed previously. A thorough peritoneal exploration is performed and multiple peritoneal biopsies are obtained from suspicious lesions, adhesions, and normal-appearing peritoneum in sites with prior disease residual. The omental remnant should be removed and submitted as multiple specimens. In patients without gross evidence of disease, random biopsy from high-risk peritoneal sites should be obtained, including the anterior and posterior cul-de-sac, pelvic sidewalls, pericolic gutters, and the right hemidiaphragm.

If lymph node biopsies were not performed or were positive at primary surgery, bilateral pelvic and para-aortic lymphadenectomy should be performed. Lymphatic chains that were previously biopsied with negative results at primary surgery do not need to be resampled because the yield of resampling in this situation is minimal. If gross disease is encountered, every effort should be made to completely resect the disease to microscopic disease residual.

Clinicopathological findings at primary surgery correlate with positive findings at second-look laparotomy. Increasing stage and amount of disease residual are inversely correlated with the proportion of negative second-look procedures, while histological grade has weaker correlations with findings.[24, 27, 129, 172] In contrast to the low rates of positive findings at second-look procedures in patients with carefully evaluated disease who are in stages I and II,[185, 246] only approximately 33 % of patients with stages III and IV disease have negative second-look laparotomies.[24, 27, 129, 172] Furthermore, the rate of negative second-look procedures among patients with advanced disease decreases from 62–77 % in women with no gross residual disease, to 30–55 % in those with optimal (< 1–2 cm) disease, and 7–28 % in those with suboptimal (> 2 cm) residual disease after primary debulking.[24, 27, 129]

The prognostic significance of findings at second-look laparotomy is considerable. In most series, survival of patients with gross persistent disease is extremely poor, with approximately 80% expiring within 2–3 years of the procedure.[35] In contrast, patients with microscopic persistent disease have a more favorable survival. Copeland and associates[39] reported survival of 96% and 71% at 2 and 5 years after second-look laparotomy, in a series of patients who had microscopic persistent disease. The majority of their patients, however, had received prior non-platin regimens, and almost all received further chemotherapy after their second-look procedure. Their results are superior to the majority of series, which included only patients who had received prior platin. The results should not be interpreted as reflecting only the natural history of microscopic persistent disease after contemporary therapy.

Because it is impossible to sample the peritoneal cavity completely, and because ovarian cancer can recur outside of the areas sampled at second-look laparotomy, it is not surprising that a negative second-look laparotomy does not guarantee cure. Series of patients with negative second-look laparotomies after treatment with nonplatin regimens, which included all stages of disease, reported overall recurrence rates of 18% with 26% for patients with stages III and IV disease.[183] In contrast, series comprised of patients with advanced-stage disease, who received platin-based regimens prior to negative second-look laparotomies, reported recurrence rates as high as 50% with relatively short follow-up.[183] It is therefore useful to consider these patients as having occult microscopic residual disease. The risk of recurrence is certainly sufficient to warrant trials of consolidation therapy in patients who have negative second-look laparotomy after platin induction regimens. The GOG is currently conducting a randomized trial of intraperitoneal P-32 versus no further therapy in patients with negative second-look laparotomies, after primary adjuvant chemotherapy for advanced epithelial ovarian carcinoma.

Secondary Debulking Procedures

There are several situations in which secondary debulking procedures may be considered. These procedures may be utilized with patients who have disease progression during primary therapy, at planned interval debulking after brief induction chemotherapy in patients with bulky disease residual, at the time of second-look procedures, and at the time of reucrrence after a clinical remission. There have been no satisfactory studies conducted of secondary debulking procedures in patients with germ cell malignancies, stromal tumors, or tubal carcinomas. Morris et al.[150] recently reported that there was no survival advantage for secondary debulking in patients who underwent these procedures for progression of disease during therapy. However, studies that note the efficacy of secondary debulking in other clinical situations need to be considered to evaluate the role of these procedures in the management of patients with epithelial ovarian carcinoma (Table **11**).

Table **11** Potential survival benefit after secondary debulking in patients with advanced epithelial ovarian carcinoma

Setting	Benefit
Interval debulking after response to initial chemotherapy	Yes (van der Berg, 1993)
Debulking at second-look laparotomy	
Complete	Yes (Hoskins, 1989; Creasman, 1992)
< 2 cm residual	Possible (Creasman, 1992)
Debulking at recurrence	
Complete or > 12 month remission	Yes (Janicke, 1992)
Debulking during progression on initial chemotherapy	No (Michel, 1989; Morris, 1989)

Planned Interval Debulking

Patients with advanced, suboptimally debulked epithelial ovarian cancer may respond to initial chemotherapy used in a neoadjuvant setting. This would allow optimal debulking after a brief induction, with limited exposure to chemotherapy. Preliminary results of a randomized trial in patients with advanced, suboptimally debulked epithelial ovarian carcinoma suggest a survival benefit for interval debulking procedures in responders to platin-based chemotherapy.[243] This strategy of the neoadjuvant use of chemotherapy followed by interval debulking has been discussed previously (Fig. **3**).

Debulking at Second-Look Laparotomy

There have been no randomized studies that evaluate the effect of secondary debulking at the time of second-look laparotomy. Several retrospective studies have suggested feasibility for optimally debulking patients with gross persistent disease in 24–84% of cases at second-look laparotomy.[8, 30, 80, 124, 127, 174] Part of the wide variance noted may reflect differences in effort of maximal cytoreductive surgery during the primary procedure; in some centers, patients were not initially explored by gynecologic oncologists and a substantial proportion of these patients might have had disease that could have been optimally debulked during the initial procedure. Morbidity of secondary debulking in this setting is not significantly different from that observed during primary debulking.

The survival benefit of secondary debulking performed at second-look laparotomy has been controversial, with studies by Chambers et al.[30] and Luesley et al.[127] suggesting no survival benefit for even complete debulking to microscopic disease residual. In contrast, Podratz and colleagues[174] noted a survival rate of 55% in patients debulked to microscopic residual versus 19% in those left with macroscopic residual. Likewise, Hoskins et al.[80] reported that patients debulked to microscopic residual at second-look laparotomy had a survival rate of 51%, similar to survival in patients who had microscopic disease without debulking, and significantly better than the survival of patients who were left with gross residual disease. Furthermore, Lippman and associates[124] reported that even debulking to optimal disease status (<2 cm largest residual)

with gross residual disease improved survival among patients who had bulky implants at the time of second-look laparotomy.

Creasman reviewed the secondary debulking reported in 16 series comprised of 1207 patients with epithelial ovarian cancer.[41] Survival was 71% for 414 patients with a negative second-look laparotomy and 47% for 192 patients with microscopic persistent disease. One hundred eighteen patients with macroscopic disease that was debulked to a microscopic residual had a survival of 31%, significantly increased from 15% for the 482 patients with macroscopic residual. However, there was also a nonsignificant trend in survival improvement among patients with macroscopic disease that was reduced to a residual of <1 cm at greatest diameter. Limitations to interpreting these studies include possible inconsistent efforts at secondary debulking, heterogeneous populations in regard to preoperative and salvage regimens, and failure to take into account the differences in biological aggressiveness of tumors in different patients. On the basis of these retrospective data, however, it appears that efforts to completely debulk patients at second-look laparotomy are justified by improved survival in those who can be maximally debulked.

Seondary Debulking at the Time of Recurrence

Patients who recur after a disease-free interval following platin-based chemotherapy have a significant chance of achieving a secondary response to additional platin-based regimens. Theoretically, secondary debulking in this setting could impart many of the benefits of primary tumor cytoreductive surgery. Morris et al.[150] reported no survival advantage for patients undergoing debulking in this setting, using diameter of residual tumor <2 cm to define optimal cytoreductive status. However, in a recent report by Janicke et al.[94] where 30 patients undergoing secondary debulking of relapsing ovarian cancer were studied, significant prolongation in survival related to residual disease volume was found. Fourteen patients were completely debulked and 12 were debulked to <2 cm residual disease. The experimentors performed 19 (63%) intestinal resections; one postoperative death occurred. Among patients who were completely debulked, median survival was 29 months, versus 9 months for those with macroscopic disease residual (p = 0.004). The recurrence-free interval prior to clinical relapse was also significantly related to median survival, with 29 and 8 months, respectively, for patients with intervals of > 12 months and < 12 months. In multivariate analysis, the amount of residual disease, recurrence-free interval before debulking, and provision of any secondary therapy were independent prognostic factors. Although this retrospective study is relatively small, it suggests that attempts at secondary debulking are worthwile in patients who have a significant relapse-free interval and can undergo complete debulking.

Palliative Procedures

Despite advances in primary surgery and chemotherapy of ovarian cancer, the majority of patients with advanced disease will ultimately experience disease progression and die due to complications caused by their disease. Refractory ovarian cancer often results in symptoms caused by intraperitoneal carcinomatosis and intestinal obstruction. Because the majority of these patients are not in severe pain and have normal mentation, palliation of intestinal obstruction might add weeks or months of quality life. Surgical attempts to correct intestinal obstruction in this setting must be balanced by the possibility of serious complications or the potential of putting the patient through a major procedure that is not successful in relieving symptoms. It is also important to realize that between 5 – 24 % of patients presenting with bowel obstruction after therapy for ovarian carcinoma will have the obstruction due to complications of prior surgery or radiation therapy, rather than from progressive disease.[35] Therefore, therapeutic options must be approached on a case-by-case basis after the patient's overall functional status, disease status, and the wishes of the patient and her family, have been considered.

Krebs and Gopelrud[105] found that 96 (46 %) of 208 patients who died of ovarian cancer had had one or more episodes of small-bowel obstruction requiring hospitalization, surgery, or both. They found that only 32 % had had sufficient relief of symptoms with prolonged nasogastric intubation to allow discharge, and 86 % of these patients returned to the hospital with recurrent intestinal obstruction within a mean of 5.5 weeks after discharge. Therefore, medical management has

little to offer for prolonged palliation in these patients, unless they have not received an adequate trial of potentially effective chemotherapy.

It is difficult to determine whether a patient will benefit from palliative surgery to relieve intestinal obstruction caused by persistent ovarian cancer. Arbitrary definitions of "benefit" have included discharge from the hospital for 2-month with the ability to eat at least a low-residue diet.[184] These rather modest definitions of benefit must be weighed against the outcome in patients who fail medical management and do not undergo surgery, where the expected median survival is only 13.5 days.[105]

The most common anatomic sites of obstruction in these patients collected from several series are the small intestine (57 %), colon (30 %), and combined small and large bowel (13 %) with benefit from surgery achieved in between 32 – 80 % of patients, when defined as survival > 60 days after surgery.[35] Median postoperative survival has ranged between 10 – 33 weeks. Therefore, several investigators have attempted to retrospectively analyze clinical factors that might predict success or failure of palliation in patients with ovarian cancer who present with bowel obstruction.

Krebs and Gopelrud[105] developed a scoring system based on age, nutritional assessment, clinical tumor spread, ascites, previous chemotherapy, and previous radiation therapy. Each factor was given a graduated score from 0 to 2. Patients with total scores of seven or more had only a 20 % chance of benefit, compared to 80 % in patients with scores of < 7. Other authors found no correlation between this scoring system or components of this scoring system when applied to their patient population.[128, 184] Fernandes et al. evaluated factors associated with 12-month survival after surgery for obstruction.[52a] They reported that the interval from primary diagnosis to obstruction, initial stage, prior radiation therapy, the presence of ascites, and a variety of radiographical studies and nutritional laboratory values were correlated with prolonges survival.

Clarke-Pearson et al.[34] retrospectively evaluated 21 preoperative variables, seven nutritional parameters, and eight intraoperative or postoperative variables to determine associations with survival of 60 days or longer from surgery. Clinical tumor status and serum albumin level were the only significant independent prognostic variables on multivariate analysis. Although tumor status cannot be modified in patients with refractory malignancy, perioperative total parenteral nutrition might be an appropriate adjunct for individual patients as an attempt to improve tolerance of surgery. Several studies have documented increased morbidity in patients who are nutritionally depleted before undergoing pallitaive surgery for intestinal obstruction caused by ovarian cancer.[28, 33, 105]

Major operative morbidity has ranged between 30–64% with an operative mortality of 14–32%.[35] Complications and mortality are increased in patients who cannot undergo definitive surgical correction of their obstruction. Rubin and associates[184] attempted to correlate operability to preoperative clinical factors, but were not able to retrospectively identify factors that would significantly discriminate between operable and inoperable patients.

Therefore, the decision to operate on a patient with bowel obstruction in the setting of persistent, advanced ovarian carcinoma must be made on the basis of good clinical judgement, with the acitve participation of the patient and her family in an informed discussion of the nature of the problem. Radiographical studies of both large and small bowel should be performed preoperatively to diagnose a possibly significant but silent large-bowel obstruction that is clinically obscurred by a proximal small-bowel obstruction. The surgeon must exercise good clinical judgement during the procedure because of the wide range of procedures that may need to be performed, including small or large-bowel diversion, bowel resection or bypass, tumor resection, or simple gastrostomy in patients with little chance of benefit from a more extensive procedure. In patients who are not candidates for surgical exploration, percutaneous gastrostomy tube placement can often effectively palliate the patient with chronic bowel obstruction who wishes removal of her nasogastric tube.[131]

▓ Secondary Chemotherapy

Epithelial Ovarian and Tubal Carcinoma

Patients with recurrent or refractory epithelial malignancies of the ovary comprise a heterogeneous group, with a substantial proportion having tumor that retains sensitivity to platin

and a second group that has platin-refractory disease. Patients who have had a remission of > 12 months after initial chemotherapy tend to have platin-sensitive disease. Likewise, a significant proportion of patients who have had a response to induction chemotherapy with platin regimens, but have small (< 1 cm) peritoneal disease may respond to dose intensification of platin using intraperitoneal cisplatin chemotherapy. In contrast, patients whose disease has progressed during primary platin induction therapy or who have had short-duration remissions after initial platin chemotherapy will rarely have significant responses to second-line platin regimens. Even dose intensification with intravenous platin rarely results in significant responses among patients with platin-refractory disease, and those who do not have significant responses to platin induction regimens do not respond to dose intensification with intraperitoneal platin therapy. The integration of secondary surgery and chemotherapy is presented in Fig. **5**.

Platin-Sensitive Recurrences

Patients who have a long interval between primary chemotherapy with platin-based regimens and relapse will often respond to a second platin regimen. Seltzer et al.[196] demonstrated this phenomenon first. They reported that 72% of their patients responded to secondary cisplatin regimens after having achieved a complete response to initial platin therapy. The exact agents in either the primary or secondary platin regimen did not seem to make a difference in the frequency of responses to second-line platin regimens, as long as there was a complete response to initial therapy. Markman and colleagues[134] reported that the response rate was dependent upon the interval from primary remission to relapse. In their series, only 30% of patients who relapsed within 24 months of initial chemotherapy responded to secondary platin regimens, compared to 59% of those who had a disease-free interval of more than 24 months. Some patients will have responses to a third or fourth platin regimen, but the duration of each subsequent response tends to be shorter than the response to the primary treatment.

Intraperitoneal Platin Chemotherapy

Many studies have reported significant secondary response rates to intraperitoneal administration of cisplatin among patients with persistent ovarian cancer who received primary intravenous platin chemotherapy. The intraperitoneal administration of cisplatin is theoretically, appealing, given the predominant intraperitoneal distribution of disease and pharmacokinetics of intraperitoneal instillation that result in approximately a 10-fold increase of intraperitoneal platin concentration compared to intravenous administration.[135] Ideally, intraperitoneal administration would allow dose intensification of cisplatin delivery to tumors that had previously responded to a lower delivered platin dose.[163] Many different intraperitoneal platin regimens have been utilized in phase II trials, but it is questionable whether combination regimens have any better activity than single-agent cisplatin administered at doses of 100–150 mg/m²/cycle.

Unfortunately, cisplatin only diffuses into the most superficial layers of intraperitoneal tumor. The result of this is that there is a significant pharmacological advantage over intravenous administration only in tumor implants that are < 2–3 mm at their greates diameter. Furthermore, intraperitoneal distribution may be problematic in patients who have undergone several previous surgeries, and up to 20% of patients will have infectious complications of an indwelling intraperitoneal catheter. Based on the studies by Markman et al.,[135] the only patients likely to benefit from intraperitoneal administration of cisplatin are those who have small (<5 mm) intraperitoneal nodules and are those presumed to have responded to primary platin regimens at second-look procedures. In these patients, approximately 20–30% will have complete responses to intraperitoneal therapy. Unfortunately, failures both within and outside of the peritoneal cavity are common after even short-term follow-up. Because of these disappointing results, many have questioned the applicability of intraperitoneal therapy in the management of patients with ovarian carcinoma.[163]

Paclitaxel

Several phase II trials have evaluated the activity of paclitaxel in patients with persistent ovarian cancer after initial platin-based combination therapy. This natural plant alkyloid extracted from the bark of the Pacific yew (*Taxus brevifolis*) has a unique mechanism of action. By stabilizing cellular microtubules, it inhibits both interphase and mitosis. Initial phase I and phase II studies have suggested responses in approximately 30% of previously treated ovarian cancer patients.[141, 189, 237] Unlike the majority of phase II trials with other agents, significant responses are observed among similar proportions of patients with platin-sensitive and platin-resistant disease. In the National Cancer Institute (NCI) Treatment Referral Center Trial,[236] 86% of patients received three or more treatments regimens, with responses observed in 22% of 619 evaluable patients.

Dose-limiting toxicity of Paclitaxel is significant granulocytopenia of brief duration. Toxicities observed in the NCI study included severe granulocytopenia in 77%, thrombocytopenia in 3%, infection in 13%, and anaphylaxis in only 0.3% when a standard prep was used. This consisted of two doses of oral decadron (20 mg) every 12 hours beginning 24 hours prior to therapy, combined with an immediate pretherapy infusion of 300 mg cimetidine and 50 mg diphenhydramine.[236] Although earlier studies suggested a high incidence of cardiac arrhythmias, significant arrhythmias were infrequently observed. In less heavily treated patient populations, severe myelosuppression was less common in doses of < 150 mg/m² administered over 24 hours.[232] Based on these studies, the Food and Drug Administration has recommended a starting dose of 135 mg/m² administered over 24 hours for paclitaxel as secondary therapy for ovarian cancer. However, the previously cited randomized trial indicates that 175 mg/m² given as the three-hour infusion can be safely administered as salvage therapy.[227]

Future research is needed to determine whether dose escalation of paclitaxel results in significant improvement in response rates and whether a shorter infusion schedule results in any reduction in the response rate. Currently, paclitaxel is the most active single second-line agent for patients with platin-refractory ovarian cancer.

Other Agents

Unfortunately, conventional doses of other chemotherapy agents are not likely to result in significant responses in patients with platin-refractory disease. Among recent GOG phase II trials in previously treated patients with ovarian cancer, ifosfamide was the only agent other than paclitaxel to produce responses in more than 20% of patients.[222] In this study, 46 patients recieved 1.2–2.5 g/m² daily for 5 days along with mesna 300 mg/m² every 4 hours (for three doses) following the ifosfamide. Three (8.1%) patients had a complete response and five (13.5%) had a partial response with a median duration of response of approximately 7 months. Most of the responders had platin-sensitive tumors or had relapsed after an initial remission. Markman and associates[135] used doses of 1.0–1.2 mg/m²/day for 5 days along with mesna. They reported only a 12% response rate in 41 patients with platin-refractory tumors and 18% response rate in 16 with platin-sensitive disease. Severe myelotoxicity, nephropathy, and central neurotoxicity were observed in a significant proportion of patients receiving secondary ifosfamide.

Early studies of hexamethylmelamine in patients who had failed platin-based chemotherapy reported discouraging response rates;[219] however, recent studies have suggested success in some patients with persistent disease after platin therapy.[133, 241] Of note, the majority of patients with favorable results in one study had nonmeasurable persistent disease after second-look laparotomy.[133] Therefore, further study is needed to define whether there is significant activity for this agent in patients with bulky refractory disease.

Etoposide also had minimal activity in early studies using 3–5-day intravenous dosing schedules.[49, 203] However, the activity of this agent is both dose and schedule dependent. Daily etoposide at doses of 50–100 mg/m², administered orally for 14–21 days, has significant activity in platin-refractory ovarian cancer.[77] Likewise, a regimen that combined oral and intravenous etoposide produced a 32% response rate.[109] Studies by the GOG are reevaluating the use of oral etoposide in patients with refractory gynecologic malignancies from multiple sites, including the ovary.

High-Dose Chemotherapy with Autologous Marrow Support

If dose intensificatin of the chemotherapeutic agents active in ovarian carcinoma is a valid means for producing increased response rates, then very high-dose chemotherapy (with rescue of hematological progenitor cells using autologous bone marrow support [ABMS] and/or peripheral stem cell support) might allow dose intensification beyond dose-limiting myelotoxicity. A few small phase I/II studies have been reported that explored this concept in ovarian cancer patients.[144, 200, 201] Although a variety of chemotherapeutic regimens were used, all series reported to date have witnessed a high proportion of responses in patients with platin-refractory and often heavily pretreated disease, ranging between 55–78% for evaluable patients. Unfortunately, the response duration was short, averaging approximately 4–6 months, with few long-term survivors in these series. Furthermore, toxicity was significant in patients who were heavily treated before receiving high-dose chemotherapy with ABMS, with a 20% incidence of mortality caused by toxicity in the series reported by Sphall et al.[201] Despite modifications of the regimen and use of peripheral stem-cell support to enhance marrow recovery, the Duke ABMS protocol has continued to have toxic deaths among patients with chemorefractory ovarian cancer, largely caused by chronic underlying cisplatin renal toxicity among patients who received a median of three regimens prior to ABMS.[168]

The high response rates reported for this technique are encouraging, but these studies indicate that there is limited application for this approach as salvage therapy for patients who have failed multiple regimens. It is possible that even with escalation of doses beyond the normal marrow tolerance, this strategy will not result in sufficient doses to overcome drug-resistant disease or improve long-term survival. The most logical place to test dose escalation supported by ABMS would be among patients with small-volume disease who have responded favorably to first-line chemotherapy. In this setting, ABMS might be able to convert a partial response into a complete response without the high mortality rate associated with this therapy in heavily pretreated patients.

Secondary Chemotherapy for Germ Cell Malignancies

Patients with recurrent or refractory germ cell malignancies of the ovary should be carefully evaluated before a salvage regimen is decided upon. If the patient has not received a prior cisplatin-based regimen, then therapy with BEP or PVB should be instituted. Patients with prior exposure to cisplatin regimens should be separated into those who relapsed after a complete remission that lasted longer than 4–6 months, and those who have disease that is truly refractory to cisplatin regimens. Patiens who have had a complete response to cisplatin-based chemotherapy should be retreated with either alternate cisplatin combination or the testicular salvage regimen that incorporates daily ifosfamide 1–1.5 gm/m^2 and mesna with either cisplatin-vinblastine or cisplatin-etoposide.[125] The prognosis for patients with disease that is clearly refractory to cisplatin-based regimens is usually poor when conventional regimens (such as VAC) are used. Therefore, high-dose chemotherapy with autologous marrow and/or peripheral stem-cell support should be considered in these patients.[157]

Secondary Chemotherapy for Stromal Cell Tumors

Just as there is no consensus for a "superior" primary chemotherapeutic regimen for patients with stromal cell tumors, secondary chemotherapy options are also poorly defined. Individualized treatment with combination regimens that employ cisplatin, adriamycin, or components of VAC should be considered, depending upon earlier drug exposure.

▨ Secondary Radiation Therapy

Both whole abdominopelvic radiotherapy and intraperitoneal chromic phosphate have been used following primary induction with surgery and chemotherapy in an attempt to consolidate the results of therapy in patients with epithelial ovarian carcinoma. In general, these efforts have had limited success, largely because of problems with serious bowel toxicity in patients who received multiple surgical procedures and chemotherapy prior to whole abdominoplevic radiotherapy. Additionally, patients with gross residual disease have relatively poor long-term disease-free survival after consolidation with radiotherapy. Finally, patients with small-volume disease, who have favorable survival after consolidation with radiotherapy, may have biologi-

cally indolent disease and their survival might not reflect an effect of the radiation. However, in selected patients with minimal residual disease (consisting of microscopic persistence or < 5 mm residual tumor at second look laparotomy), whole abdominopelvic radiation therapy is a viable option for secondary therapy.

Unfortunately, the majority of studies reported to date have been small single-arm trials of sequential therapy, without randomization to a control arm.[69, 70, 79, 210] Of note, a randomized trial of whole abdominopelvic radiotherapy, which was compared to chemotherapy after cisplatin induction chemotherapy, reported equivalent survival results.[118] Studies have attempted to reduce toxicity of consolidation abdominopelvic radiotherapy by reducing the total dose given to the upper abdominal fields below 2250 cGy and/or reducing the pelvic dose below 4500 cGy. Others have attempted to both increase the biological effectiveness of the radiation therapy and decrease the toxicity by using hyperfractionation techniques, giving two or three small daily fractions to higher total doses. Studies by Morgan et al.[148] and Kong et al.[101] used hyperfractionation to deliver upper abdominal doses of approximately 30 Gy, with relatively low rates of bowel morbidity during short-term follow-up. Although these studies indicate feasibility of this approach, randomized studies are needed to determine whether there is any survival benefit with consolidation radiotherapy in patients with small-volume persistent disease after primary chemotherapy.

Palliative radiotherapy may be useful in managing complications of localized disease, such as vaginal bleeding, pelvic pain, or partial colonic obstruction. The majority of the patients treated with palliative radiation therapy have advanced disease at other sites. This limits the effect of localized treatment on long-term survival. It should be noted that a recent meta-analysis indicated that the combination of radiotherapy with surgical extirpation and/or chemotherapy resulted in improved survival among patients with brain metastases from epithelial ovarian carcinoma compared to radiotherapy alone.[179] Although this retrospective analysis was biased to favor combination therapy because patients with higher functional status and more limited brain metastases received more aggressive therapy, median survival of 18 months in the combination modality group suggests that aggressive palliation is beneficial in selected patients with brain metastases.

Hormonal Therapy

Hormonal therapy of ovarian epithelial cancers and tubal cancers has a long history of empirical use, but even though many of these malignancies have sex-steroid hormone receptors, response rates to various forms of hormonal manipulation have been disappointing. Taken together, progestins and antiestrogens have objective response rates of approximately 10% in patients with previously treated ovarian cancer, with an additional 20–30% of patients having stable disease.[231] Furthermore, a randomized trial of cisplatin-adriamycin with or without tamoxifen in patients with untreated epithelial ovarian cancer resulted in equivalent progression-free and overall survival in the two arms.[190] Gonadotropin-releasing hormone analogue therapy trials with leuprolide acetate and cyproterone acetate in women with previously treated ovarian cancer resulted in similar response rates of 17% and 7%, respectively.[95, 234] Although there have been anecdotal reports of response to hormonal therapy in women with tubal carcinomas, there are no trials that support significant activity for these agents in tubal cancers.

Despite the low response rates cited above, hormonal therapy of patients with epithelial ovarian or tubal cancer remains a reasonable option in women who have failed or cannot tolerate second-line chemotherapy. Medroxyprogesterone acetate (160 mg/day orally) has few side effects and often results in a subjective sense of well-being or stimulates appetite in these patients. Other histological types of ovarian malignancy do not respond to hormonal manipulation. Finally, there are no data to indicate that estrogen replacement therapy has an unfavorable effect on the survival of patients with epithelial ovarian carcinoma. Hormonal replacement is offered to premenopausal patients who have estrogen deficiency symptoms after ovarian removal.

Future Research

Clinical

The need for well-designed clinical trials in the clinical management of ovarian epithelial malignancies was emphasized in previous sections of this chapter. Some of the issues that need to be resolved include maturation of the results of studies randomizing patients with early disease to observation or P-32 versus platin-based chemotherapy, and integration of taxol into the management of patients with advanced disease. The role of primary adjuvant and consolidation treatment using modern techniques of radiotherapy and dose-intense chemotherapy with autologous hematological stem-cell support need to be evaluated in future randomized trials. The role of surgical debulking and radical lymphadenectomy at various points in the management of advanced-stage disease need to be studied further. Despite chemosensitivity of most primary epithelial ovarian malignancies, phase II trials will continue to be needed to identify agents with significant activity in patients with platin-resistant disease. As discussed below, determination of chemotherapy activity based on in vitro testing of the sensitivity of individual tumors to chemotherapeutic agents correlates to clinical responses in retrospective studies.[198] Prospective trials to determine whether in vitro chemosensitivity assays aid in the individualized selection of primary and salvage regimens are currently being conducted in the United States and Europe.

Due to small patient numbers, randomized trials of the management of germ cell and stromal cell malignancies are not possible. Phase II trials of management, based upon testicular chemotherapy regimens, will continue to be evaluated in patients with ovarian germ cell malignancies, and well-designed phase II trials are needed to identify active regimens in patients with stromal tumors. The small number of fallopian tubal malignancies limits the feasibility of conducting formal trials of treatment regimens outside of large multi-institutional settings; future management of patients with tubal cancer will continue to mirror the therapy of ovarian cancer because the tumor biology of these malignancies is so similar.

Basic Science

A comprehensive review of the current status of research on the molecular biology and immunology of ovarian carcinoma is beyond the scope of this chapter. Although identification of the breast ovarian cancer BRCA-1 and -2 genes may directly benefit only a few patients with familial epithelial malignancies, the advances in our understanding of the interactions of tumor suppressor and pro-motor genes may make genetic manipulation a feasible future treatment strategy for epithelial malignancies of the ovary and other sites.[153]

The largest family of oncogenes is comprised of tyrosine kinases.[153] A large proportion of tyro-sine kinases are transmembrane receptors for growth factors which function in the signal trans-duction for these growth factors. Binding with growth factors internalizes the protein-ligand complex and results in the phosporylation of tyrosines in a variety of intracellular proteins. This type of tyrosine kinase is down regulated after binding with its growth factor. In contrast, many of the tyrosine kinases produced by onco-genes are membrane associated (but do not func-tion as receptors) and are not down regulated by interaction with growth factors. HER-2/*neu* oncogene is typical for this type of oncogene. Expressed by approximately 30% of epithelial ovarian cancers,[7, 202] its expression is associated with a higher incidence of positive findings at second-look laparotomy and a worsened progno-sis.[7] Preliminary in vitro experiments suggest that anti-HER-2/*neu* antibodies inhibit anchor-age independence and proliferation of cells that express HER-2/*neu*.[153] Clinical trials of anti-HER-2/*neu* antibody are in progress.

Tumor suppressor genes encode proteins that result in an antiproliferative effect in cells. Loss of function in both alleles of a tumor suppressor gene appears to result in malignant transforma-tion.[153] The tumor suppressor gene most closely associated with epithelial gynecological malig-nancies is the p53 gene. The p53 tumor suppres-sor gene probably encodes a regulator of DNA transcription, and mutation or overexpression of this gene is observed in approximately one-third of epithelial ovarian cancers.[137, 160] Sequencing of the p53 gene raises the possibility of using intro-duction of wild-type p53 or inactivation of mu-tated p53 in malignant cells to produce redif-ferentiation.

The interactions of oncogenes and suppressor genes, and the function of native growth factors on the development of malignant are currently the subject of intense research. Furthermore, the mechanisms by which malignant cells invade normal tissues and produce metastasis are poor-ly understood. Research into the biology of tissue invasion and metastasis is in its infancy.

As noted previously, ovarian epithelial car-cinomas are initially sensitive to a variety of dif-ferent chemotherapeutic agents, but usually develop resistance or even cross-resistance to other drugs after repeated exposure to chemo-therapy. The mechanisms of membrane-associat-ed, intracellularly mediated, and nuclear-asso-ciated resistance are currently areas of intense research.[153] One promising avenue of research is investigating the use of buthionine sulfoximine (BSO) as an intracellular glutathione inhibitor to enhance response to platin chemotherapy. Elevated levels of glutathione correlate with cis-platin resistance in ovarian cancer cell lines.[6, 84] Based on in vitro studies,[71, 167] clinical phase I studies of BSO are being conducted.

In vitro testing for chemosensitivity (using the human tumor clonogenic assay) has been applied to ovarian malignancies since the 1970s.[1] Although modifications of this technique have a low evaluability rate (ranging between 40–70%), and retrospective analyses have been hampered by methodological difficulties, the positive and negative predictive values for correlation with response or resistance to subsequent chemo-therapy have ranged between 40–77% and 80–99%, respectively.[1, 17] Short-term radiolabeled DNA precursor uptake assays (using tritiated thy-midine or uridine), fluorescent cytoprint assays comparing serial photographic analysis of reten-tion of fluorescein before and after exposure to cytotoxic drugs, and ATP-bioluminescence assays have been developed in an attempt to overcome some of the limitations of the human tumor clonogenic assay.[198] Of these, the largest experi-ence with ovarian and other gynecological malig-nancies has been the ATP-bioluminescence assay.[198, 199]

The initial experience with this assay in 31 gynecological malignancies had a 100% correla-tion with response and a 75% correlation with resistance when results of the assay were compared with the clinical response, and at least one of the drugs tested in the assay was used in the subsequent chemotherapy regimen.[198] Evalu-ability of the assay appears to average 90% for primary and recurrent ovarian cancer.[198] This assay is undergoing prospective evaluation among ovarian cancer patients enrolled in a GOG primary chemotherapy trial in addition to evalu-ation as an adjunct for selection of drug(s) most likely to be active for individual patients who have not responded to initial therapy. In addition, there is currently an ongoing randomized trial in Switzerland testing this assay in primary ovarian carcinoma stage III and IV with promising preliminary results. Further potential applications include the evaluation of new cytotoxic agents using established cell lines or fresh tumor tissues prior to clinical testing.[99]

The development of modern molecular biology techniques has resulted in a greater understanding of the mechanisms of malignant transformation, tumor growth and metastasis, and the mechanisms of chemotherapeutic sensitivity and resistance in malignancies. However, more information in these areas of basic science is required before these have a significant impact on the clinical care of patients with ovarian and tubal malignancies.

References

1. Alberts DS, Chen HSG, Salmon SE et al. Chemotherapy of ovarian cancer directed by the human tumor stem cell asay. Cancer Chemother Pharmacol. 1981; 6:279–285.
2. Alberts DS, Green S, Hannigan EV et al. Improved therapeutic index of carboplatin plus cyclophosphamide verus cisplatin plus cyclophosphamide: Final report by Southwest Oncology Group of a phase III randomized trial in stages III and IV ovarian cancer. J Clin Oncol. 1992; 10:706–717.
3. Bajorin DF, Sarosdy MF, Bosl GJ et al. A randomized trial of etoposide plus carboplatin versus etoposide plus cisplatin in patients with metastatic germ cell tumors. J Clin Oncol. 1993; 11:598–607.
4. Barnes W, Johnson J, Waggoner S et al. Reverse hysterocolposigmoidectomy (RHCS) for resection of panpelvic tumors. Gynecol Oncol. 1991; 42:151–155.
5. Bast RC Jr, Klug TL, St John E et al. A radioimmunoassay using a monoclonal antibody to monitor the course of epithelial ovarian cancer. N Engl J Med. 1983; 309:883–887.
6. Batist G, Behrens B, Makuch R et al. Serial determinations of glutathione levels and glutathione related enzyme activities in human tumor cells in vitro. Biochem Pharmacol. 1986; 35:2257–2259.
7. Berchuck A, Kamel A, Whitaker R et al. Overexpression of HER-2/neu is associated with poor survival in advanced epithelial ovarian cancer. Cancer Res. 1990; 50:4087–4091.
8. Berek JS, Hacker NF, Lagasse LD et al. Survival of patients following secondary cytoreductive surgery in ovarian cancer. Obstet Gynecol. 1983; 61:189–197.
9. Berek JS, Hacker NF, Lagasse LD. Rectosigmoid resection colectomy and reanastomosis to facilitate resection of primary and recurrent gynecologic cancer. Obstet Gynecol. 1984; 64:715–720.
10. Bjorkholm E, Silfversward C. Prognostic factors in granulosa cell tumors. Gynecol Oncol. 1981; 11:261–268.
11. Bolis G, Colombo N, Favalli G et al. Randomized multicenter clinical trial in stage I epithelial ovarian cancer. Proc Am Soc Clin Oncol. 1992; 11:225.
12. Blythe JG, Wahl TP. Debulking surgery: Does it increase the quality of survival? Gynecol Oncol. 1982; 14:396–408.
13. Boente MP, Godwin AD, Hogan WM. Screening, imaging, and early diagnosis of ovarian cancer. Clin Obstet Gynecol. 1994; 37:377–391.
14. Boring CC. Cancer statistics, 1993. CA 1993; 43:7–50.
15. Bostwick DG, Tazelaar HD, Ballon SC et al. Ovarian epithelial tumors of borderline malignancy. Cancer. 1986; 58:2052–2065.
16. Bourne T, Campbell S, Steer C et al. Transvaginal color flow imagery: A possible new screening technique for ovarian cancer. Brit Med J. 1989; 299:1367–1370.
17. Bradley EC, Issell BF, Hellman R. The human tumor colony-forming assay: a biologic and clinical review. Invest New Drugs. 1984; 2:59–70.
18. Brand E, Pearlman N. Electrosurgical debulking of ovarian cancer: a new technique using the argon beam coagulator. Gynecol Oncol. 1990; 39:115–119.
19. Buchsbaum HJ, Brady MF, Delgado G et al. Surgical staging of carcinoma of the ovaries. Surg Gynecol Obstet. 1989; 169:226–232.
20. Burghart E, Hellmuth P, Lahousen M et al. Pelvic lymphadenectomy in operative treatment of ovarian cancer. Am J Obstet Gynecol. 1986; 155:315–321.
21. Burns BL, Rutledge F, Smith JP et al. Management of ovarian carcinoma. Am J Obstet Gynecol. 1967; 98:374–382.
22. Buttram VC, Vaquero C. Post-ovarian wedge resection adhesive disease. Fertil Steril. 1975; 26:874–878.
23. Byrne J, Mulvihill JJ, Meyers MH et al. Effects of treatment on fertility in long-term survivors of childhood or adolescent cancer. N Engl J Med. 1987; 317:1315–1318.
24. Cain J, Saigo P, Piersce V et al. A review of second look laparotomy for ovarian cancer. Gynecol Oncol. 1986; 23:14–20.
25. Calvert AH, Newell DR, Gumbrell LA et al. Carboplatin doseage: Prospective evaluation of a simple formula based on renal function. J Clin Oncol. 1989; 7:1748–1756.
26. Carlson RW, Sikic BI, Turbow MM et al. Combination cisplatin, vinblastine, and bleomycin chemotherapy (PVB) for malignant germ cell tumors of the ovary. J Clin Oncol. 1983; 1:645–651.
27. Carmichael JA, Shelley WE, Brown LB et al. A predictive index of cure versus no cure in advanced ovarian carcinoma patients–Replacement of second-look laparotomy as a dignostic test. Gynecol Oncol. 1987; 269–278.

28. Castaldo TW, Petrilli ES, Ballon SC et al. Intestinal operations in patients with ovarian carcinoma. Am J Obstet Gynecol. 1981; 139:80–84.
29. Chambers JT, Merino MS, Kohorn EI et al. Borderline ovarian tumors. Am J Obstet Gynecol. 1988; 159:1088–1094.
30. Chambers SK, Chambers JT, Kohorn EI et al. Evaluation of the role of second-look surgery in ovarian cancer. Obstet Gynecol. 1988; 72:404–410.
31. Chapman RM, Sutcliffe SB, Malpas JS. Cytotoxic-induced ovarian failure in women with Hodgkin's disease. I. Hormonal function. JAMA. 1979; 1877–1882.
32. Childers JM, Hatch KD, Tran A-N et al. Laparoscopic para-aortic lymphadenectomy in gynecologic malignancies. Obstet Gynecol. 1993; 82:741–747.
33. Clarke-Person DL, Chin NO, DeLong ER et al. Surgical management of intestinal obstruction in ovarian cancer: Clinical festures, postoperative complications, and survival. Gynecol Oncol. 1987; 26:11–18.
34. Clarke-Person DL, DeLong ER, Chin NO et al. Intestinal obstruction in patients with ovarian cancer: Variables associated with surgical complications and survival. Arch Surg. 1988; 123:42–45.
35. Clarke-Person DL, Kohler MF, Hurteau JA et al. Surgery for advanced ovarian cancer. Clin Obstet Gynecol. 1994; 37:439–460.
36. Colombo N, Sessa C, Landoni F et al. Cisplatin, vinblastine, and bleomycin combination chemotherapy in metastatic granulosa cell tumor of the ovary. Obstet Gynecol. 1986; 67:265–268.
37. Colombo N, Bonazzi C, Chiari S et al. Fertility in young patients after limited surgery with or without chemotherapy for ovarian tumors. In: Meerphol HG, Pfleiderer A, Profous ChZ (eds). Das Ovarialkarzinom, 2 Therapie. Springer-Verlag, Berlin, 1993; pp 24–30.
38. Colon-Otero G, Malkasian G, Edmonson JH. Secondary myelodysplasia and acute leukemia following carboplatin-containing chemotherapy for ovarian cancer. J Natl Cancer Inst. 1993; 85:1858–1859.
39. Copeland LJ, Gershenson DM, Sharton JT et al. Microscopic disease at second-look laparotomy in advanced ovarian cancer. Cancer. 1985; 55:472–480.
40. Creasman WT, Soper JT. Assessment of the contemporary management of germ cell malignancies of the ovary. Am J Obstet Gynecol. 1985; 153:828–836.
41. Creasman WT. Evaluation of debulking surgery at second-look laparotomy. In: Sharp F, Mason WP, and Creasman WT (eds): OVARIAN CANCER. Chapman and Hall Medical, London 1992; 375–383.
42. Currie JL, Bagne F, Harris C et al. Radioactive chomic phosphate suspension: Studies on distribution, dose absorbtion and effective therapeutic radiation in phantoms, dogs, and patients. Gynecol Oncol. 1981; 12:193–218.
43. Decker DG, Fleming TR, Malkasian GD. Cyclophosphamide plus cisplatin in combination: Treatment program for stage III or IV ovarian carcinoma. Obstet Gynecol. 1982; 60:481–487.
44. Dembo AJ, Bush RS, Beale FA et al. The princess Margaret Hospital study of ovarian cancer: Stage I, II, and asymptomatic III presentations. Cancer Treat Rep. 1979; 63:249–254.
45. Dembo AJ, Bush RS, Beale FA et al. A randomized clinical trial of moving strip versus open fiel whole abdominal irradiation in patients with invasive epithelial cancer of the ovary. Int J Radiat Oncol Biol Phys. 1983; 9:97–104.
46. Dembo A, Davy M, Stenwig AE et al. Prognostic factors in patients with stage I epithelial ovarian cancer. Obstet Gynecol. 1990; 75:263–273.
47. Deppe G, Malviya VK, Boike G et al. Use of Cavitron surgical aspirator for debulking of diaphragm metastases in patients with advanced carcinoma of the ovaries. Surg Gynecol Obstet. 1989; 168:455–458.
48. Dottino PR, Plaxe SC, Cohen CJ. A phase II trial of adjuvant cisplatin and doxorubicin in stage I epithelial ovarian cancer. Gynecol Oncol. 1991; 43:203–205.
49. Edmonson J. Phase II evaluation of VP-16213 (NSC 141540) in patients with advanced ovarian carcinoma resistant to alkylating agents. Gynecol Oncol. 1978; 6:7–9.
50. Edmonson JH, McCormack GM, Wieand HS et al. Cyclophosphamide-cisplatin versus cyclophosphamide carboplatin in stage III–IV ovarian cancer: A comparison of equally myelosuppressive regimens. J Natl Cancer Inst. 1989; 81:1500–1504.
51. Ehrlich CE, Einhorn L, Williams SD et al. Chemotherapy for stage III–IV epithelial ovarian cancer with cis-dichlorodiamine-platinum (II), adriamycin, and cyclophosphamide: A preliminary report. Cancer Treat Rep. 1979; 63:282–288.
52. Evans AF III, Gaffey TA, Malkasian GD Jr et al. Clinicopathologic review of 118 granulosa and 82 theca tumors. Obstet Gynecol. 1980; 55:231–236.
52a. Fernandes JR, Seymour RJ, Suissa S. Bowel obstruction in patients with ovarian cancer: a search for prognostic factors. Am J Obstet Gynecol. 1988; 158(2):244–249.
53. Finkler NJ, Benacerraf B, Lavin PT et al. Comparison of serum CA 125, clinical impression, and ultrasound in the preoperative evaluation of ovarian masses. Obstet Gynecol. 1988; 72:659–664.
54. Fox H, Agrawal K, Langley FA. A clinicopathologic study of 92 cases of granulosa cell tumor of the ovary with special reference to the factors influencing prognosis. Cancer. 1975; 35:231–242.
55. Freidman JB, Weiss NS. Sounding board. Second thoughts about second-look laparotomy. N Engl J Med. 1990; 322:1079–1080.
56. Gerbie MV, Brewer JI, Tamimi U. Primary choriocarcinoma of the ovary. Obstet Gynecol. 1975; 46:720–728.

57. Gershenson DM, Copeland JL, Del Junco G et al. Second-look laparotomy in the management of malignant germ cell tumors of the ovary. Obstet Gynecol. 1986; 67: 789–794.

58. Gershenson DM, Kavanaugh JJ, Copeland JL et al. Treatment of malignant nondysgerminomatous germ cell tumors of the ovary with vinblastine, bleomycin, and cisplatin. Cancer. 1986; 57: 1731–1737.

59. Gershenson DM, Copeland JL, Kavanagh JJ et al. Treatment of metastatic stromal tumor of the ovary with cisplatin, doxorubicin, and cyclophosphamide. Obstet Gynecol. 1987; 70: 765–769.

60. Gershenson DM. Menstrual and reproductive function after treatment with combination chemotherapy for malignant ovarian germ cell tumors. J Clin Oncol. 1988; 6: 270–275.

61. Gershenson DM, Morris M, Cangir A et al. Treatment of malignant germ cell tumors of the ovary with bleomycin etoposide, and cisplatin. J Clin Oncol. 1990; 8: 715–720.

62. Goldie JH, Coldman AJ. A mathematical model for relating the drug sensitivity of tumors to their spontaneous mutation rate. Cancer Treat Rep. 1979; 63: 1727–1735.

63. Goldstein SR, Subramanyam B, Snyder JR et al. Postmenopausal cystic adnexal mass: The potential role of ultrasound in conservative management. Obstet Gynecol. 1989; 73: 8–12.

64. Gordon A, Lipton D, Woodruff JD. Dysgerminoma: A review of 158 cases from the Emil Novak Ovarian Tumor registry. Obstet Gynecol. 1981; 58: 497–504.

65. Granberg S, Norstrom A, Wikland M. Comparison of endovaginal ultrasound and cytological evaluation of cystic ovarian tumors. J Ultrsound Med. 1991; 10: 9–14.

66. Green MH, Boice JD Jr, Greer BE et al. Acute non-lymphocytic leukeima after therapy with alkylating agents for ovarian cancer: A study of five randomized clinical trials. N Engl J Med. 1982; 307: 1416–1421.

67. Griffiths CT. Surgical resection of tumor bulk in the primary treatment of ovarian cancer. Monogr Natl Cancer Inst. 1975; 42: 101–104.

68. Guthrie D, Davy MLJ, Phillips PR. Study of 656 patients with "early" ovarian cancer. Gynecol Oncol. 1984; 17: 363–375.

69. Hacker NF, Berek JS, Brunison CM et al. Whole abdominal radiation therapy as salvage therapy for epithelial ovarian cancer. Obstet Gynecol. 1985; 65: 60–66.

70. Hainsworth JD, Malcolm A, Johnson DH et al. Advanced minimal residual ovarian cancer: Abdominopelvic irradiation following combination chemotherapy. Obstet Gynecol. 1983, 61: 619–625.

71. Hamilton T, Winker M, Louie K. Augmentation of melphalan, adriamycin, and cisplatin cytotoxicity in drug-resistant and – sensitive human ovarian cancer cell lines by buthione sulfoximine mediated glutathione depletion. Biochem Pharmacol. 1985; 34: 2583–2586.

72. Hart WR, Norris HJ. Borderline and malinant mucinous tumors of the ovary. Histologic criteria and clinical behavior. Cancer. 1973; 31: 1031–1043.

73. Hawkis RE, Roberts K, Wiltshaw E et al. The prognostic significance of the half-life of serum CA-125 in patients responding to chemotherapy for epithelial ovarian carcinoma. Br J Obstet Gynecol. 1989; 96: 1395–1398.

74. Hellstrom A-C, Silfversward C, Nilsson B, Pettersson. Carcinoma of the fallopian tube. A clinical and histopathologic review. The Radiumhemmet series. Int J Gynecol Cancer. 1994; 4: 395–400.

75. Henderson SR, Harper RC, Salazar OM et al. Primary carcinoma of the fallopian tube: Difficulties in diagnosis and treatment. Gynecol Oncol. 1977; 5: 168–175.

76. Herrmann UJ, Locher GW, Goldhirsch A. Sonographic patterns of ovarian tumors: Prediction of malignancy. Obstet Gynecol. 1987; 69: 777–781.

77. Hillcoat BL. Phase II evaluation of VP-16213 in advanced ovarian carcinoma. Gynecol Oncol. 1985; 22: 162–166.

78. Hoskins PJ, O'Reilly SE, Swenerton KD et al. Ten-year outcome of patients with advanced epithelial ovarian carcinoma treated with cisplatin-based multimodality therapy. Jclin Oncol. 1992; 10: 1561–1568.

79. Hoskins WJ, Lichter AS, Whittington R et al. Whole abdominal and pelvic radiation in patients with minimal disease at second-look surgical reassessment for ovarian cancer. Gynecol Oncol. 1985; 20: 271–277.

80. Hoskins WJ, Rubin SC, Dulaney E et al. Influence of secondary cytoreduction at the time of second-look laparotomy on the survival of patients with epithelial ovarian carcinoma. Gynecol Oncol. 1989; 34: 365–370.

81. Hoskins WJ, Bundy BN, Thigpen JT et al. The influence of cytoreductive surgery on recurrence-free interval and survival in small-volume stage III epithelial ovarian cancer: A Gynecologic Oncology Group study. Gynecol Oncol. 1992; 47: 159–166.

82. Hoskins WJ, Bundy WP, Brody MF et al. The effect of diameter of larger residual disease on survival after primary cytoreductive surgery in patients with suboptimal residual epithelial ovarian carcinoma. Am J Obstet Gynecol. 1994, 170: 974–979.

83. Hoskins WJ. Surgical staging and cytoreductive surgery of epithelial ovarian cancer. Cancer. 1993: 71s: 1534–1540.

84. Hosking L, Whelan R, Shellard S et al. An enaluation of the role of glutathione and its associated enzymes in the expression of differential sensitivities to antitumor agents shown by a range of human tumour cell types. Biochem Pharmacol. 1990; 40: 1833–1842.

85. Houlston RS. Genetic epidemiology of ovarian cancer: Segregation analysis. Ann Hum Genet. 1991; 55: 291–297.

86. Hreshchyschyn MM, Park R, Blessing JA et al. The role of adjuvant therapy in stage I ovarian cancer. Am J Obstet Gynecol. 1980; 138: 139–145.

87. Hudson CN. Surgical treatment of ovarian cancer. Gynecol Oncol. 1973; 1:370–375.

88. Hunter RW, Alexander NDE, Soutter WP. Meta-analysis of surgery in advanced ovarian carcinoma: Is maximum cytoreductive surgery an independent determinant of prognosis? Am J Obstet Gynecol. 1992; 166:504–510.

89. Hunter VJ, Daly L, Helms M et al. The prognostic significance of CA 125 half-life in patients with ovarian cancer who have received primary chemotherapy after surgical cytoreduction. Gynecol Oncol. 1990; 36:1164–1167.

90. International Federation of Obstetrics and Gynecology: FIGO revised staging for ovarian cancer. Am J Obstet Gynecol. 1989; 156:263–264.

91. Jacobs AJ, Deppe G, Cohen CJ. Combination chemotherapy of ovarian granulosa cell tumors with cis-platinum and doxorubicin. Gynecol Oncol. 1982; 14:294–300.

92. Jacobs AJ, McMurray EH, Parham J et al. Treatment of carcinoma of the fallopian tube using cisplatin, doxorubicin, and cyclophosphamide. Am J Clin Oncol. 1986; 9:436–442.

93. Jacobs I, Oram D, Fairbanks J et al. A risk of malignancy index incorporating CA-125, ultrasound and menopausal status for accurate preoperative diagnosis of ovarian cancer. Brit J Obstet Gynaecol. 1990; 97:922–929.

94. Janicke F, Holscher M, Kuhn W et al. Radical surgical procedure improves survival time in patients with recurrent ovarian cancer. Cancer. 1992; 70:2129–2136.

95. Kavanagh JJ, Roberts W, Townsend P et al. Leuprolide acetate in the treatment of refractory or persistent epithelial ovarian cancer. J Clin Oncol. 1989; 7:115–120.

96. Kaye SB, Lewis CR, Paul J et al. Randomized study of two doses of cisplatin and cyclophosphamide in epithelial ovarian cancer. Lancet. 1992; 340:329–333.

97. Kerlikowske K, Brown JS, Grody DG. Should women with familial ovarian cancer undergo prophylactic oophorectomy? Obstet Gynecol. 1992; 80:700–707.

98. Kistner RW. Peritubal and peri-ovarian adhesions subsequent to wedge resection of the ovaries. Fertil Steril. 1969; 20:35–41.

99. Koechli OR, Sevin B-U, Haller U (eds). Chemosensitivity Testing in Gynecologic Malignancies and Breast Cancer. Basel, Karger, 1994.

100. Kohn E, Reed E, Link C et al. A pilot study of taxol, cisplatin, cyclophosphamide and GCSF in newly-diagnosed stage III/IV ovarian cancer patients. Proc Am Soc Clin Oncol. 1993; 12: 257.

101. Kong JS, Peters LJ, Wharton JT et al. Hyperfracionated split-course whole abdominal radiotherapy for ovarian carcinoma: Tolerance and toxicity. Int J Radiat Oncol Biol Phys. 1988; 14: 737–745.

102. Klassen D, Shelley W, Staareveld A et al. Early stage ovarian cancer: A randomized clinical trial comparing whole abdominal radiotherapy, melphalan, and intraperitoneal chromic phosphate: A National Cancer Institute of Canada clinical trials group report. J Clin Oncol. 1988; 1254–1263.

103. Kliman L, Rome RM, Fortuen DW. Low malignant potential tumors of the ovary: a study of 76 cases. Obstet Gynecol. 1986; 68:338–346.

104. Krebs HB, Gopelrud DR. Surgical management of bowel obstruction in advanced ovarian carcinoma. Obstet Gynecol. 1983; 61:327–330.

105. Krebs HB, Gopelrud DR. The role of intestinal intubation in obstruction of the small intestine due to carcinoma of the ovary. Surg Gynecol Obstet. 1984; 158:467–471.

106. Krebs H, Gopelrud ER, Kilpatrick SJ et al. Role of CA 125 as tumor marker in ovarian carcinoma. Obstet Gynecol. 1986; 67:473–480.

107. Krepart G, Smith JP, Rutlege F et al. The treatment for dysgerminoma of the ovary. Cancer. 1978; 41:986–990.

108. Krigman H, Bentley R, Robboy SJ. Pathology of epithelial ovarian tumors. Clin Obstet Gynecol. 1994; 37:475–491.

109. Kuehnle H. Etoposide in cisplatin-refractory ovarian cancer. Proc Am Soc Clin Oncol. 1988; 7:137–145.

110. Kurjak A, Zalud I, Jurkovic D et al. Transvaginal color Doppler for the assessment of pelvic circulation. Acta Obstet Gynecol Scand. 1989; 68:131–135.

111. Kurman RJ, Norris HJ. Embryonal carcinoma of the ovary: a clinicopathologic entitiy distinct from endodermal sinus tumor resembling embryonal carcinoma of the adult testis. Cancer. 1976; 38:2420–2425.

112. Kurman RJ, Norris HJ. Endodermal sinus tumor of the ovary: A clinical and pathological analysis of 71 cases. Cancer. 1976; 38:2204–2219.

113. Kurman RJ, Norris HJ. Malignant mixed germ cell tumors of the ovary: A clinical and pathologic analysis of 30 cases. Obstet Gynecol. 1976; 48:579–587.

114. Kurman RJ, Scardino PT, Waldman TA et al. Malignant germ cell tumors of the ovary and testis: An immunologic study of 69 cases. Ann Clin Lab Sci. 1979; 9:462–465.

115. Kuwai M, Kano T, Kikkawa F et al. Transvaginal Doppler ultrasound with color flow imaging in the diagnosis of ovarian cancer. Obstet Gynecol. 1992; 79:163–167.

116. Lack EE, Perez-Atayde AR, Murthy ASK et al. Granulosa theca cell tumors in premenarchal girls: A clinical and pathologica study in ten cases. Cancer. 1981; 48:1846–1854.

117. Lapolla JP, Benda J, Vigliotti AP et al. Dysgerminoma of the ovary. Obstet Gynecol. 1987; 70:268–275.

118. Lawton F, Luesley D, Blackledge G et al. A randomized trial comparing whole abdominal radiotherapy with chemotherapy following cisplatinum cytoreduction in epithelial ovarian cancer. West Midlands Ovarian Cancer Group Trial II. J Clin Oncol. 1990; 2:4–10.

119. Lawton FG, Redman CW, Luesley DM et al. Neo-adjuant (cytoreductive) chemotherapy combined with intervention debulking surgery in advanced, unresected epithelial ovarian cancer. Obstet Gynecol. 1989; 73:61–65.

120. Leake JF, Rader RS, Woodruff JD et al. Retroperitoneal lymphatic involvement with epithelial ovarian tumors of low malignant potential Gynecol Oncol. 1991; 42:124–130.

121. Levin L, Hyrniuk WM. Dose intensity analysis of chemotherapy regimens in ovarian carcinoma. J Clin Oncol. 1987; 5:756–757.

122. Levin L, Simon R, Hryniuk WM. Importance of multi-agent chemotherapy regimens in ovarian carcinoma: Dose intensity analysis. J Natl Cancer Inst. 1993; 85:1732–1742.

123. Lim-Tan SK, Cajigas HE, Scully RE. Ovarian cystectomy for serous borderline tumors: A follow-up study of 35 cases. Obstet Gynecol. 1988; 72:775–780.

124. Lippman SM, Alberts DS, Slaymen DJ et al. Second-look laparotomy in epithelial ovarian carcinoma. Prognostic factors associated with survival duration. Cancer. 1988; 61:2571–2578.

125. Loehrer PJ, Lauer R, Roth BJ et al. Salvage therapy with VP-16 or vinblastine plus iphosphamide plus cisplatin in recurrent germ cell cancer. J Clin Oncol. 1988; 109:540–546.

126. Loehrer PJ, Elson P, Johnson DH et al. A randomized trial of cisplatin plus etoposide with or without bleomycin in favorable prognosis disseminated germ cell cancer: An ECOG study. Proc Am Soc Clin Oncol. 1991; 10:540.

127. Luesley DM, Chan KK, Fielding JW et al. Second-look laparotomy in the management of epithelial ovarian carcinoma: An evaluation of fifty cases. Obstet Gynecol. 1984; 64:421–427.

128. Lund B, Hansen M, Lundvall F et al. Intestinal obstruction in patients with advanced carcinoma of the ovaries treated with combination chemotherapy. Surg Gynecol Obstet. 1989; 169:213–218.

129. Lund B, Williamson P. Prognostic factors four outcome and survival in patients with advanced ovarian carcinoma. Obstet Gynecol. 1990; 76:617–623.

130. Luxman D, Bergman A, Sagi J et al. The postmenopausal mass: Correlation between ultrasonic and pathologic findings. Obstet Gynecol. 1991; 77:726–728.

131. Malone JM, Koonce T, Larson DM et al. Palliation of small bowel obstruction by percutaneous gastrostomy in patients with ovarian carcinoma. Obstet Gynecol. 1986; 68:431–433.

132. Malkasian GD, Knapp RC, Lavin PT et al. Preoperative evaluation of serum CA 125 levels in premenopausal and postmenopausal patients with pelvic masses: Discrimination of benign from malignant disease. Am J Obstet Gynecol. 1988; 159:341–347.

133. Manetta A, MacNeill C, Lyter JA et al. Hexamethylmelamine as a single second-line agent in ovarian cancer. Gynecol Oncol. 1990; 36:93–96.

134. Markman M, Rothman R, Reichman B et al. Second line platinum therapy in patients with ovarian cancer previously treated with cisplatin. J Clin Oncol. 1991; 9:389–393.

135. Markman M, Berek JB, Blessing JA et al. Characteristics of patients with small-volume residual ovarian cancer unresponsive to cisplatin-based chemotherapy: Lessons learned from a Gynecologic Oncology Group phase II trial of ip cisplatin and recombinatn a-interferon. Gynecol Oncol. 1992; 45:3–8.

136. Markman M, Hakes T, Reichman B et al. Ifosfamide and mesna in previously treated advanced ovarian cancer: Activity in platinum-resistant disease. J Clin Oncol. 1992; 10:243–248.

137. Marks JR, Davidoff AM, Kerns BJ et al. Overexpression and mutation of p53 in epithelial ovarian cancer. Cancer Res. 1991; 51:2979–2964.

138. Massad LS, Hunter VJ, Szpak CA et al. Epithelial ovarian tumors of low malignant potential. Obstet Gynecol. 1991; 78:1027–1032.

139. Maxon WZ, Stehman FB, Ulbright TM et al. Primary carcinoma of the fallopian tube. Evidence for activity of cisplatin combinatin therapy. Gynecol Oncol. 1987; 26:305–310.

140. McGowan L, Lesher LP, Norris HJ et al. Misstaging of ovarian cancer. Obstet Gynecol. 1985; 65:568–573.

141. McGuire WP, Rowinsky EK, Rosenshein NB et al. Taxol: A unique antineoplastic agent with significant activity in advanced ovarian epithelial neoplasms. Ann Intern Med. 1989; 111:273–279.

142. McGuire WP, Hoskins WJ, Brady MF et al. A phase III trial of dose-intense versus standard dose cisplatin and cytoxan in advanced ovarian cancer. Proc Am Soc Clin Oncol. 1992; 11:226.

143. McGuire WP, Hoskins WJ, Brady MF et al. A phase III trial comparing cisplatin/cytoxan and cisplatin/taxol in advanced ovarian cancer. Proc Am Soc Clin Oncol. 1993; 12:225.

144. McKenzei RS, Alberts DA, Bishop MR et al. Phase I trail of high-dose cyclophosphamide, mitoxantrone, and carboplatin with autologous bone marrow transplantation in female malignancies: Pharmacologic levels of mitoxantrone and high response rate in refractory ovarian cancer. Proc Am Soc Clin Oncol. 1991; 10:186.

145. Meire HB, Farrant P, Guha T. Distinction of benign from malignant ovarian cysts by ultrasound. Brit J Obstet Gynaecol. 1978; 85:893–899.

146. Michel G, Zarea D, Castigne D et al. Cytoreductive surgery in ovarian cancer. Eur J Surg Oncol. 1989; 15:201–204.

147. Monga M, Carmichael JA, Shelley WE et al. Surgery without adjuvant chemotherapy for early epithelial ovarian carcinoma after comprehensive surgical staging. Gynecol Oncol. 1991; 43:195–197.

148. Morgan L, Chafe W, Mendenhall W et al. Hyperfractionation of whole-abdomen radiation therapy: Salvage treatment of persistent ovarian carcinoma following chemotherapy. Gynecol Oncol. 1988; 31:122–129.

149. Morris M, Gershenson D, Wharton T et al. Secondary cytoreductive surgery in epithelial ovarian cancer: Nonresponders to first-line therapy. Gynecol Oncol. 1989; 33 : 1 – 5.

150. Morris M, Gershenson D, Wharton T et al. Secondary cytoreductive surgery for recurrent epithelial ovarian cancer. Gynecol Oncol. 1989; 34 : 334 – 338.

151. Moyle JW, Rochester D, Sider L et al. Sonography of ovarian tumors: Predictability of tumor type. Am J Roentgenol. 1983; 141 : 985 – 991.

152. Munnell EW. The changing prognosis and treatment in cancer of the ovary: A report of 235 patients with primary ovarian cancer 1952 – 1961. Am J Obstet Gynecol. 1968; 100 : 790 – 805.

153. Mutch DG, Williams S. Biology of epithelial ovarian cancer. Clin Obstet Gynecology. 1994; 37 : 406 – 422.

154. Neijt JP, ten Bokkel-Huinink WW. Randomized trial comparing two combination chemotherapy regimens (HEXA-CAF versus CHAP-5) in advanced ovarian carcinoma. Lancet. 1984; 2 : 594 – 600.

155. Neijt J, ten Bokkel-Huinink WW, van der Berg et al. Randomized trial comparing two combination chemotherapy regimens (CHAP-5 vs CP) in advanced ovarian carcinoma. J Clin Oncol. 1987; 5 : 1157 – 1168.

156. Nelson BE, Rosenfield AT, Schwartz PE. Preoperative abdominopelvic computed tomographic prediction of optimal cytoreduction in epithelial ovarian carcinoma. J Clin Oncol. 1993; 11 : 166 – 172.

157. Nicosi SV, Matus-Ridley M, Meadows AT. Gonadal effects of cancer therapy in girls. Cancer. 1985; 55 : 2364 – 2369.

158. Nichols CR, Tricot G, Williams SD et al. Dose-intensive chemotherapy in refractory germ cell cancer: A phase I/II trial of high-dose carboplatin and etoposide with autologous bone marrow transplantatin. Ann Intern Med. 1989; 7 : 932 – 939.

159. Norris HJ, Zirkin HJ, Benson WL. Immature (malignant) teratoma of the ovary: a clinical and pathologic study of 58 cases. Cancer. 1976.; 37 : 2359 – 2365.

160. Okamoto A, Sameshima Y, Yokoyama S et al. Frequent allelic losses and mutations of the p53 gene in human ovarian cancer. Cancer Res. 1991; 51 : 5171 – 5176.

161. Omura GA, Bundy BN, Berek JS et al. Randomized trial of cyclophosphamide plus cisplatin with or without doxorubicin in ovarian carcinoma: A GOG study. J Clin Oncol. 1989; 7 : 457 – 465.

162. Ozols R, Louie K, Plowma et al. Enhanced melphalan cytotoxicity in human ovarian cancer in vitro and in tumor bearing nude mice by butothione sulfoximine depletion of glutathione. Biochem Pharmacol. 1987; 36 : 147 – 153.

163. Ozols R. Intraperitoneal salvage chemotherapy in ovarian cancer: Who is left to treat? Gynecol Oncol. 1992; 45 : 1 – 2.

164. Ozols RF, Kilpatrick D, O'Dwyer P et al. Phase I and pharmacokinetic study of taxol and carboplatin

165. Parker RT, Parker CH, Wilbanks GD. Cancer of the ovary: Survival studies based on operative therapy, chemotherapy, and radiotherapy. Am J Obstet Gynecol. 1970; 108 : 878 – 888.

166. Peters WA, Anderson WA, Hopkins MP. Results of chemotherapy in advanced carcinoma of the fallopian tube. Cancer. 1989; 63 : 836 – 838.

167. Peters WA, Anderson WA, Hopkins MP et al. Prognostic features of carcinoma of the fallopian tube. Obstet Gynecol. 1988; 71 : 757 – 762.

168. Peters WP: personal communication, 1994.

169. Piver MS, Barlow JJ, Lele SB. Incidence of sublcinical metastases in stage I and II ovarian carcinoma. Obstet Gynecol. 1978; 52 : 100 – 104.

170. Piver MS, Maltefano J, Baker TR et al. Adjuvant cisplatin-based chemotherapy for stage I ovarian adenocarcinoma: A preliminary report. Gynecol Oncol. 1989; 35 : 69 – 72.

171. Piver MS, Maltefano J, Hempling RE et al. Cisplatin-based chemotherapy for stage II ovarian adenocarcinoma: A preliminary report. Gynecol Oncol. 1990; 39 : 249 – 252.

172. Podczaski ES, Stevens CJ, Manetta A et al. Use of second look laparotomy in the management of patients with epithelial ovarian malignancies. Gynecol Oncol. 1987; 28 : 205 – 214.

173. Podratz KC, Podczaski ES, Gaffey TA et al. Primary carcinoma of the fallian tube. Am J Obstet Gynecol. 1986; 254 : 1319 – 1330.

174. Podratz KC, Schray MF, Wieand HA et al. Evaluation of treatment and survival after positive second-look laparotomy. Gynecol Oncol. 1988; 31 : 9 – 21.

175. Purola E, Nieminen U. Does rupture of cystic carcinoma during operation influence the prognosis? Ann Chir Gynaecol Fenn. 1968; 57 : 615 – 617.

176. Requard CK, Mettler FA, Wicks JD. Preoperative sonography of malignant ovarian neoplasms. Am J Radiol. 1981; 137 : 79 – 82.

177. Reich H, McGlynn F, Wilkie W. Laparoscopic management of stage I ovarian cancer: A case report. J Reprod Med. 1990; 35 : 601 – 605.

178. Robinson WR, Curtin JP, Morrow CP. Operative staging and conservative surgery in the management of low malignant potential ovarian tumors. Int J Gynecol Cancer. 1992; 113 – 118.

179. Rodriguez GC, Soper JT, Berchuck A et al. Improved palliation of cerebral metastases in epithelial ovarian cancer using a combined modality approach including radiation therapy, chemotherapy, and surgery. J Clin Oncol. 1992; 10 : 1553 – 1560.

180. Rosenschein NB, Leichner PK, Vogelsang G. Radiocolloids in the treatment of ovarian cancer. Obstet Gynecol Surv. 1979; 34 : 708 – 720.

181. Roth LM, Anderson MC, Gocan ADT et al. Sertoli-Leydig cell tumors: A clinicopathologic study of 34 cases. Cancer. 1981; 48 : 187 – 199.

182. Rowinsky EK, Gilbert M, McGuire WP et al. Sequences of taxol adn cisplatin: A phase I and

in previously untreated patients with advanced ovarian cancer: A pilot study of the GOG. Proc Am Soc Clin Oncol. 1993; 12 : 259.

pharmacologic study. J Clin Oncol. 1991; 9:1692–1703.

183. Rubin SC, Hoskins WJ, Hakes TB et al. Recurrence after negative second look laparotomy for ovarian cancer: Analysis of risk factors. Am J Obstet Gynecol. 1988; 159:1094.

184. Rubin SC, Hoskins WJ, Benjamin I et al. Palliative surgery for intestinal obstruction in advanced ovarian cancer. Gynecol Oncol. 1989; 34:16–19.

185. Rubin SC, Jones WB, Curtin JP et al. Second-look laparotomy in stage I ovarian cancer following comprehensive surgical staging. Obstet Gynecol. 1993; 82:139–142.

186. Rubin SC, Wong GYC, Curtin JP et al. Platinum-based chemotherapy of high-risk stage I epithelial ovarian cancer following comprehensive surgical staging. Obstet Gynecol. 1993; 82:143–147.

187. Rulin MC, Preston AL. Adnexal masses in postmenopausal women. Obstet Gynecol. 1987; 70:578–581.

188. Samanth KK, Black WC. Benign ovarian stromal tumors associated with free peritoneal fluid. Am J Obstet Gynecol. 1970; 107:538–548.

189. Sarosy G, Kohn E, Link C et al. Taxol dose intensification in patients with recurrent ovarian cancer. Proc Am Soc Cancer Res. 1992; 11:226.

190. Schwartz PE. Combination chemotherapy in the management of ovarian germ cell malignancies. Obstet Gynecol. 1984; 64:564–572.

191. Schwartz PE, Chambers JP, Kohorn EI et al. Tamoxifen in combination with cytotoxic chemotherapy in advanced epithelial ovarian cancer. Cancer. 1989; 63:1074.

192. Scully RE. Tumors of the ovary and maldeveloped gonads. In Atlas of Tumor Pathology, Fascicle 16. Washington, DC, Armed Forces Institute of Pathology, 1979.

193. Sedlis A. Carcinoma of the fallopian tube. Surg Clin North Amer. 1978; 58:121–140.

194. Seligman AM, Rutenburg AM. Effect of 2-chlorohydroxydiethyl sulfide (hemisulfur mustard) on carcinomatosis with ascites. Cancer. 1952; 5:1354–1368.

195. Sell A, Bertelsen K, Anderson JE et al. Randomized trial of whole abdomen irradiation versus pelvic irradiation plus cyclophosphamide in treatment of early ovarian cancer. Gynecol Oncol. 1990; 37:367–373.

196. Seltzer V, Vogl S, Kaplin BH. Retreatment of advanced ovarian cancer with diammine dichloroplatinum-based combination chemotherapy after replase from complete remission: High overall and complete response rates of substantial value. Gynecol Oncol. 1985; 21:167–176.

197. Sevelda P, Vavra N, Schemper M et al. Prognostic factor for survival in stage I epithelial ovarian carcinoma. Cancer. 1990; 65:2349–2352.

198. Sevin B-U, Perras JP, Averette HE et al. Chemosensitivity testing in ovarian cancer. Cancer. 1993; 71s:1613–1620.

199. Sevin BU, personal communication, 1994.

200. Shea TC, Flaherty M, Elias A et al. A phase I clinical and pharmacokientic study of carboplatin and autolotous bone marrow support. J Clin Oncol. 1989; 7:651–661.

201. Shpall EJ, Clarke-Pearson DL, Soper JT et al. High-dose alkylating agent chemotherapy with autologous bone marrow support in patients with stage III/IV epithelial ovarian cancer. Gynecol Oncol. 1990; 38:386–392.

202. Slamon DJ, Godolphin W, Jones L et al. Studies of HER-2/neu proto-oncogene in human breast and ovarian cancers. Science. 1989; 244:707–709.

203. Slayton R. Phase II trial of VP-16213 in the treatment of advanced squamous carcinoma of the cervix and adenocarcinoma of the ovary: A Gynecologic Oncology Group strudy. Cancer Treat Rep. 1979; 63:2089–2092.

204. Slayton RE. Management of germ cell and stromal tumors of the ovary. Semin Oncol. 1984; 11:299–325.

205. Slayton RE, Park RC, Silverberg SG et al. Vincristine, dactinomycin, and cyclophosphamide in the treatment of malignant germ cell tumors of the ovary: A Gynecologic Oncology Group study (a final report). Cancer. 1985; 56:243–248.

206. Smith JP, Rutledge F. Chemotherapy in the treatment of cancer of the ovary. Am J Obstet Gynecol. 1970; 107:691–703.

207. Smith JP, Rutledge F, Delclos L. Post-operative treatment of early cancer of the ovary: A random trial between post-operative irradiation and chemotherapy. Natl Cancer Inst Monogr. 1975; 42:149–153.

208. Snider DD, Stuart GC, Nation JG et al. Evaluation of surgical staging in stage I low malignant potential ovarian tumors. Gynecol Oncol. 1991; 40:129–132.

209. Sonnendecker EW. Is routine second look laparotomy for ovarian cancer justified? Gynecol Oncol. 1988; 31:249.

210. Soper JT, Wilkerson RH, Bandy LC et al. Intraperitoneal chromic phosphate P-32 as salvage therapy for persistent carcinoma of the ovary after surgical restaging. Amer J Obstet Gynecol. 1987; 156:1153–1158.

211. Soper JT, Couchman G, Berchuck A et al. The role of partial sigmoid for debulking epithelial ovarian carcinoma. Gynecol Oncol. 1991; 41:239–244.

212. Soper JT, Hunter VJ, Daly L et al. Preoperative serum tumor-associated antigen levels in women with pelvic masses. Obstet Gynecol. 1990; 75:249–254.

213. Soper JT, Berchuck A, Clarke-Pearson DL. Adjuvant intraperitoneal chromic phosphate therapy for women with apparent early ovarian carcinoma who have not undergone comprehensive surgical staging. Cancer. 1991; 68:725–729.

214. Soper JT, Berchuck A, Doge R et al. Adjuvant therapy with intraperitoneal chromic phospate (32P) in women with early ovarian carcinoma after comprehensive surgical staging. Obstet Gynecol. 1992; 79:993–997.

215. Soper JT, Johnson P, Johnson V et al. Comprehensive restaging laparotomy in women with apparent early ovarian carcinoma. Obstet Gynecol. 1992; 80:949–953.

216. Soper JT, Management of early-stage epithelial ovarian cancer. Clin Obstet Gynecol. 1994; 37: 423–438.

217. Spanos WJ. Preoperative hormonal therapy of cystic adnexal masses. Am J Obstet Gynecol. 1973; 116:551–558.

218. Stellar MA, Soper JT, Szpak CA et al. The importance of determining kayotype in premenarchal females with gonadal dysgerminoma: two case reports. Int J Gynecol Cancer. 1991; 1 : 141–143.

219. Stehman FB, Ehrlich CE, Callangan MF. Failure of hexamethylmelamine as salvage therapy in ovarian epithelial adenocarcinoma resistant to combination chemotherapy. Gynecol Oncol. 1984; 17:189–194.

220. Stenwig JT, Hazelcamp JT, Beecham JB. Granulosa cell tumors of the ovary: A clinicopathologic study of 118 cases with long-term follow-up. Gynecol Oncol. 1979; 7:136–148.

221. Stillman RJ, Schinfeld J, Schiff I et al. Ovarian failure in long-term survivors of childhood malignancy. Am J Obstet Gynecol. 1981; 139:62–68.

222. Sutton GP, Blessing JA, Holmesley HD et al. Phase II trial of ifosfamide and mesna in advanced ovarian carcinoma: A Gynecology Oncology Group study. J Clin Oncol. 1989; 7:1672–1676.

223. Sutton GP, Stehman FB, Einhorn LH et al. Ten-year follow-up of patients receiving cisplatin, doxorubicin and cyclophosphamide chemotherapy for advanced epithelial ovarian cancer. J Clin Oncol. 1989; 7:223–229.

224. Sutton GP. Ovarian tumors of low malignant potential. In: Rubin SC, Sutton GP (eds): OVARIAN CANCER. McGraw-Hill Inc, New York, 1993; 425–450.

225. Sutton GP. Chemotherapy of epithelial ovarian cancer. An overview. Clin Obstet Gynecol. 1994; 37:461–474.

226. Swenerton KD, Hilsop TG, Spinelli J et al. Ovarian carcinoma: A multivariate analysis of prognostic factors. Obstet Gynecol. 1985; 65:264–269.

227. Swenerton K, Eisenhauser E, ten Bokkel-Huinink W et al. Taxol in relapsing ovarian cancer: high versus low dose and short versus long infusionl A European-Canadian study coordinated by the NCI Canada Clinical Trials Group. Proc Am Soc Clin Oncol. 1990; 12:256.

228. Talerman A, Haije WG, Baggerman L. Serum alpha-fetoprotein (AFP) in patients with germ cell tumors of the gonads and extragondal sites: Correlation between endodermal sinus (yolk sac) tumors and raised serum AFP. Cancer. 1980; 46:380–389.

229. Tamimi HK, Figge DC. Adenocarcinoma of the uterine tube: potential for lymph node metastases. Am J Obstet Gynecol. 1981; 141 : 132–144.

230. Taylor MD, DePetrillo AD, Turner AR. Vinblastine, bleomycin, and cisplatin in malignant germ cell tumors of the ovary. Cancer. 1985; 56:1341–1349.

231. Thigpen JT, Vance RB, Balducci L et al. New drugs and experimental approaches in ovarian cancer treatment. Semin Oncol. 1984; 11 : 314–333.

232. Thigpen T, Blessing JA, Ball H et al. Phase II trial of taxol as second-line therapy for ovarian carcinoma: A Gynecologic Oncology Group Study. Proc Am Soc Clin Oncol. 1990; 9:604.

233. Thomas GM, Dembo AJ, Hacker NF et al. Current therapy for dysterminomas of the ovary. Obstet Gynecol. 1987; 70:268–275.

234. Thompson P, Osborne R, Slevin M et al. A phase II study of cyproterone acetate in advanced ovarian cancer. London Gynecology Oncology Group. Proc Am Soc Clin Oncol. 1990; 9:160.

235. Tobias JS, Griffith CT. Management of ovarian cancer. N Engl J Med. 1976; 294; 877–882.

236. Trimble EL. Taxol in platinum-refractory ovarian cancer. J Clin Oncol. 1993; 11 : 2405–2410.

237. Trimbos JB, Scheuler JA, van Lent M et al. Reasons for incomplete surgical staging in early ovarian carcinoma. Gynecol Oncol. 1990; 37:374–377.

238. Trimbos JB, Scheuler JA van der Burg M et al. Watch and wait after careful surgical treatment and staging in well-differentiated early ovarian cancer. Cancer. 1991; 67:597–602.

239. Vasilev S, Schlaerth J, Campeau J et al. Serum CA-125 levels in pre-operative evaluation of pelvic masses. Obstet Gynecol. 1988; 71 : 751–756.

240. Vergote IB, Gormer OP, Abeler VM. Evaluation of serum CA 125 levels in the monitoring of ovarian cancer. Gynecol Oncol. 1987; 157:88–94.

241. Vergote I, Himmelmann A, Frankendal B et al. Hexamethylmelamine as second-line therapy in platin-resistant ovarian cancer. Gynecol Oncol. 1992; 47:282–286.

242. Vergote IB, Vergote-De Vos LN, Abeler VM et al. Randomized trial comparing cisplatin with radioactive phosphorous or wholeabdominal irradiation as adjuant treatment of ovarian cancer. Cancer. 1992; 69:741–749.

243. van der Burg MEL, van Lent M, Kobiersha A et al. Interval debulking surgery (IDS) does improve survival in advanced epithelial ovarian cancer (EOC): An EORTC Gynecological Cancer Cooperative Group (GCCG) study. Proc Am Soc Clin Oncol. 1993; 29:818.

244. Vogl SE, Bevenzweig M, Kaplan B et al. The CHAD and HAD regimens in advanced ovarian cancer: Combination chemotherapy including cyclophosphamide, hexamethylmelamine, adriamycin, and cisplatin. Cancer Treat Rep. 1979; 63:311–317.

245. Warne GL, Fairley KF, Hobbs JB et al. Cyclophosphamide-induced ovarian failure. N Engl J Med. 1973; 289:1159–1153.

246. Walton L, Ellenberg SS, Major FJ et al. Results of second-look laparotomy in early-stage ovarian carcinoma. Obstet Gynecol. 1987; 70:139–142.

247. Webb MJ, Decker DG, Mussey E et al. Factors influencing survival in stage I ovarian cancer. Am J Obstet Gynecol. 1973; 116:222–228.

248. Weiner Z, Thaler I, Beck D et al. Differentiating malignant from benign ovarian tumors with transvaginal color flow imaging. Obstet Gynecol. 1992; 79:159–162.

249. Williams SD, Birch R, Einhorn LH et al. Disiminated germ cell tumors: chemotherapy with

cisplatin plus bleomycin plus either vinblastine or etoposide. N Engl J Med. 1987; 316:1435–1440.

250. Williams SD, Blessing JA, Moore DH et al. Cisplatin, vinblastine, and bleomycin in advanced and recurrent ovarian germ-cell tumors. Ann Intern Med. 1989; 111:22–27.

251. Williams SD, Blessing JA, Liao SY et al. Adjuvant therapy of ovarian germ cell tumors with cisplatin etoposide, and bleomycin: A trial of the Gynecologic Oncology Group. J Clin Oncol. 1994; 12:701–706.

252. Williams TJ, Dockerty MB. Status of the contra-lateral ovary in encapsulated low grade malignant tumors of the ovary. Surg Gynecol Obstet. 1976; 143:763–766.

253. Williams TJ, Symmonds RE, Litwak O. Management of unilateral and encapsulated ovarian cancer in young women. Gynecol Oncol. 1973; 1:143–148.

254. Wiltshaw E, Kroner T. Phase II study of cisdichlorodiammine platinum (NSC 119875) in advanced adenocarcinoma of the ovary. Cancer Treat Rep. 1976; 60:55–68.

255. Xu F, Luppu R, Rodriguez GC et al. Antibody-induced growth inhibition is mediated through immunohistochemically and functionally distinct epitopes on the extracellular domain of the c-erbB-2 (HER-2/neu) gene product p185. Int J Cancer. 1993; 53:410–408.

256. Young RC, Chabner BA, Hubbard SP et al. Advanced ovarian adenocarcinoma: A prospective clinial trial of melphalan (L-PAM) versus combination chemotherapy. N Engl J Med. 1978; 299:1261–1266.

257. Young RC, Decker DG, Wharton JT et al. Staging laparotomy in early ovarian cancer. JAMA. 1983; 250:3072–3076.

258. Young RC, Walton LA, Ellenberg SS et al. Adjuvant therapy in stage I and stage II epithelial ovarian cancer: Results of two randomized trials. N Engl J Med. 1990; 322:1021–1027.

259. Young RH, Scully RE. Ovarian sex-cord stromal tumors: Recent progress. Int J Gynecol Pathol. 1982; 1:101–112.

260. Young RC, Dickerson GR, Scully RE. Juvenile granulosa cell tumor of the ovary. Am J Surg Pathol. 1984; 8:575–581.

261. Young RC, Scully RE. Ovarian Sertoli-Leydig cell tumors: A clinicopathologic analysis of 23 cases. Am J Surg Pathol. 1985; 9:543–548.

262. Zambetti M, Escabo A, Pilotti S et al. Cisplatinum/vinblastine/bleomycin combination chemotherapy in advanced or recurrent granulosa cell tumors of the ovary. Gynecol Oncol. 1990; 36:317–320.

7 Carcinoma of the Breast

R. Kreienberg and V. Schneider

Introduction and Historical Review of the Development of Multimodality Treatment Concepts

Cancer of the breast and its treatment have concerned physicians since antiquity. There are reports on breast cancer in the ancient Egyptian, Greek, and Roman medical literature.[32] Only toward the end of the 19th century, however, were treatment concepts developed, which are, in part, still valid today. It was then recognized that a sufficiently wide margin of resection and removal of the axillary lymph nodes were essential for a successful surgical approach. Therefore, since patients around the turn of the century usually presented with large tumors in late stages and surgery was the only treatment modality available, emphasis was placed on extensive, surgical resection. Thus, the breast, axillary nodes of all three levels, and both pectoral muscles were removed en bloc by the classic radical mastectomy developed by Halsted and Rotter in the 1880s.[118, 119] As with cancer surgery of other organ sites, the more radical the surgical approach, the higher the chances of survival were considered at that time. Radical mastectomy remained the standard for surgical treatment of carcinoma of the breast until well into the 1960s.

Other treatment modalities were slow to develop. Although radiotherapy was in use at the turn of the century, it remained an adjuvant to radical surgery, but decreased in significance because no clear-cut benefit for survival could be demonstrated. Likewise, the acceptance of chemotherapy and hormone therapy as components of a multimodality approach was slow. Several factors finally precipitated the revolution that has taken place in the treatment of carcinoma of the breast over the last 25 years.

First, the more aggressive and surgical techniques did not result in any improvement in the survival. Irrespective of operative approach, more than 50% of the patients died of metastatic disease within 10 years after diagnosis.

Second, the serious side effects techniques of hormonal therapy, such as oophorectomy, adrenalectomy, and hypophysectomy, were replaced by newly developed, highly effective, hormonal antagonists and agonists, which are reversible in their action and have only minor side effects.

Third, the development of multidrug regimens showed chemotherapy to be effective in an adjuvant setting.

Fourth, the recognition of breast-conserving surgery as equivalent to mastectomy when combined with postoperative radiotherapy, represented a major turning point in breast cancer treatment. It also attracted much attention and raised many hopes in the public.

Fifth, the necessity of a multidisciplinary treatment brought the surgeon, gynecologist, medical oncologist, radiation therapist, and pathologist together into a close working relationship.

Finally, the collaboration of national and international multicenter study groups, such as the National Surgical Adjuvant Breast Project (NSABP), the European Organization for Research on Treatment of Cancer (EORTC), and the International Breast Cancer Study Group (formerly Ludwig study group), allowed for the rapid testing of new concepts and regimens in statistically meaningful ways. The communication within the international community was considerably improved by consensus conferences, which established standards and guidelines as a framework for treatment.

Today, the principles of multimodality treatment of carcinoma of the breast are remarkably uniform throughout the world.

Primary Disease

Diagnosis

If carcinoma of the breast is suspected, the diagnosis must be confirmed morphologically. Generally, a breast biopsy will be necessary to obtain material on which a pathological diagnosis will be possible. Positive cytologic findings are in most institutions not sufficient to warrant ablative tumor treatment. In experienced hands, however, the results of fine-needle aspiration approach those of biopsy and frozen-section examination.[104, 158]

Excisional Biopsy

A suspicious lesion should always be excised in its entirety. If malignancy is suspected, a margin of uninvolved tissue should be included in the wide excision. In general, the skin incision should be placed directly over the lesion. The incision of the skin should be curvilinear and follow Langer's lines to achieve better cosmetic results.[168] With the exception of the inframammary area, radial incisions are not recommended. In the inframammary region, a curvilinear incision may cause a cosmetically disturbing tilt of the nipple, inferiorly.[168] In young patients with unquestionably benign disease, a circumareolar incision may be chosen. Clearly, this approach gives the best cosmetic results. It requires, however, blunt dissection and the breast tissue must be tunnelled through in order to reach the lesion. In case of malignancy, this technique is contraindicated.

The fresh, unfixed specimen should be delivered immediately to the pathology laboratory.[188] The surgeon is discouraged from cutting the specimen before sending it to pathology because orientation, determination of size, and evaluation of the margins of resection may be rendered impossible. Instead, sutures to mark the medial, lateral, and superior surfaces of the excised tissue should be inserted to ensure proper orientation. These sutures may be coded by various colors or lengths. Material for receptor analysis should be taken from the unfixed specimen within 30 minutes of tissue removal.[49] It is the responsibility of the pathologist to obtain tumor tissue for receptor assay, freeze it in liquid nitrogen, and store it at minus 70°C or below. Shipment, if necessary, should be done on dry ice.[138]

Incisional Biopsy

With this technique, only a portion of the suspected lesion is removed. This approach is undertaken only when the suspected mass is too large for complete removal and a morphological diagnosis has to be established. Incisional biopsy

allows for diagnosis and receptor determination under inoperable circumstances, such as large ulcerating tumors or inflammatory carcinoma of the breast.

Needle Biopsy

Transcutaneous biopsy, which uses a larger bore needle (drill, core, or trucut), is an alternative to incisional biopsy, since it provides a tissue core for histological examination. However, the small amount of tissue usually obtained, the blind approach of the biopsy, and possible crush artifacts, render this a less than optimal specimen for the pathologist.

Fine-needle Aspiration

Synonymous terms for this technique are aspiration biopsy, fine-needle biopsy, and thin-needle aspiration. It has to be clearly understood that this technique provides material for cytologic examination only; no tissue is available. This technique has seen a remarkable rebirth in the last 20 years,[104] after having been long neglected following its initial description at the Memorial Hospital in New York in 1933. The advantages are dispensability of anesthesia, minimal preparation, and easily repeatable performance. Although pathologists in the United States have become quite familiar with the technique, it is absolutely essential that the surgeon and pathologist have a clear understanding about the significance of a positive cytologic report on carcinoma of the breast. In particular, there must be distinct guidelines on whether an unequivocal cytologic diagnosis on malignancy warrants major surgery. Fine-needle aspiration is clearly the method of choice in suspected cystic lesions. In this instance, the aspiration is therapeutic, as well as diagnostic. In solid tumors, a firm diagnosis may be rendered, in most cases, in an outpatient setting. Layfield et al.,[158] have recently compiled all of the published 83 series on fine-needle aspiration of solid tumors of the breast, and found in 63 000 patients a cumulative false-negative rate of 2.8% and a false-positive rate of 0.3%, a figure certainly comparable with the results of frozen section examination.

In view of the increasingly complex, preoperative decision-making process in carcinoma of the breast, a firm diagnosis of malignancy allows the surgeon, as well as the patient, to focus on the various aspects of breast preservation versus mastectomy, without being distracted by the hope for a still benign biopsy result. For this purpose, fine-needle aspiration is the method of choice.

The Nonpalpable Lesion

The increasing use of mammography as a screening procedure to detect early breast cancer has rendered excision of a nonpalpable lesion a fairly common problem. In the past, removal of the corresponding quadrant, without localization, was occasionally performed. This is no longer acceptable because it removes an unnecessarily large amount of breast tissue, without even ensuring complete excision of the suspicious lesion. Similarly, placement of a needle under mammographic control, and injection of a dye or contrast material during surgery to mark the lesion, is no longer a technique to be recommended. The mobile position of the needle and the diffuse spread of the dye after the incision was made, also caused larger than necessary excisions. The superior technique for localization of a nonpalpable lesion is clearly the use of a springhook wire, which is passed into the breast through a needle guide using fenestrated, mammographic compression plates. The wire tip is anchored firmly in the vicinity of the lesion under mammographic vision. The surgeon may then use the wire as a guide to the lesion, making either an incision directly overlying the tumor, or choosing the cosmetically superior circumareolar approach. The mammographic pictures that show the wire in place should be on hand for the surgeon to allow optimal adaptation of sample size.

Intraoperative specimen mammography is absolutely essential to ensure complete removal of the suspected tissue. Comparison with the preoperative mammography determines whether all microcalcifications have been removed. Specimen radiography should be carried out in the radiology department, and the biopsy incision should only be closed after communication between the surgeon and the radiologist has taken place. If in doubt, the radiologist may ask the surgeon to remove additional tissue. If the lesion has been completely removed, the biopsy should then be transported immediately to the pathology department for further processing. Frozen-section examination of nonpalpable lesions should *not* be undertaken, as it is unreliable. Instead, the tissue should be generously sampled and embedded in paraffin for further investigation. Any tissue removed for either frozen-section examination, or hormone-receptor assay, may unintentionally remove the entire lesion, and the diagnosis will be missed.[188]

Based on preliminary work by Swedish study groups,[189] several companies have recently developed mammographic equipment for stereotactic fine-needle aspiration of nonpalpable lesions. Although published results have been encouraging so far, it remains to be seen whether negative results are reliable, or should be followed up by biopsy.

As previously illustrated, only close cooperation of surgeon, radiologist, and pathologist ensures optimal results in the management of nonpalpable lesions.

One-Step or Two-Step Surgery

Over the last couple of years, there has been a distinct shift from one-step to two-step surgery. One-step surgery combines excisional biopsy (possibly with a margin of resection), frozen-section examination, and definitive surgical treatment of breast and axilla in one procedure. In our experience, this is still the preferred option for patients with established malignancy, who understand the available treatment modalities, and who prefer to have one single operation and anesthesia. Many patients, however, opt for biopsy as a first step. They are then able to discuss the various aspects of definitive surgery with their physician. With the choice between preservation of the breast on one hand, and mastectomy on the other, the two-step procedure allows for careful consideration of the pros and cons by the patient and her family. There has been no conclusive proof that the two-step procedure increases the risk of systemic spread of cancer cells, as was suspected earlier. Likewise, there are no data available which prove that an undue time lag between the first and second step of the operation is detrimental to survival.

As will be discussed later in the section on breast-conserving surgery, some of the possible contraindications against conservative surgery, such as multicentricity of the tumor, extensive intraductal carcinoma, or extensive lymphatic spread, can only be established after careful histopathologic examination of the tumor.[3, 93, 95, 151] This is another reason for selecting the two-step procedure.

Pathologic Classification

In view of the increasingly recognized heterogeneity of carcinoma of the breast, a uniform and consistent pathologic classification of malignant breast tumors is of utmost importance. To reduce interobserver variability to a minimum, multi-center studies usually establish a panel of pathologists or a central pathology laboratory, where the original sections are reviewed. Basis for an internationally binding, unified terminology is provided by the World Health Organization (WHO) Classification on Histological Typing of Breast Tumors, second edition of 1981.[256] The WHO Classification differs only minimally from previous classification systems, such as the Atlas of Tumor Pathology, second series, by the Armed Forces Institute of Pathology,[171] and the Syllabus of the National Surgical Adjuvant Breast Project on Pathology of Invasive Breast Cancer.[96]

Table **1**   Histopathological typing

Cancer, NOS[a]
   Intraductal (in situ)
   Invasive with predominant intraductal component
   Invasive
   Comedo
   Inflammatory
   Medullary with lymphocytic infiltrate
   Mucinous (colloid)
   Papillary
   Scirrhous
   Tubular
   Other

Lobular
   In situ
   Invasive with predominant in situ component
   Invasive

Nipple
   Paget disease, NOS[a]
   Paget disease with intraductal carcinoma
   Paget disease with invasive ductal carcinoma

---

[a] Not otherwise specified.
Compiled from Hermanek P, Sobin LH, eds. TNM classification of malignant tumors. 4th ed. Berlin: Springer, 1987; and Bealus OH, et al., eds. Manual for Staging of cancer. 3rd ed. Philadelphia: JB Lippincott; 1988.

For optimal results, a number of precautions must be taken. Electrocautery instruments should not be used for obtaining breast biopsies. Cautery artifacts may not only prevent proper tumor classification, but also make further investigations, such as hormonal assays, electron microscopy, or histochemical examination impossible. Cuts made into the tumor by the surgeon for orientation purposes will make it difficult or impossible for the pathologist to record the correct size of the lesion and to evaluate the margins of resection. Delay in delivering the specimen to the laboratory will prevent reliable hormone receptor assays.[49]

As a rule, the pathology report on carcinoma of the breast should state tumor size (in diameter or in three dimensions), tumor type according to WHO, tumor grade, margins of resection, extent of an in situ component (in percent of the entire lesion), and possible lymphatic spread. Since many carcinomas of the breast contain minor components of specific subtypes, it is important to classify the tumor according to the predominant pattern. It has been found that the favorable prognosis of some of the rare subtypes only applies to tumors that are almost entirely composed of one specific pattern. The pathologist should, therefore, denote in the histopathologic classification, only those tumors as composite that show an extensive mixture of patterns. Terms not specifically listed in the WHO Classification, but commonly used in the past, such as scirrhous carcinoma, or carcinoma simplex, should be avoided.[256]

Carcinoma in Situ

The two distinct epithelial-structural units of the breast are duct and lobule. Accordingly, two intraepithelial forms of carcinoma are distinguished.[210] Intraductal carcinoma ("ductal carcinoma in situ") is characterized by a proliferation of neoplastic cells within an adjacent group of mammary ducts.[8] The basement membrane remains intact. Proliferation of uniform appearing cells with bland nuclei surrounding evenly spaced and perfectly round lumina is typical of the cribriform pattern of intraductal carcinoma. In the comedo type, enlarged ducts are stuffed with distinctly atypical cancer cells. Typical of this type is the small central core of necrotic tissue, which extrudes from the cut surface like a comedo of the skin when the lesion is compressed. The term "comedo carcinoma," therefore, should be restricted to this well-defined subtype of intraductal carcinoma that can be recognized grossly. The third and least common type, micropapillary carcinoma, shows delicate strands of malignant cells covering the duct walls in a semicircular fashion, reminiscent of "Roman bridges." Mixtures of the three subtypes are common.[97] The central necrotic core of the comedo type regularly shows foci of calcification. This is of major diagnostic significance because these calcifications serve as an important sign of malignancy in the mammogram, in the form of clustered microcalcifications.

The vast majority of carcinoma in situ is detected through mammographic calcifications. By contrast, the cribriform and micropapillary form of intraductal carcinoma generally lack microcalcifications. In most instances, they represent incidental findings. In about 10% of cases, intraductal carcinoma may grow to reach palpable size.[228] Lesions of up to 4 centimeters may still remain intraepithelial. Obviously, only complete histopathologic examination with extensive recutting will allow ruling out foci of microinvasion in such instances. By definition, intraductal carcinoma has a theoretical cure rate of 100%. There is, therefore, no indication for axillary node dissection in patients with intraductal carcinoma once invasion has been ruled out.[228] Nevertheless, there have been reports of axillary metastases in 1–2% of patients with in situ breast cancer.[33] It must be assumed that in these cases, foci of minimal invasion were missed by the histologic examination.[155]

The traditional treatment recommendation for intraductal carcinoma has been total mastectomy. If the lesion is less than 2 centimeters, some authors recommend wide excision.[288] In two papers on long-term follow-up of ductal carcinoma in situ treated by biopsy only because of an erroneous "benign" diagnosis,[18, 91] there was development of invasive carcinoma in only 25%. A conservative treatment in nonpalpable duct-cell carcinoma in situ appears, therefore, justified. For the conservatively treated patient, recurrence based on the multifocal growth pattern of intraductal carcinoma remains a serious threat. Careful, mammographic follow-up is therefore mandatory.

The second type of intraepithelial neoplasia of the breast is lobular carcinoma in situ. This type of lesion is much less commonly detected than intraductal carcinoma because it is never palpable and does not show any calcifications. As a rule, it is an incidental finding in breast tissue that has been removed for other reasons. Histologically, the acinar structures of the lobule are extended and completely filled with bland looking, uniform cells of small size. There is a spectrum of changes ranging from lobular atypia through lobular hyperplasia to lobular carcinoma in situ. This lesion is notorious for its multifocality and bilaterality.[156] Multifocal development of lobular carcinoma in situ is reported in up to 35% of the cases, including the opposite breast. The risk of subsequent development of invasive carcinoma ranges from 10% to 30%. Since these subsequent invasive carcinomas may not only occur in the opposite breast, but may even be of the duct-cell type, the relationship between lobular carcinoma in situ and invasive carcinoma seems to be that of an indicator of potential malignant disease, rather than that of a precursor lesion. The significance of lobular carcinoma (or lobular neoplasia, as some authors have preferred to term this lesion) has been debated for years. In view of the described risk pattern, the choice of therapy in lobular carcinoma in situ seems to be limited to either close follow-up examination or bilateral mastectomy.[5] Currently, most authors recommend clinical and mammographic follow-up examinations. Attempts to discover bilateral disease by so-called mirror-image biopsies of the opposite breast have generally been abandoned.[211, 230]

Invasive Carcinoma

Proper histopathologic classification of invasive carcinoma is essential because there are well established and significant differences in growth rates, recurrence rates, and multifocality of the various types of carcinoma of the breast. For initial orientation, it can be stated that 80% of the invasive carcinomas of the breast are of the duct-cell type, or not otherwise specified (NOS), 10% are of lobular type, and 10% are of special subtypes including inflammatory carcinoma and Paget disease.

Invasive duct-cell carcinoma is by far the most common malignancy of the breast. It presents as a firm, poorly delineated nodule, which is invariably solid. The cut surface of the lesion is white and gritty due to microcalcifications. The firmness is a result of reactive fibrosis.

There is an inverse relationship between the amount of benign connective tissue and the firmness of the lesion. The malignant tumor cells extend into the surrounding tissue, following the fibrous strands. This growth pattern, in turn, is responsible for the fixation to the surrounding tissue and the stellate appearance in mammography and ultrasound examination. Since the size of the lesion is still one of the most important parameters for prognosis, care should be taken to record the exact measurements. In general, the greatest diameter in millimeters serves as tumor size and is preferable to a three-dimensional measurement. The size should be determined in fresh state, as fixation may cause shrinkage, and before tissue is removed for receptor assays.

In most major series, invasive lobular carcinoma represents between 5% and 10% of cases. Although a number of subtypes have been described,[77] their significance is limited because mixtures are common and no prognostic differences have been reported. Common to all types is a linear growth pattern (so-called "Indian filing"), a strict single-cell occurrence with an absence of acinar structures and a predominance of remarkably uniform, small tumor cells. Additional classic signs for invasive lobular carcinoma are occasional signet ring cells and a socalled "targetoid" growth pattern surrounding minor benign duct structures. As with lobular carcinoma in situ, calcification is not a sign of this tumor type. Differences in gross appearance, survival figures, and receptor content have not been described for invasive lobular carcinoma, in comparison with the more common duct-cell type. However, the propensity for multifocality and bilaterality is significant because the diagnosis of invasive lobular carcinoma precludes, for some authors, breast-preserving surgery.[227]

Rare Subtypes of Invasive Carcinoma

A number of well-recognized variants of invasive duct-cell carcinoma, representing about 5% of invasive carcinomas of the breast, may be grouped together because they are all characterized by a significantly better prognosis.[96] Representatives of this group are tubular (well differentiated), medullary (circumscribed), mucinous (colloid), papillary, apocrine, and adenoid-cystic carcinoma. Not only is this group of rare lesions characterized by a significantly

lower rate of axillary metastases and a higher 5-year survival rate, but it is also well known for it's benign appearance in clinical and radiographic examination. The medullary and mucinous variants almost always appear as round, well circumscribed, and soft lesions, lacking any calcifications. It should be kept in mind that only the pure forms, being defined as containing at least 70% of a specific growth pattern, are associated with a better prognosis. So-called mixed or atypical forms approach the survival rate of the invasive duct-cell carcinoma (NOS).[96] Medullary carcinoma must be viewed as the most enigmatic of these special subtypes of invasive carcinoma because, with its high mitotic rate, its rapid growth rate, and its undifferentiated tumor cell characteristics, it has the appearance of a classic, grade III lesion, yet it carries a better prognosis than the better differentiated duct-cell carcinoma (NOS).[206] The remaining rare forms of invasive carcinoma of the breast, such as pure squamous, metaplastic, and secretory carcinoma are not dealt with in this overview.

Inflammatory Carcinoma

This tumor type is not a histopathologic, but rather a clinical entity. It carries the worst prognosis of all known types of breast cancer and almost always leads to death within 2 years after diagnosis.[73, 248] Clinically, inflammatory carcinoma is characterized by an enlarged edematous breast with elevated temperature. Usually, no mass is palpable, rendering diagnosis difficult. By the less experienced, inflammatory carcinoma may be mistaken for nonpuerperal mastitis. Nonresponse to antibiotic therapy after a week should raise the suspicion for inflammatory carcinoma in such an instance. The erythematous skin changes often show signs of "peau d'orange," and axillary and supraclavicular lymph node involvement can often be established by palpation alone. The diagnosis may be established by an incisional biopsy, occasionally by fine-needle aspiration, if a deep-seated mass is palpated. The prominent skin changes are the result of a diffuse, subdermal involvement of lymphatics by tumor emboli, which may be detected by random skin biopsy.[73]

Primary surgical treatment by mastectomy is obsolete because no survival benefits have been demonstrated.[35, 76, 162, 224] The treatment of choice is aggressive chemotherapy and/or endocrine treatment followed by mastectomy and irradiation to the thoracic wall.[117, 199, 216] This may be followed by another cycle of chemotherapy with anthracycline containing regimens.

Paget Disease of the Breast

Paget disease of the breast has been known since its initial description by Sir James Paget in 1874, as a diffuse eczema with crust formation of the areola and nipple. Often, there is fluid oozing or breast secretion. It is now almost universally accepted that this condition is a rare but typical manifestation of an underlying duct-cell carcinoma, which may be in situ or invasive. A palpable mass is only present in about 50 % of cases. It is assumed that the underlying duct-cell carcinoma spreads continuously as an in situ extension to the nipple, where it is found as intra-epidermal clusters of malignant cells in biopsy material. These large Paget cells show histo-chemical and immuno-histochemical character-istics of duct cells. They will be most easily identified by the cytologic examination of a scraping of the nipple.

The logical choice for the treatment of Paget disease is mastectomy. If no intramammary lesion can be located, it may be difficult to convince a patient that the entire breast has to be removed for a simple crust of the nipple area. There have been a few series on breast-conserv-ing surgery for Paget disease.[157, 207] It appears that a group of highly selected patients, with no palpable tumor and negative mammography, may benefit from this type of treatment.

Staging

Staging describes the extent of a malignant disease at the time of diagnosis. For this purpose, a standardized, internationally recognized system is being used. The oldest staging systems for breast carcinoma, such as the Columbia Classification System in the United States, the Manchester System in England, and the Steinthal System in Germany, described only four tumor stages to which the various signs and manifesta-tions of breast cancer were assigned. The T-N-M System, now in use, independently describes primary tumor, regional lymph nodes, and distant metastases (see Table **2**). The latest up-date of the T-N-M Classification of tumors was

Table **2**   pTNM classification

pT—Primary Tumor
The pathological classification requires the examina-tion of the primary carcinoma with no gross tumor at the margins of resection. A case can be classified pT if there is only microscopic tumor in a margin.
The pT categories correspond to the T-categories

pN—Regional Lymph Nodes
The pathological classification requires the resection or examination of at least the low axillary lymph nodes (Level I) and the lymph nodes behind the pectoralis muscle (Level II). Such a resection ordinarily includes ten or more lymph nodes

pNx	Regional lymph nodes cannot be assessed (not removed for study or previously removed)	
pN0	No regional lymph node metastasis	
pN1	Metastases to mobile ipsilateral axillary node(s)	
	pN1a	Only micrometastasis (none larger than 0.2 cm)
	pN1b	Metastasis to lymph node(s), any larger than 0.2 cm
	pN1bi	Metastasis in 1–3 lymph nodes, any more than 0.2 cm and less than 2.0 cm in greatest dimension
	pN1bii	Metastasis to four or more lymph nodes, any more than 0.2 cm and all less than 2.0 cm in greatest dimension
	pN1biii	Extension of tumor beyond the capsule of a lymph node metastasis less than 2.0 cm in greatest dimension
	pN1biv	Metastasis to a lymph node 2.0 cm or more in greates dimension
pN2	Metastasis to ipsilateral axillary lymph nodes that are fixed to one another or to other structures	
pN3	Metastasis to ipsilateral internal mammary lymph node(s)	

pM—Distant Metastasis
The pM categories correspond to the M categories

Modified from Hermanek P, Sobin LH (eds.): TNM Classification of malignant Tumors, ed. 4. Berlin Springer Verlag, 1987; and Bealus OH et al. (eds.) Manual for Staging of cancer. 3rd ed. Philadelphia J.B. Lippincott; 1985

published by the UICC in 1992 (Third Edition, second revision).[244] Only the invasive component of the tumor should be considered while mea-suring tumor size. Involvement of the pectoral muscle, as well as skin and nipple retraction, have no influence on the staging of the primary tumor.

T-Staging

In palpable breast tumors, physical examination gives a fairly accurate estimation of tumor size. In oblong or oval lesions, the largest tumor diameter is used as tumor size. Although mammography is not always able to determine the benign or malignant nature of a lesion, it is highly accurate in size estimation. The possible distortion of the lesion by the compression of the breast during mammography is of no practical significance. Care should be taken not to make measurements on magnified images. Another highly accurate technique for measuring tumor size is ultrasonography. Lesions may be measured with an accuracy of plus or minus 1 millimeter. Unfortunately, not all carcinomas of the breast are visible by ultrasonography. All other parameters going into the clinical staging system, such as fixation to muscle or chest wall and skin changes, such as ulceration or peau d'orange, may be easily recognized during physical examination.

N-Staging

The preoperative clinical examination determines whether the axillary nodes are free of tumor (N0), are thought to contain metastases (N1), or contain metastases and are also matted together (N3). It should be remembered that palpable axillary lymph nodes are common. Clinically negative lymph nodes are usually less than one centimeter in diameter. They are mobile and soft. In this situation, there may be inflammatory or allergic reactions on the lower arms, hands, or fingers detectable. Clinically suspicious axillary lymph nodes are usually larger than one centimeter, firm, with an irregular surface, and not as mobile as benign lymph nodes. However, the clinical evaluation of axillary lymph nodes is highly inaccurate. The false positive and false negative rate is around 30%.[94]

There have been recent attempts to use ultrasound for the clinical staging of axillary node involvement.[34, 194, 242] It is not currently clear whether this approach is of any significance. In the case of clinically suspicious nodes in the lower axillary region, the diagnosis may be confirmed by fine-needle aspiraton. This is the only method for a preoperative morphologic confirmation of axillary disease.

M-Staging

Carcinoma of the breast most commonly metastasizes to bone, liver, and lung. Supraclavicular node metastasis is considered a distant metastasis, as are bone, lung etc. Distant metastases (M) at the time of primary diagnosis are uncommon (< 5%). It is, therefore, a well-established practice to rule out distant metastases to these organs by bone scan, ultrasound examination of the liver, and chest X-ray. In the case of suspicious findings, clarification by other imaging techniques, are necessary, such as tomography or CT-scanning. These examinations also establish important baselines for later follow-up.

Postoperative Staging

Since clinical staging is fraught with error, the UICC has adopted a postoperative or pathologic staging system for almost all tumor sites (Table 2). For carcinoma of the breast, the criteria for the postoperative T-staging are identical with the preoperative staging system, differentiating between clinical (cTNM) and pathological (pTNM) stages. The establishment of a diagnosis of carcinoma in situ is a tyical postoperative event. It should be kept in mind that pathological tumor size refers only to the invasive component of the lesion.

Postoperative N-staging is based on isolation and removal of all lymph nodes from the axillary fat pad in the laboratory, followed by microscopic examination. For diagnostic accuracy, a minimum of ten nodes should be removed. On average, 15–20 lymph nodes are found in level I to III. There should be no difference in the number of removed nodes with breast conserving surgery in comparison with modified radical mastectomy.[87]

"Node sampling" (removing only easily accessible nodes or less than ten), is not sufficient to obtain a representative specimen and is therefore unacceptable. The number of involved axillary lymph nodes is the single, most important prognostic parameter in carcinoma of the breast. The postoperative staging system separates the N1b group, into four subgroups, according to the number of involved nodes and the size of metastases (see Table 2). The number of involved nodes have been grouped into one to three, and four or more. The classification N2 for matted lymph nodes remains unchanged.

Prognostic Factors

Prognostication on an individual basis is one of the most important goals of current breast cancer research. It would allow for the definition of patient subgroups that may or may not benefit from adjuvant therapy.[172] Ultimately, it would enable the physician to tailor treatment exactly to the individual patients needs. It would eliminate both overtreatment and undertreatment. Although there have been exciting new research directions, a breakthrough has not occured from a practical point of view. In the following, the accepted prognostic parameters, such as lymph node status, tumor size, tumor grading, and hormone receptor status will be discussed. Other factors will be described in the section in current research.

Lymph Node Status (Fig. 1)

Among the accepted prognostic parameters, the number of histologically proven positive axillary lymph nodes is the single most important indicator for prognosis.[90] About half of all patients operated upon have histologic evidence of axillary lymph node involvement. If the axillary lymph nodes are tumor free, 5-year survival rate is 80%. With a single node involved, this figure

drops to 63%. With four nodes involved; only 50% of patients survive, and only 29% live for 5 years with more than ten lymph nodes involved. There is evidence that axillary nodes are more commonly involved with tumors located in the lateral portion of the breast, while drainage of the medial breast partially flows into the internal mammary node chain.

The axilla is divided into three levels (Figure 1). Level I is represented by tissue located lateral and inferior to the lateral border of the pectoralis minor muscle, level II directly beneath the muscle, and level III superior and medial to the pectoralis minor. Although axillary node involvement by level gives some important information, it was found that survival correlates best with total number of involved nodes.

Tumor Size

The size of the primary tumor is an important indicator of prognosis. Size also correlates closely with lymph node status. According to several studies,[91, 249] it is an independent prognostic factor and retains its value for prognostication if the lymph node status has been accounted for. If lymph nodes are negative, tumors less than two centimeters (T1) carry a particularly good prognosis. In patients with negative nodes, size of the primary tumor seems to be the best predictor for of local recurrence.

Tumor Grade

Grading the degree of differentiation of the primary tumor is a well-established means of prognostication for malignant lesions of all sites. First attempts to grade carcinoma of the breast were made by Greenough in 1925.[111] The basis of the currently used grading system was laid by Bloom and Richardson in 1957.[23] They introduced a scoring system evaluating three parameters. This system is still in use today with minor modifications. The three parameters examined are formation of tubules, nuclear pleomorphism, and mitotic rate. Grading should be applied to all invasive carcinomas. Grading of an in situ carcinoma is not useful.[244] Preferably, the periphery of the invasive tumor should be used for grading. If there is heterogeneous differentiation, the area with the highest degree of malignancy should be used. The scoring system of Bloom and

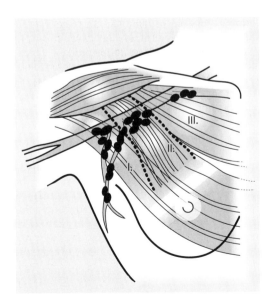

Fig. 1   Levels I – III of axillary lymph nodes

Richardson assigns one to three points to the three parameters mentioned above. By convention, the three grades of well-differentiated (grade I), moderately well-differentiated (grade II), and poorly differentiated (grade III) tumors are formed.[21–23]

Histologic grade correlates highly with the rate of recurrent disease and with overall survival.[59] Grade III carcinomas carry a significantly higher risk of treatment failure. Tumor grade serves as a basis in some ongoing studies to separate patients into high and low-risk groups.

Tumor grading is a subjective evaluation of three microscopic criteria by the pathologist. A fairly high interobserver variability of up to 30% has been documented.[41, 64, 237, 238] Tumor grade can, therefore, be seen only as a rough estimate of the degree of malignancy. Attempts have been made to quantify tumor grade by more advanced techniques, such as measurement of nuclear DNA content and estimation of growth rates of breast cancer cells. These techniques must still be seen as experimental and are dealt with in the section on current research.[11, 24]

Black et al.[20] introduced the term nuclear grading, which has lead to some confusion. The nuclei of breast cancer cells in histologic sections are compared with normal duct cells and graded according to their degree of atypia. Unfortunately, the classification of the three groups (well-differentiated, moderately well-differentiated, and poorly differentiated), runs opposite to the system used in histologic grading, so that the well-differentiated form is reported as grade III, the intermediate group as grade II, and the poorly differentiated group as grade I. There is no conclusive evidence that nuclear grading is more accurate or has a higher prognostic value than histological grading. It is, therefore, not routinely used in the evaluation of carcinoma of the breast.[82]

Hormone Receptor Status

Although hormone dependency in carcinoma of the breast has been recognized for many years, only the development of new techniques has allowed for the determination of hormone dependency at the time of surgery.[110] Hormone receptor status is a powerful prognostic indicator, regardless of tumor stage.[65] The receptor status is, however, inversely related to tumor grade.[82]

Grade III tumors (poorly differentiated) usually have a very low or nonexistent receptor content. Likewise, some tumor types, such as medullary carcinoma, are always receptor negative. Preliminary results indicate that receptor content also correlates with cell growth rate. The faster growing tumors tend to have lower receptor content than the more slowly growing carcinomas.[133]

Currently, both estrogen receptor and progesterone receptor are determined in human breast cancer tissue. They are used as independent prognostic indicators. Since expression of progesterone receptor activity requires a functioning estrogen receptor, PR positivity is more significant than ER positivity and correlates better with prognosis.

It should be mentioned that there are currently two methods for receptor assay available.[49, 141, 170, 205] The conventional dextran-coated charcoal method (DCC) is still the most widely used technique. It requires approximately 500 milligrams of tumor tissue and uses radioactive binding methods. The results are reported as hormone binding capacity in fmol per milligram cytosol protein. The cut-off point for a negative result has been arbitrarily put at less than 20 fmol/mg cytosol. The second, more recent technique for measuring receptor content, is an immunohistochemical assay.[62, 240] In the late 1980s, monoclonal antibodies were successfully cloned against the receptor proteins.[110] It then became possible to demonstrate the receptors directly in histological section using the well-established peroxidase–antiperoxidase technique.[61] The immunohistochemical detection of receptor proteins has several advantages. It allows for receptor determination even in very small tumors, which could not have been measured with the biochemical assays. No tumor tissue has to be removed before histological examination of the lesion. The heterogeneity of receptor expression in the same tumor tissue can be recognized. The technique may even be applied to cytological specimens, such as fine-needle aspirations and malignant effusions.[100] Finally, it became apparent that active receptor protein is not located in the cytoplasm as previously assumed, but within the nucleus.[142]

▨ Radical Surgery

Mastectomy

The common feature of all radical operative procedures is the removal of the entire mammary gland including the overlying skin with nipple and areola (mastectomy). The various procedures and their numerous modifications differ only in the amount of surrounding tissues being removed. These tissues include the axillary and internal mammary lymph nodes, as well as both pectoral muscles.

The most radical procedure, *extended radical mastectomy*, was performed in a few institutions in Europe and in the U.S. in the 1950s and is today only of historic interest.[174, 217] It added the removal of the internal mammary lymph node chain to the then standard procedure of radical mastectomy. There was no survival benefit in a large international prospective study.[153, 154] The published series give, however, some important information on involvement patterns of internal mammary nodes. According to Veronesi et al.,[251, 254] metastases to the internal mammary lymph node chain are not related to the location of the primary tumor within the breast, as was suspected, but on tumor size and extent of axillary lymph node involvement.

Radical mastectomy was the standard operative treatment for carcinoma of the breast for almost a century. Most published reports are still based on radical mastectomy, and the procedure still serves as baseline against which all other techniques are measured. Today, it must also be considered obsolete, and even in radically oriented departments, it is essentially no longer performed.[165] The characteristic feature of this technique is the removal of both major and minor pectoral muscle.[5]

Thus, it assures a free margin of resection in tumors involving pectoral fascia or muscles. After transection of the origins of these two muscles, the entire axillary fossa and infraclavicular area is broadly exposed, so that a complete axillary dissection is assured. A significantly higher number of axillary lymph nodes are removed with radical mastectomy than with any other procedure. The specimen is obtained en bloc and consists of both pectoral muscles, mammary gland with overlying skin, and axillary content. The division of axillary lymph nodes in level I, II, and III was originally devised for the radical mastectomy

specimen because the pectoralis minor muscle serves as an easily recognizable structure on the reverse side of the specimen for the separation into three groups of lymph nodes. Clinically patients after radical mastectomy may be easily identified by the missing anterior axillary fold. The main reason for abandoning this procedure as standard treatment for carcinoma of the breast was the lack of evidence of a survival advantage for patients treated by this approach.[80, 86] Cosmetically, it is clearly inferior to the modified radical mastectomy. Breast augmentation, with most of the currently available techniques, is not possible because of the missing pectoral muscle. In prospective randomized trials, it was shown that even local control of the disease was not improved with this more radical approach.[83]

Modified radical mastectomy is characterized by preservation of the pectoralis major muscle. After an oblique incision, the mammary gland and axillary contents are removed. Because of numerous modifications, this technique is not standardized to the same degree as radical mastectomy. The most commonly quoted technique, reported by Patey and Dyson in 1948,[196] solves the problem of the limited access to the axillary fossa by removal of the pectoralis minor muscle. Other modifications allow for partial or complete preservation of this muscular structure. With these techniques, however, a complete dissection of levels II and III is no longer assured. The most commonly performed procedure is total mastectomy with preservation of both pectoral muscles and an axillary node dissection of level I and II. Nodes from level III can be removed by further retracting the pectoral muscles. This is indicated when macroscopic nodes are found.

Modified radical mastectomy is currently the standard operative treatment for carcinoma of the breast. Breast preserving procedures, as discussed in below, are only indicated if certain requirements are fulfilled.

Total (simple) mastectomy is the least aggressive form of mastectomy and consists of the removal of the mammary gland with an ellipse of skin, including the nipple-areola complex. Both pectoral muscles are preserved, no axillary lymph nodes are removed. There are a number of well-defined indications for this technically rather simple procedure. It is the treatment of choice for in situ carcinoma, if invasion has definitely been ruled out. After breast preserving surgery, total mastectomy is performed in patients with recurrent disease. This so-called salvage mastectomy carries a fairly favorable prognosis. As a palliative procedure, total mastectomy may be performed in selected patients with histologically proven distant mestastases to prevent ulceration of the primary tumor. In exceptional situations, it may also be indicated as a preventive measure, such as the development of atypical hyperplasia in the contralateral breast in patients with successfully treated breast cancer.

Reconstructive Surgery

The recent decision by the Food and Drug Administration (FDA) in 1991, to ban silicone breast implants for breast augmentation, has created considerable confusion and irritation in patients and physicians alike.[6, 18, 99, 140] According to the FDA, silicone implants may still be used in patients treated for cancer, but these patients need to be registered as part of a clinical study of silicone implants. Other techniques of reconstruction, such as skin flaps, are not affected by the FDA decision. In most countries, silicone implants are currently banned for breast augmentation in nonmalignant conditions.

Reconstructive surgery of the breast is indicated in patients not qualifying for breast preserving surgery, who wish to restore their physical appearance to an acceptable degree.[25, 57] There is no detrimental effect of this elective procedure on prognosis. Although a primary reconstruction at the time of mastectomy is possible in most instances, reconstruction is usually performed as a second procedure after completion of treatment. In general, at least 3 to 6 months should have elapsed. The objectives of breast reconstruction are restoration of the contour of the breast, compensation of the skin deficit, restoration of the nipple and areola, and creation of symmetry by adjusting the size and shape of the contralateral breast. For this purpose, a number of techniques are available.[30, 31] The placement of a silicone implant into the retropectoral space is rarely possible, due to insufficient skin. Therefore, an expander implant is necessary in most patients to create sufficient skin surface and space for placement of a secondary silicone implant. In a stepwise fashion, the expander is filled with saline until an optimal form has been obtained. Finally, the expander implant is exchanged by a permanent implant, using a smaller volume to obtain a natural contour of the breast.

Other reconstructive procedures include the use of myocutaneous flaps and free transplants, but these are fairly extensive procedures requiring considerable expertise. They should only be performed by experienced plastic surgeons.[125, 190]

■ Breast-Conserving Surgery

The almost universal acceptance of breast-preserving surgery as surgical treatment for selected patients with carcinoma of the breast, is based on three key prospective, randomized studies that were performed in the last 20 years. All three studies arrived at essentially the same conclusion: There is no significant 5 and 7-year survival disadvantage for patients treated with this technique. Radiotherapy of the remaining breast tissue is an essential component, if the breast is to be preserved.[123] Finally, patients treated with breast-conserving techniques have to be carefully selected, based on a number of well-defined criteria.

These trials were performed at the National Cancer Institute in Milan, Italy,[252, 253] in the United States by the National Surgical Adjuvant Breast and Bowel Project (NSABP),[81, 87] and at the Institute Gustave Roussy in France.[220–222] In these three studies, a total of approximately 2000 patients with stage I or II carcinoma of the breast were randomly assigned to either breast preserving surgery and postoperative radiation, or to mastectomy. In the NSABP trial, one group of patients was treated with breast preserving surgery and no radiation.[81] Although the Milan trial was initiated in June of 1973, the majority of the patients in the three centers have to date been followed for approximately ten years only, which means that final conclusions are not yet available. The preliminary results of these studies have, however, been so convincing, that breast conserving surgery has been accepted by the medical community and the media with the publication by the NSABP 5-year results in 1985.[81] In the meantime, further specifications as to technique, indications, contraindications, and follow-up, were agreed upon in two consensus conferences held at the National Cancer Institute in Bethesda in September 1985 and in June 1990.[51, 53] The following discussion will be based on these recommendations.

There are essentially three types of breast preserving operations.[10] The *tumorectomy (simple excision)* removes the tumor without regard to margins of resection. It is not sufficient as a cancer operation. The *wide excision (lumpectomy, tylectomy or partial mastectomy)* removes the lesion with grossly free margins of resection of approximately one centimeter. The *quadrantectomy*, which was the preferred technique in the Milan trial, consisted of the complete removal of the respective breast quadrant, in which the primary tumor was located the overlying skin was partly resected as well. In general, quadrantectomy was considered to give poor cosmetic results, due to excessive skin excision, but may yield lower local recurrences than wide excisions. Guidelines for the technical performance were published by the NSABP and are summerized as follow:[168] The incision should be placed directly over the palpable mass; curvilinear incisions are to be preferred; an ellipse of skin is only resected if the tumor is located superficially. These general recommendations are modified if the tumor is located in the lower quadrants of the breast. If skin is to be resected, the ensuing skin deficit will shorten the distance from nipple to inframammary fold, and the breast will be cosmetically distorted. In this situation, therefore, a radial incision is indicated. If no skin is removed, a curvilinear incision is preferrable. Constant digital control of the lesion guides the operating physician through the procedure, ensuring a sufficiently wide line of excision. After the placement of sutures to orient the specimen, it should be sent to the pathologist for histology and hormone receptor analysis. At this point, frozen section assessment of the margins of resection may be necessary if gross inspection finds tumor within a few millimeters of the line of excision. Mobilization and adaptation of the remaining breast tissue is usually not recommended but should be considered for resections larger than 2 cm in diameter. The defect fills with blood and fibrin and usually gives a good cosmetic result. Drainage without suction may be applied. The wound should be closed with an intracutaneous suture, to obtain a thin and barely visible scar.

Axillary dissection is performed by a separate incision, which may be transverse or longitudinal. For cosmetic reasons, the incision line in the axilla can be drawn on the skin with a marker pen in the evening before the operation to ensure that the incision can be hidden by the arm. If the primary lesion is in the tail area of the upper–outer quadrant, a single incision suffices. A complete level I and II (III) dissection should be performed. Axillary lymph node sampling is strongly discouraged. Level II excision is facilitated by elevating the pectoralis minor muscle. According to the NSABP data, the mean and total number of lymph nodes removed by this lateral approach does not significantly differ from the modified radical mastectomy.[87]

Careful selection of patients for breast-preserving surgery is of major importance.[93,151] There are a number of clearly defined criteria which exclude patients from breast preserving surgery (see Table **3**a). Tumor size plays an important role in determining whether breast-conserving surgery is indicated. Whereas the Milan trial accepted only tumors of up to 2 centimeters in diameter, the NSABP study went up to 4 centimeters as the upper limit. Lately, the relative size of tumor to breast is considered to be of prime importance to assure cosmetically acceptable results. According to current data, tumor size in itself does not seem to be an important factor for local recurrence. More important seem to be multicentricity of the lesion[95] and, interestingly enough, the amount of in situ carcinoma accompanying the invasive lesion.[93,151] Thus, multicentric carcinoma with diffuse microcalcifications is an absolute contraindication. Relative contraindications are either an extensive intraductal component of the invasive tumor or the unquestionable involvement of lymphatic vessels. Other lesions better treated by mastectomy, are centrally located carcinomas, with or without Paget disease, histologically involved margins of resection, and those found in patients with collagen vascular diseases. Similarly, T4 lesions are not candidates for breast preserving surgery because involvement of skin, fixation to muscle, or thoracic wall preclude successful treatment by limited surgery. In the NSABP study,[81] patients with distant metastases were also excluded. Whether involvement of a margin of resection, as demonstrated by intraoperative frozen section, is an absolute contraindication, is controversial. In the NSABP study, these patients were excluded.[81] In the experience of other investigators,[3,46] the risk of local recurrence was not increased for patients with involved margins if proper postoperative radiotherapy was applied. Finally, it

Table **3**   Surgical treatment

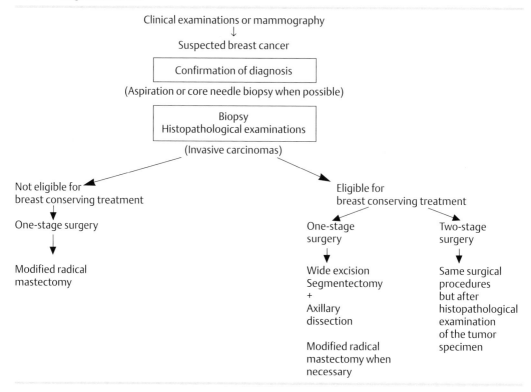

Table **3a**   Contraindications for breast-conserving surgery[a]

The following criteria identify breast cancers that should not be treated by breast-preserving modalities:

a) Morphological criteria:
  – Positive surgical margins
  – Lymphvascular space invasion of the breast tissue or the skin
  – Multicentricity

A concomitant intraductal component should not be considered an absolute contraindication for breast conserving surgery, except if the intraductal involvement is very extensive. The presence of lobular carcinoma in-situ (LCIS) is not a contraindication

b) Technical considerations:
  – If mammograms are inadequate for follow-up, e.g., in the presence of diffuse microcalcifications or mastopathia

_____
[a] Modified according to the NIH Consensus report (1990).

should be emphatically stated that the axillary lymph node status is *not* a criterion for the selection of patients for breast conserving surgery.

▓ Radiation after Limited and Radical Surgery

The use of postoperative radiotherapy after mastectomy on the one hand, and after breast conserving surgery on the other hand, has been developing in opposite directions. Whereas adjuvant radiation after mastectomy is steadily decreasing in significance, the necessity for postoperative treatment after breast conservation is being confirmed by all ongoing studies. Postoperative radiotherapy to the remaining ipsilateral breast tissue is a mandatory component of conservative treatment of carcinoma of the breast. According to current standards, conservative treatment by surgery alone is incomplete.[93]

The role of radiation as an adjuvant form of treatment after mastectomy was already recognized at the turn of the century, shortly after the discovery of X-rays. With the successive development of vastly improved new radiation equipment, from ortho-, to mega-, and finally supervoltage machines, it became possible to deliver significantly higher doses at deeper levels, preventing the severe side effects at the skin level seen in the early days. Conversely, the constant development of new equipment made it impossible to compare published treatment series, delaying the final assessment of benefits from postoperative radiation after mastectomy for many years. Nevertheless, a number of well-designed studies (NSABP Trial B-02, Manchester, Stockholm and Oslo Trial) were conducted[92, 258] and recently summarized.[58] There is no survival benefit for patients treated with postoperative radiation at the 5 and 10 year level. There is, however, a significant reduction of the local recurrence rate in the order of 30%.[92] Since there is no benefit to survival, local radiation therapy *for* recurrence has essentially the same effect as prophylactic postoperative irradiation. It appears that the number of patients benefiting from prophylactic postoperative radiotherapy is small, since treatment failure is mainly the result of distant metastases. Similarly, the subset of patients benefiting from axillary radiation treatment is essentially limited to those patients with remaining microscopic tumor foci in the axilla without distant spread. Since, according to our current understanding, axillar disease is an indicator of systemic spread, the number of patients falling into this category is extremely small. In both the Stockholm and the Oslo Trial, there was, however, a small survival advantage for patients with positive axillary nodes and primary breast tumors located in the inner and central portions of the breast. In this subset of patients, involvement of the internal mammary chain of lymph nodes was in the order of 50%. Treatment by radiotherapy of these lymph nodes is indicated in this situation.

As to the prevention of local recurrence, there is general agreement that radiotherapy is an effective means to prevent recurrent disease of the thoracic wall. Therefore, it has been common practice, particularly in Europe, to add postoperative radiotherapy routinely. This practice is currently changing. There are a number of institutions selecting patients carrying a high risk for local recurrence for postoperative radiotherapy. These high-risk factors include large primary tumors (T3), skin involvement (T4), incomplete excision, extensive axillary involvement with tumor extension through the lymph node capsule, and proven supraclavicular tumor extension. Patients not falling into these risk categories are not treated by prophylactic radiation. Rather, this type of treatment is applied at the time of proven recurrence.

The rationale for postoperative radiotherapy after breast preserving surgery is two-fold: sterilization of microscopic remnants of the primary tumor unintentionally left behind, and elimination of multicentric tumor foci in the remaining breast tissue. According to current data, the vast majority of local recurrences after conservative surgery are caused by relapsing primary tumors and not by multicentric tumor development. Breast irradiation (applying levels of 50 gray to the whole breast and a boost to the primary site), has been shown to be an effective means of significantly reducing local recurrence. In the NSABP study B06, the rate of recurrence was reduced from 28% in patients who did not receive postoperative radiation, to 8% in patients with postoperative radiotherapy.[81] These data at the 5-year level were confirmed at the 8-year level, the figures being 35% and 10%, respectively.[87] Results from a large nonrandomized study indicate that recurrences after breast preserving surgery and postoperative radiation accumulate rather constantly at a level of 1.5% for the first 10 postoperative years.[152] The ongoing prospective trials seem to confirm these data. Risk factors for recurrence and clinical patterns will be discussed in the section on recurrent disease.

Details of radiotherapeutic technique are beyond the scope of this review. In general, current standard equipment consists of a linear accelerator, allowing the delivery of a homogeneous dose throughout the breast from three tangential fields. The standard treatment consists of 45 gray in 25 fractions over 5 weeks. As discussed, the total dose to the site of the primary tumor is boosted to 63 gray, which significantly reduces the recurrence rate.

Adjuvant Therapy

As previously outlined, better local control of carcinoma of the breast by more aggressive sur-

Table **4** Adjuvant systemic therapy modalities (Refs. 39, 149)

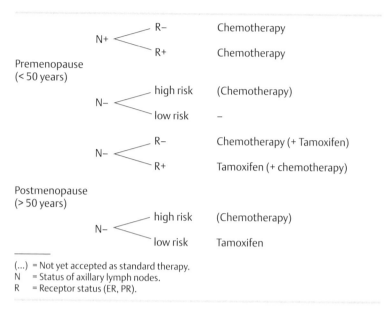

Premenopause (< 50 years)	N+	R–	Chemotherapy
		R+	Chemotherapy
	N–	high risk	(Chemotherapy)
		low risk	–
Postmenopause (> 50 years)	N–	R–	Chemotherapy (+ Tamoxifen)
		R+	Tamoxifen (+ chemotherapy)
	N–	high risk	(Chemotherapy)
		low risk	Tamoxifen

(...) = Not yet accepted as standard therapy.
N   = Status of axillary lymph nodes.
R   = Receptor status (ER, PR).

gery is unable to improve survival.[85] It is logical to assume that those patients who ultimately succumb to their disease already harbor occult micromestastases at distant sites at the time of diagnosis. It is increasingly accepted that any modifications in the treatment of the primary tumor (be it more, or less, aggressive) have no bearing on the ultimate fate of this large group of patients, representing more than 50% of all women afflicted with carcinoma of the breast. Any improvement in cure rates of the disease may only be achieved by systemic treatment of distant micrometastases at the time of initial diagnosis.[85, 130] This concept of "adjuvant," i.e., supportive treatment after surgery, has been tested with initial success in experimental animals and subsequently applied to a number of human cancers, especially in the pediatric age group. For carcinoma of the breast, first attempts of a "perioperative chemotherapy" were conducted in the 1960s.[109] Subsequently, extensive clinical trials with the prolonged use of intermittent multidrug regimens showed a significant improvement of the 5-year survival rate.[26] From these studies, the basic concepts of adjuvant chemotherapy were developed: adjuvant chemotherapy is only indicated in a selected group of patients; combination chemotherapy is more effective than monotherapy; perioperative application has no advantage over a postopera-

tive treatment; 6 monthly cycles are sufficient in most patients.[39, 88, 146, 184, 185]

Carcinoma of the breast is a hormone responsive tumor. It was tempting to test adjuvant hormone treatment, in particular since its toxicity is minor in comparison with chemotherapy. The earliest trials of adjuvant oophorectomy failed to show any advantage of survival, mainly because at that time, no knowledge of the estrogen-receptor protein existed. A preselection of patient subgroups, based on this powerful prognostic indicator, was not yet possible. After the description of estrogen and progesterone receptors as mediators of hormonal influence by Jensen,[65] a positive effect of adjuvant hormone therapy was rapidly established. Further progress was dependent on the development and propagation of technology to measure receptor protein content on a large-scale basis, and on the introduction of an essentially toxicity-free receptor blocker, such as tamoxifen. The first prospective, randomized trial of tamoxifen as adjuvant therapy was initiated in 1975, in Denmark.[193] Further studies rapidly followed. It became apparent that adjuvant hormone therapy is most beneficial for postmenopausal patients with positive axillary lymph nodes. The treatment should last at least 2 years, and that although the benefit is most pronounced in patients with receptor positive carcinomas, there is also marginal improvement in the recurrence-free survival in patients with negative tumors.[14, 70, 71, 81]

New statistical methods making so called metaanalyses possible are of major significance for the evaluation of the effectiveness of adjuvant therapy in carcinoma of the breast. Data on breast cancer were compiled by Richard Peto and collaborators at Oxford University in England.[70-72] In short, the expected and observed numbers of deaths are evaluated for the different treatment protocols of trials with similar designs, which were conducted by different investigators. As statistically significant results are obtained even from minor therapeutic effects, if the number of patients is sufficiently high, meta-analysis is a highly effective technique for detecting treatment advantages, which may not be significant in an individual trial. The first publication by Peto's group in 1985 summarized a total of 32 prospective trials on adjuvant therapy in 13000 patients. It represented an important data base for the recommendations of the NIH consensus statement on adjuvant therapy for breast cancer in September 1985. The latest publication of 1992 draws conclusions based on 75000 patients, including approximately 90% of all patients ever treated in randomized studies. For most trials, not only 5-year, but also 10-year survival data were available.

The following recommendations on current adjuvant treatment standards are based on the NIH consensus statements of 1985 and 1990,[51, 53] and the two published reports by Peto's group of 1985 and 1992.[70-72] (See Table **4**.) These recommendations are stratified according to three criteria: extent of axillary lymph node involvement, hormone receptor status, and menopausal status. It is therefore essential that these data are available before any decision on adjuvant therapy is made. Whereas axillary lymph node count and ER and PR levels are provided by the laboratory report, there may be occasional problems in determining the menopausal status, particularly in periclimacteric women. To simplify matters, some studies use the age of 50 as an arbitrary line to divide patients into pre- and postmenopausal. More correctly, determination of serum-FSH levels may be used to determine menopausal status. FSH values higher than 50 IU/L are a reliable indicator of postmenopausal status, values below this level indicate premenopausal status.

Adjuvant Chemotherapy

Adjuvant chemotherapy is now considered standard treatment for premenopausal patients with positive lymph nodes.[39, 70-72, 88, 104] Combination chemotherapy is clearly superior to single-agent chemotherapy. Most commonly, the CMF protocol (cyclophosphamide, methotrexate, 5-fluorouracil) is used.[250] For further details of dosage and timing, see Table **9**. CMF therapy should not extend over 6 monthly cycles. Treatment for longer periods has not been shown to offer any survival advantage. Best results are obtained in patients with limited axillary lymph node involvement, one to three positive nodes. The higher the number of involved axillary lymph nodes, the less effective is adjuvant chemotherapy. In patients with more than ten involved axillary lymph nodes, standard adjuvant chemotherapy is no longer recommended.

According to Peto's data,[71] 5-year survival rates in premenopausal women with positive axillary lymph nodes and no stratification as to number of involved nodes, is 73% in women receiving adjuvant chemotherapy, compared with 65% in women without adjuvant treatment. These figures translate into a more optimistic sounding reduction of disease related deaths, by 30% at the 5-year level. Realistically, while recommending patients for adjuvant chemotherapy, it should be remembered that out of 100 patients receiving this type of treatment, 65 patients do not benefit, because they are alive at 5 years even without treatment, and 25 patients do not benefit because they succumb to their disease with or without adjuvant chemotherapy. Only less than ten patients out of 100 actually benefit from adjuvant chemotherapy.

The role of adjuvant chemotherapy for node negative premenopausal patients is currently under investigation.[27, 135] Preliminary results of three prospective randomized studies were presented in a single issue of the New England Journal of Medicine 1989.[84, 163, 167] These studies (NSABP B13; Ludwig Trial 5 and Eastern Cooperative Oncology Group) arrived at essentially the same conclusion. Although the follow-up period was relatively short (3 to 4 years), there was a significant prolongation of disease-free survival among women receiving adjuvant chemotherapy. Risk factors for selection of patients included estrogen receptor negativity and tumors larger than 3 centimeters in diameter. Because of the short follow-up period, an effect on survival was not observed. Therefore, no final recommendations can be made at this point in time. The subgroup of patients carrying a high risk of recurrence and possibly benefiting from adjuvant chemotherapy include node negative patients with negative receptor status, large primary tumors, grade III lesion, and rapidly proliferating tumors. If treatment in such a situation is considered, patients and their physicians are strongly encouraged to participate in controlled clinical trials. It should be emphasized that at the present time, current data on survival benefits are not yet sufficient to recommend adjuvant chemotherapy in node negative patients.

Similarly, postmenopausal patients with positive axillary lymph nodes and *negative-*hormone receptor status represent a group of patients who may benefit from adjuvant chemotherapy. Again, data from controlled clinical trials are not yet conclusive enough to justify chemotherapy. For the time being, outside of clinical studies, an individual decision should be made after careful discussion with the patient considering age, tumor grade, size of the lesion, and possibly indicators of proliferative activity.

Among the side effects associated with adjuvant chemotherapy, short and long-term effects have to be separated. Among the short term effects, myelosuppression with white blood cell counts of less than 2000 and thrombocytopenia are most common. From a patients point of view, nausea and vomiting, as well as alopecia, are most troubling. Long-term toxicity, such as an increased incidence of second malignancy or chronic suppression of the immune system, is more difficult to ascertain. Final data, particularly on the most commonly used CMF regimen, are not yet available.[126] It appears, however, that an increased rate of leukemia and other secondary malignancies has to be expected. The NSABP is essentially the only study group with enough patients recruited and a long enough observation time to provide preliminary data on secondary malignancies. The NSABP experience was summarized in 1985, and consisted of 27 cases of leukemia (0.5%) among over 5000 patients treated by adjuvant chemotherapy.[89]

Finally, there are only a few data available on preoperative "neoadjuvant" chemotherapy. Preoperative chemotherapy is currently standard treatment only for inflammatory breast cancer and in selected cases of locally advanced breast cancer with extensive skin involvement.

Adjuvant Hormone Therapy

Tamoxifen treatment of postmenopausal patients with positive axillary lymph nodes and *positive* receptor status is currently considered standard therapy. There have been seven prospective randomized trials, each of them showing a significant increase in the recurrence-free survival rate. Again, this positive outcome was confirmed by the meta-analysis of Peto, who summarized the effects on close to 30000 patients, who were examined in 72 individual trials on the effectiveness of tamoxifen.[71] Overall, a reduction in the annual mortality rate by 20% was observed in patients over 50 years of age. Similarly the recurrence rate was reduced in postmenopausal patients by 29%. Considering the essentially toxicity-free application of this drug, adjuvant hormone therapy with tamoxifen in postmenopausal, node positive patients has been a major achievement in the treatment of carcinoma of the breast.

Surprisingly, there was also a significant reduction in recurrence rate and mortality in node positive, postmenopausal patients with low (less than 10 fmol-mg) or negative receptor content. There was a reduction in the recurrence rate of 16% in these patients. Possible reasons for this discrepancy may be due to problems with receptor assays, transport delay of tumor tissue, or a theoretical induction of receptors.

According to current standards, antiestrogen treatment with tamoxifen in adjuvant form is not indicated in premenopausal patients.[184] It is ineffective and may induce estrogen and progestorone hormone production via stimulation of FSH and LH and thus possibly stimulate tumor cell growth in premenopausal patients with ovarian function. There are currently a number of clinical studies using LHRH agonists or antagonists for adjuvant hormone treatment in premenopausal patients. Preliminary results of a randomized, multicenter, international trial comparing this type of adjuvant hormone therapy with standard CMF adjuvant chemotherapy, indicate that receptor-positive premenopausal patients may benefit from this treatment.[137] Outside of clinical trials, such treatment cannot yet be recommended. Agonists of pituitary gonadotropine releasing hormones initially cause an increased secretion of LH and FSH. Subsequently, with the depletion of storage levels, the stimulatory effect on the ovary subsides, resulting in a temporary, reversible blockage of ovarian estrogen function. Currently available drugs of this type are buserelin and goserelin.

Biological and other Therapies

Treatment of carcinoma of the breast by immunological or biological means is strictly investigational. None of these methods are currently accepted as part of a standard treatment protocol. Immunologic and biologic treatment of carcinoma of the breast should, therefore, be restricted to well defined and supervised clinical trials at larger medical centers. In the last couple of years, these new techniques have raised new hopes because they may represent a breakthrough in cancer treatment in general. Clinical trials so far conducted[131, 132, 212–215] and published have not yet provided convincing data to support these expectations. Further progress depends on a better understanding of the complex interaction of the human immune system.

First attempts to manipulate the immune system in order to interfere with malignant tumor growth date back to the turn of the century. It was, however, not until the 1960s that it became possible to eliminate malignant cells by immunologic means in experimental animals. For this purpose, a number of nonspecific immunostimulants, such as BCG (Bacillus Calmette-Guerin) and corynebacterium parvum were used.[120] Unfortunately, these experimental data could never be confirmed by clinial studies in humans. Lately, new developments in immunology have precipitated a new wave of immunologic treatment protocols in human cancer. First, there have been major advances in our understanding of the human immune system. Secondly, newly developed techniques of genetic engineering allowed the production of an essentially unlimited number of highly specific substances interacting with the immune system.[143, 144, 145] Thus, the term biological response modifiers (BRM) was created for a class of proteins that are able to modify the inflammatory and immune response. Most prominent among these are cytokines, which include interferon gamma, interleukins, and tumor necrosis factor. Cytokines are the most important

and most promising biological response modifiers.[178, 179] Further details of this group of substances are given in the section on current research.

In a further development, some of the specific biologic response modifiers, such as interleukins, are used to stimulate specific subpopulations of autologous lymphocytes in vitro, in order to enhance their tumor destroying capacity.[2, 4, 38, 131, 132, 150, 212–215, 246] Again, more details on these experimental approaches will be furnished in the section on current research.

Follow-up Management

Although the necessity for follow-up examinations in breast cancer patients at regular intervals is undisputed, the extent of such follow-up has become a matter of debate.[169] Over the last 20 years, standardized follow-up schedules of patients with carcinoma of the breast have been instituted in a number of countries. It was the intention of these schemes to detect recurrent disease at an early stage by a medical history, physical examination, a series of lab tests, X-rays, and isotope examination. It is becoming increasingly clear that this has no benefit for the patient.[67] There is no improvement of survival by early detection of metastases.[245] As discussed earlier, once metastatic disease has developed, a cure is no longer possible. Therefore, the recognition of distant spread at an asymptomatic stage a few months before clinical manifestation has no bearing on the ultimate outcome. The critical view that the overzealous compilation of large numbers of follow-up data is irrelevant, is accepted by an increasing number of investigators. Instead, new emphasis is being put on quality of life, psychosocial assistance, and occupational rehabilitation.[37, 44]

According to current standards, patients should be seen by their physician every 3 months for the first 2 years after the completion of therapy. Subsequently, follow-up examinations at 6 month intervals are recommended. Prime objectives should be guidance, advice, and support in the difficult process of accepting the disease. There should be particular emphasis on history and physical examination. Laboratory testing should be reduced to a minimum.[147] It has been shown that the majority of recurrences are detected by history and examination alone. Specifically, questions directed at typical symptoms, such as pain, cough, lymph-node enlarge-ment, or skin alterations should be asked.[262] According to current understanding, there is little if any use for laboratory tests, X-rays, and bone scans. Of the tumor markers, only CEA and CA15/3 (MCA) may be of help because of reasonable specificity and sensitivity. They are most valuable, however, for monitoring therapeutic success after initiation of treat-ment.

Of all radiographic examinations, only mammography of the contralateral breast and the ipsilateral breast after breast preserving surgery are of unquestionable significance. Metachronous carcinoma in the contralateral of the breast develops in 4% to 6% of cases. The significance of newly detected calcifications in the ipsilateral breast after conservative surgery has already been emphasized. Mammog-raphy at yearly intervals is, therefore, rec-ommended. Ultrasound examination of the breast is not recommended as an isolated technique without mammography. In con-trast, bone scans are only indicated in symp-tomatic patients.[19] Routine bone scans as a screening procedure are costly and usually create more anxiety than benefit because of low specificity.[42, 186] For the evaluation of pos-sible liver disease, ultrasound is the method of choice. It is a fairly accurate technique for detecting metastases of 1 cm in size and larger.

Recurrent Disease

Of all patients afflicted by carcinoma of the breast, about half will develop a recurrence within 10 years after diagnosis (Table **6**). At present, recurrent breast cancer cannot be cured. Ultimately, all of these patients will die of their disease. The goal of treatment of metastatic breast cancer is, therefore, pal-liation of symptoms. Whether a prolongation of survival is at all possible, is currently a mat-ter of debate. The experienced clinician will use the available modalities wisely and prudently, to alleviate symptoms and to op-timize the quality of life. It should be kept in mind that with currently available techniques, all symptoms can effectively be influenced, including bone pain, ulcerating skin lesions, and shortness of breath from to pleural effu-sion. The guiding principal for treatment of metastatic breast cancer is palliation and not cure.

Recurrent disease after breast conserving surgery, limited to the remaining ipsilateral breast tissue, is the only exception to this rule.[116] In the well defined situation of a strictly local recurrence, disease-free survival of close to 70% may be achieved by the so-called salvage mastec-tomy. The discrepancy between local recurrence after mastectomy and local recurrence after breast conserving surgery cannot be overem-phasized.

Table **5** Combined modality approach for local–regional recurrence

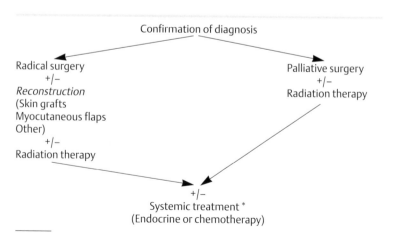

Confirmation of diagnosis

Radical surgery
+/–
Reconstruction
(Skin grafts
Myocutaneous flaps
Other)
+/–
Radiation therapy

Palliative surgery
+/–
Radiation therapy

+/–
Systemic treatment *
(Endocrine or chemotherapy)

* only in cases with proven distant metastases.

Table **6** Cumulative recurrence rates (%) in node negative and node-positive breast cancer patients after 10 years (Refs. 249, 250)

Site of first relapse	Percentage of patients	
	N–	N+
Local/regional* only	6.0	17.8
Distant	10.0	28.2
bone	6.2	14.4
visceral	2.6	10.9
soft tissue	1.2	2.9
Multiple sites	7.2	23.3
local/regional and distant	2.0	9.1
multiple distant	5.2	14.2
Contralateral	4.7	6.2
Total	27.9	75.5

▓ Diagnostic and Surgical Procedures

Local Recurrence after Breast Conserving Surgery [124]

Recurrent disease in the treated breast after breast-conserving surgery, is only associated with distant metastases in a minority of patients.[102] Since axillary dissection has already been performed at the time of primary treatment, a so-called salvage mastectomy is the standard treatment in this situation. Only limited experience is currently available with a repeat wide excision for local recurrence after breast-conserving therapy.[152] The 10-year survival rate of patients after salvage mastectomy, is reported to range between 69% and 81%, and does not significantly differ from those patients treated conservatively and without recurrence after breast conserving surgery and radiotherapy (as reported by Kurtz from the Marseille Cancer Institute in 1989).[152] Among 1600 patients treated between 1963 and 1982, the overall recurrence rate was 11%. There was a fairly constant yearly actuarial risk of breast recurrence, averaging 1.5% for the first 10 years. For the third 5-year period, the risk decreased to 1.1% per year. Of particular importance was the rare entity of uncontrolled local recurrence after conservative treatment.[13] It paralleled the clinical signs and the prognosis of inflammatory carcinoma and led to rapid demise of the patient. It was reported to

occur in 14%[95] to 21%[152] of all recurrences. It is interesting to note that there was a significant reduction in the likelihood of local recurrence in premenopausal patients with positive lymph nodes who did receive adjuvant chemotherapy.[208] It is assumed that a possible interaction between radiation therapy and chemotherapy is additive in it's effect on local tumor control.

The diagnosis of recurrent disease in an operated and irradiated breast requires particular attention. In the majority of patients, the recurrence will be suspected by clinical investigation alone. In the differential diagnosis, fat necrosis, suture granuloma, and radiation fibrosis are of particular significance under these circumstances. Biopsy confirmation is, therefore, mandatory. The significance of new calcification in the postirradiated breast, detected by mammography, has recently been emphasized.[235] In 19 patients who had developed new mammographic calcification without an associated palpable mass, 11 (58%) showed evidence of malignancy in the subsequent biopsy. Prognostic factors for patients with breast recurrence after conservative surgery[101] included disease-free interval since primary therapy, tumor grade, and size of the recurrence. No significant influence on overall survival following recurrence was found for menopausal status, initial T- and N-stage, and estrogen receptor status. There have been no reports on increased problems with wound healing in patients treated by salvage mastectomy in a previously irradiated breast.

Local Recurrence after Mastectomy

As indicated above, local recurrence after mastectomy carries a much more ominous prognosis than local recurrence after breast conservation.[78] It represents the first manifestation of systemic disease in the vast majority of patients. Distant metastases will follow in 81% to 100%,[15, 108] usually within 2 years.[159] Although the median survival from first local relapse is significantly longer than from first systemic relapse, 5-year survival is only around 20%. The recurrence occurs in over half of all patients less than 2 years after diagnosis; about 90% of all recurrences occur within 5 years. In most cases, tumor will reappear within or around the central scar or on the chest wall. Most commonly, single or multiple nodules of up to one centimeter appear. Only a minority of tumors recurs in the axilla or in the supraclavicular fossa. In more advanced situations, induration of the entire chest wall with diffuse inflammation creates the image of the so-called cancer en cuirasse. Other signs of advanced local recurrence are edema of the arm, bone destruction of the sternum or ribs, pleural effusion, or mediastinal involvement. It is essential to confirm local recurrence by biopsy. A repeat determination of receptor status on this biopsy material is advisable. Dependent on previous surgery and irradiation, particular attention as to site and type of biopsy is necessary. If the recurrence is isolated, the biopsy should be excisional. Further management depends upon staging for distant metastases, which is essential at this point. Minimal requirements include a bone scan, chest X-ray, ultrasonography of the liver, and determination of tumor markers. If the search for distant metastases is negative, an attempt at wide excision using plastic surgical procedures may be indicated in exceptional situations.[200, 231] The method of choice for local recurrence limited to the chest wall is, however, radiotherapy.[136, 177]

Regional and Distant Metastases

Recurrence in the axillary and internal mammary chain of lymph nodes are classified as regional disease. According to the new guidelines by the UICC, the supraclavicular lymph nodes are now considered to represent distant metastases.[244] As with local recurrence, the majority of distant metastases occur within 2 years of diagnosis. The risk of relapse continues, however, in carcinoma of the breast even after 30 years of follow-up. The most common sites of distant metastases are bone, lung and pleura, soft tissue, liver, and even ovary, in this order. Once distant metastases have occurred, prognosis is poor. Median survival ranges from 5% to 18% after 5 years. For diagnostic purposes, radiologic and biochemical investigations are used. If at all possible, biopsy confirmation should be obtained. Whereas bone scanning is used to search for possible metastatic sites, X-ray verification is essential to prevent false-positive diagnosis. Among the tumor markers, the oncofetal protein CEA is the most widely used marker. Tumor markers have low specificity and, despite the large number of available markers, an increase is not sufficient evidence for a firm diagnosis of metastatic disease.

▓ Radiation Therapy

Radiation is most effective in controlling symptomatic metastases of breast cancer. Palliation can be achieved in most cases.[176] Symptoms disappear or decrease considerably. The most common indications for treatment are bone pain and risk of pathological fracture.[183] Chest wall recurrences, uncontrollable by other techniques, also lend themselves successfully to radiation. In general, 30 to 40 Gy in 10 to 15 fractions are applied over 2 to 3 weeks to achieve a response rate between 70% and 90%.[43] A wide range of dose fractionation (dependent on size and location of metastases) is used. Further details are beyond the scope of this review.

▓ Chemotherapy

When considering chemotherapy for patients with metastasizing carcinoma of the breast, it should be kept in mind that an increase in survival cannot be achieved for the group as whole. There may, however, be subgroups, not yet clearly defined, in which prolongation of survival may be achieved by chemotherapy. In general, indications for chemotherapy are nonresponse to hormone therapy in symptomatic patients, and life-threatening complications in patients with rapidly progressive tumors such as visceral metastases (see Tables **7**, **8**).[202]

Combination chemotherapy was introduced to the treatment of hormone resistent metastasizing carcinoma of the breast by Cooper in 1969.[55] He used the combination of the five drugs cyclophosphamide, methotrexate, 5-flourouracil, vincristine, and prednisone (CMFVP). Because of considerable neural toxicity, vincristine was deleted from this five drug regimen. Similarly, prednisone is not considered essential. Therefore, the regimen consisting of methotrexate, flourouracil, and cyclophoshamide is currently the most widely used regimen (see Table **9**). The introduction of anthracyclines, such as doxorubicin in 1975, increased the response rate, but at a higher rate of toxicity. These four drugs, cyclophosphamide (C), 5-flourouracil (F), methotrexate (M), and doxorubicin (A) represent the most effective and by far the most commonly used drugs for carcinoma of the breast. A partial or complete response will be achieved in about half of all patients treated with chemotherapy. A complete response, with disappearance of all

Table 7 Differentiation in low and high-risk metastatic breast cancer patients according to Posinger (Refs. 202, 203)

Criteria		Score points
Number of metastatic sites:		
bone, skin, soft tissue	each	1
Bone-marrow involvement		4
Lung metastases:		
nodular, less than 10		3
nodular, more than 10		5
diffuse lymphangiosis carcinomatosa		6
Liver metastases		6
Receptor status:		
positive		1
unknown		2
negative		3
Disease-free interval		
> 2 years		1
< 2 years		3
Score points:	low risk	< 7
	high risk	> 7

evidence of tumor is, however, seen in less than 20% of patients. It is likely that the major effect of chemotherapy in carcinoma of the breast is achieved shortly after initation. If the tumor is responsive, the maximum reduction of tumor burden is achieved within two to four cycles of chemotherapy. Clinical evidence of response is evident between 2 and 3 months. These considerations strongly recommend the use of chemotherapy in short cycles of 3 to 6 months. In contrast to hormone treatment, there is no evidence that a prolonged use of cytotoxic therapy provides any additional benefit.

Among the four core drugs mentioned, doxorubicin is the most active single drug for treating metastatic carcinoma of the breast. The toxic side effects are, however, considerable. Alopecia occurs in almost all patients within 2 to 3 weeks. The most severe side effect, cardiotoxicity, occurs frequently after an accumulative dose of 450 mg per square meter if used in combination with other drugs. In order to mitigate this severe side effect, newer drugs were developed, the most prominent being 4-epirubicin. Although alopecia occurs almost as frequently as

Table 8 Systemic therapy modalities for metastatic breast cancer

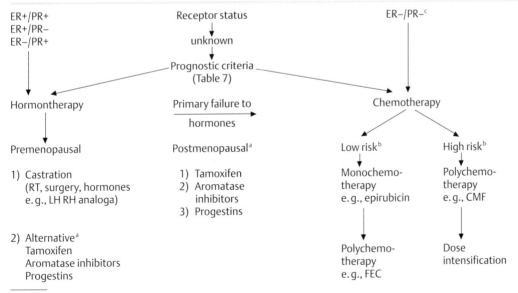

---
[a] Trial of 1st – 3rd line.
    Hormones in all cases of CR, PR, or NC to hormones.
[b] High risk, e. g., liver and lung metastases.
[c] Receptor data on primary or recurrent tumor if available.

1. Chemotherapy of breast cancer

A. Standard therapy

Premenopausal and postmenopausal adjuvant/or metastatic

Cyclophosphamide/Methotrexate/Fluorouracil				CMF
Cyclophosphamide	100 mg/m^2	p.o.	day 1–14	
Methotrexate	40 mg/m^2	i.v.	day 1 + 8	
5-Fluorouracil	600 mg/m^2	i.v.	day 1 + 8	

Every 28 days

Side effects: Nausea, vomiting, leuco-, thrombocytopenia, alopecia

Premenopausal and postmenopausal adjuvant/or metastatic

modified CMF-Protocol

Cyclophosphamide	500 mg/m^2	i.v.	day 1 + 8
Methotrexate	40 mg/m^2	i.v.	day 1 + 8
5-Fluorouracil	500 mg/m^2	i.v.	day 1 + 8

Every 28 days

Side effects: Nausea, vomiting, leucoeytopenia, thrombocytopenia, alopecia

B. Therapy for "high-risk" patients

Three-drug regimen

Fluorouracil/Adriamycin/Cyclophosphamide or Epirubicin				FAC FEC
5-Fluorouracil	500 mg/m^2	i.v.	day 1	
Adriamycin/Epirubicin	50 mg/m^2	i.v.	day 1	
Cyclophosphamide	500 mg/m^2	i.v.	day 1	

Every 28 days

Side effects: Nausea, vomiting, leucoeytopenia, thrombocytopenia, alopecia

Cave:	Cardiotoxicity	
	Adriamycin	450 mg/m^2 dose limit
	Epirubicin	750 mg/m^2 dose limit

Two-drug regimen

			AC or EC or NC
Adriamycin or	40 mg/m^2	i.v.	day 1
Epirubicin or	40 mg/m^2	i.v.	day 1
Novantrone with	12 mg/m^2	i.v.	day 1
Cyclophosphamide	600 mg/m^2	i.v.	day 1

Every 21 days

Side effects: Nausea, vomiting, leucoeytopenia, thrombocytopenia, alopecia

Cave:	Cardiotoxicity,	
	Adriamycin	450 mg/m^2 dose limit
	Epirubicin	750 mg/m^2 dose limit
	Novantrone	200 mg/m^2 dose limit

Table **9** (Continued)

Novantrone/Prednimustin			"Noste"
Novantrone	12 mg/m^2	i.v.	day 1
Prednimustin	100 mg/m^2	p.o.	day 3 – 7

Every 28 days

Side effects: Nausea, vomiting, leucocytopenia, thrombocytopenia, alopecia

Cave: Novantrone   200 mg/m^2 cumulative dose limit

C. Monotherapy ("Low-risk" patients)

Epirubicin			E "weekly"
Epirubicin	12 – 20 mg/m^2	i.v.	Once weekly

Continuously until disease progression

Side effects: Nausea, vomiting, leucocytopenia, thrombocytopenia

Cave:	Cardiotoxicity,		
	Epirubicin	750 mg/m^2 dose limit	

Mitoxantrone			N-Mono
Novantrone	12 mg/m^2	i.v.	day 1

Every 21 days

Side effects: Nausea, vomiting, leucocytopenia, thrombocytopenia

Cave: Novantrone 200 mg/m^2 cumulative dose limit

Prednimustin	40 mg/m^2	p.o.	daily

Continuously until disease progression

Side effects: Nausea, leucocytopenia, and thrombocytopenia

---

2. Hormone therapy of breast cancer

Postmenopausal adjuvant/or metastatic
Antiestrogen

Tamoxifen			TAM
Tamoxifen	20 – 30 mg	p.o.	daily

Adjuvant 2 – 5 years or continously until disease progression

Side effects: Nausea (rare), hot flushes, thrombocytopenia, and leucocytopenia

---

Postmenopausal (recurrent)
Aromatase inhibitor

Aminogluthetimide			AG
Aminogluthetimide	500 mg	p.o.	daily
+ Cortisonacetate	37.5 mg	p.o.	daily
	(25 mg a.m. + 12.5 p.m.)		

Continuously until disease progression

Side effects: Fatigue, hypotension, nausea

Table **9** (Continued)

Premenopausal and postmenopausal (recurrent)
Progestin

High dose Medroxyprogesteronacetate				HD-MPA

Medroxyprogesterone-acetate	500–1000 mg	p.o.	daily	

Continuously until disease progression
Side effects: Weight gain, hypertension, thrombosis, Cushing syndrome
Cave: hypertonic crisis, embolism, diabetes

Premenopausal and postmenopausal (recurrent)
Progestin

Megestroalcetate				MA

Megestrolacetate	160–320 mg	p.o.	daily	

Continuously until disease progression
Side effects: Weight gain, hypertonia, thrombosis, Cushing syndrome
Cave: hypertonic crisis, embolism, diabetes

Premenopausal (recurrent)
GnRH-analogues

GnRH-therapy		GnRH-Analogues	

Buserelin	1 Amp.	s.c.	every 3–4 weeks
or			
Goserelinacetate	1 Amp.	s.c.	every 4 weeks
or			
Gonadorelinacetate	1 Amp.	i.m.	every 4 weeks

Continuously until disease progression
Side effects: Hot flushes, loss of libido

Premenopausal and postmenopausal (palliative)
Androgens

Drostanolonpropionat	100 mg	i.m.	day 1, 3, 5

Continuously once a week

Testolactone (Fludestrin)

Testolactone	250 mg	i.m.	once a week

Continuously once a week

with doxorubicin, the cardiotoxic side effect of 4-epirubicin is only 50% (see Table **9**).

Hormone Therapy

If systemic therapy is indicated in patients with metastatic breast carcinoma, it is current consensus that hormone therapy is preferrable to chemotherapy. Again, indications for treatment are symptoms associated with metastatic disease; the goal of treatment is palliation. Guidelines for treatment of metastatic carcinoma of the breast were developed in a consensus conference in Munich, Juli 1988.[52] Criteria for selection of therapy are menopausal and receptor status.[50] A number of treatment modalities are availabel (hormone receptor blocker, adrenal supression with enzyme blocker and high-dose progestins in postmenopausal patients; ovarian ablation adrenal supression and high-dose progestins in premenopausal patients) (see Table **9**). A sequential application of these hormonal modalities may lead to successive remissions in responsive patients. Patients who are nonresponsive to hormonal therapy, should be treated by chemotherapy.

Tamoxifen is the treatment of choice for postmenopausal patients with positive or unknown receptor status.[186, 197] Response rates of 60% are achieved by a daily dose of 20 milligrams. A tamoxifen trial should last at least 3 months because sufficiently high serum levels are reached only after several weeks. In nonresponding or relapsing patients, the second-line treatment in postmenopausal patients is aminoglutethimide, which supresses the adrenal gland by inhibiting the enzyme aromatase.[219] The daily dose is 500 milligrams; a cortisone replacement of 30 to 40 milligrams per day is mandatory.[239] High-dose progestin treatment is the third line of this sequential–hormonal therapy in postmenopausal patients. Medroxyprogesterone acetate is administered at a dose of 500 to 1000 milligrams daily.[40, 201] MPA serum level measurements are recommended to assure levels that will achieve remission. As an alternative, megastrol acetate may be used at a dose of 160 to 320 milligrams.[243] The effective serum level of megastrol acetate is still unknown. Patients with positive-androgen receptor status or advanced breast cancer patients with catabolic metabolism may require androgen treatment, or high-dose cortisone treatment in exceptional cases.

For premenopausal patients, the traditional first-line hormonal treatment has been oophorectomy, with response rates in the order of 30%. Recently, similar response rates have been achieved with tamoxifen in premenopausal patients and with LHRH analogues.[260] These drugs are applied subcutaneously once a month, and are currently being evaluated in a number of studies. It appears that they will be replacing the oophorectomy as the first-line treatment in premenopausal patients in the near future.[137] Second and third-line hormonal therapy in premenopausal patients corresponds to the steps outlined above for postmenopausal patients.[204]

A combination of various hormonal treatment modalities is not indicated; there has been no evidence of an additive effect. Similarly, a combination of hormone therapy with chemotherapy is not indicated in the individual treatment cycle. The hormonal treatment should be continued indefinetely until progression of the disease.

Current Research

The following chapter summarizes some of the current new developments in the diagnosis and treatment of carcinoma of the breast that are not yet part of a standard treatment protocol. These new techniques are being tested in clinical trials around the world. Some of them, such as the new prognostic parameters, are about to be incorporated into standard diagnostic regimens. Others, such as the immunologic treatment modalities, are still in an experimental stage. Only those techniques are included in this short review, which may be of significance for clinical practice in the foreseeable future.[226]

Prognostic Factors

As discussed above, a major area of breast cancer research is the development of more precise parameters for prognostication of tumor behavior and relapse pattern.[172] Based on currently accepted prognostic factors, such as axillary lymph node status, tumor size and grade, and hormone receptor status, a fairly accurate estimation of survival and recurrence can be made for larger patient cohorts. However, the individual patient's personal fate remains undetermined. Treatment decisions are based on

Table **10** Prognostic factors for proliferation und growth regulation

Prognostic factor	Poor prognosis
Thymidine incorporation	high
S-Phase (%)	high
Ploidy index	aneuploid
KI-67	high
EGF receptor	positive
HER-2 neu oncogene amplification	high
P 170-Glycoprotein expression	high

Prognostic factors for invasion:

Cathepsin D	positive
Urokinase type plasminogen activator	positive
Bone marrow metastasis	positive

probabilities and not on individual tumor cell parameters. Considering the heterogeneity of human breast-cancer cell lines, the development of more sophisticated techniques to characterize tumor cell behavior is of major significance. Most of the new parameters that are being tested measure the proliferation and growth capacity of the individual patient's tumor cells (see Table **10**).[173, 181, 232]

Measurement of nuclear DNA content and determination of DNA ploidy distribution have shown that tumors with a diploid or near-diploid pattern have a significantly better prognosis than tumors with aneuploid-chromatin patterns.[11, 24, 56, 236] Initially, these studies were performed by microphotometric DNA determination on Feulgen-stained sections or imprints. Flow cytometric techniques, which are now available, have considerably simplified the study of ploidy.[47, 69] There is, however, considerable overlap with receptor content and histologic grade. Diploid tumors tend to be receptor positive and low grade, whereas aneuploid tumors are mostly receptor negative and high grade.

Cell cycle analysis is another method used for determining the proliferative fraction of a malignant tumor.[139] Determination of the S-phase fraction by flow cytometry measures the percentage of cells currently in the S-phase of the cell cycle, the phase preceding cell division. This phase fraction of the tumor cell population may also be determined by the thymidine-labelling index, a radioactive method measuring the incorporation

of DNA components. The growth fraction[161, 175] may be determined by a specific antibody directed against the antigen Ki-67,[106, 107] which is associated with all phases of the cell cycle (G1, S, G2 and M-phase).[12] This monoclonal antibody may be used on histologic sections as an immuno–histochemical reagent or, more elegantly, in an image analysis system[103] or with flow cytometry. It should be kept in mind that there are important differences between these various techniques, although all of them give an estimation of proliferative capacity of the cell. The antigen Ki-67 is expressed in all phases of the cell cycle except G0. S-phase fraction and ploidy levels are both based on DNA content analysis. Flow cytometric techniques use homogenized tissue preparations, which commonly include a mixture of benign cells that may cause an underestimation. Ki-67 immune reactivity can only be determined on frozen tissues. In contrast, flow cytometric examinations are also possible on archival paraffin embedded specimens.

The epidermal growth factor receptor (EGF receptor) is expressed in 20% to 50% of breast cancer patients as a cell surface antigen and may be demonstrated either biochemically or immunohistochemically. EGF receptor expression is associated with a significant reduction of recurrence free and total survival rate.[218]

Overexpression of an oncogene (HER-2-neu-oncogene) has been shown by Slamon et al.[234] to be correlated with early relapse and poor survival. These data were confirmed by Paik et al.[192] on the NSABP material, and by others.[16, 29, 265]

Finally, there have been attempts to determine the invasive potential of breast cancer cells at an early stage of the disease. It has been shown that the secretion of lysosomal enzymes, such as cathepsin D, represents a prognostic parameter independent of tumor size, node involvement, hormone receptor status, and grading.[241] It has been hypothesized that this enzyme enhances tumor invasion by proteolysis of the host–tissue matrix. The detection of micrometastases in bone marrow[60, 166] by highly sensitive immunocytochemical techniques, was also used as an early predictor of subsequent development of metastatic disease. Systematic bone marrow aspiration from the sternum, sacrum, and iliac crests under general anesthesia at the time of initial breast-cancer surgery, was introduced by Dearnaley et al. in 1981. Using a newly developed monoclonal antibody against the epithelial membrane antigen, they detected tumor cells in 25% of patients with no other evidence of distant metastases. Significance of these findings for therapy are still controversial.

Immunotherapy

More recent methods and developments in the past few years have given rise to some promising perspectives with regard to the use of immunotherapy in tumor disease. On the one hand, there are almost countless new substances now produced by genetic engineering for stimulation and modulation of the immune system in cancer patients. On the other hand, procedures have been developed that allow the enrichment of autologous stimulated lymphocytes, which have lately been used for interesting treatment approaches.

Biological Response Modifiers (BRM)

These complex biological substances have immuno-modulatory effects under certain conditions (see Table **11**). However, these substances cannot be used selectively for the stimulation of tumor defense mechanisms or for specific inhibition of tumor growth.

Table **11**   Biological response modifiers (BRM) (Ref. 150)

Complex biological substances
  BCG
  Corynebacterium parvum
  OK 432
  OHI
  Lentinan

Defined pharmaca
  Levamisole
  Polyribonucleotide (Poly U: Poly C)
  PG_E-inhibitors
  Tuftsin
  Bestatin
  Muramyldipeptide

Cytokines
  Interferons
  Interleukins
  Tumor necrosis factor
  Growth factors
  Thymus hormone

Differentiation factors

In the past few years, a large number of proteins have gained particular importance, modifying inflammatory and immune responses. If these proteins are produced by cells, they are called cytokines and include interferons, interleukins, and tumor necrosis factors. Cytokines are the most important and most promising biological response modifieres today, besides the growth and differentiation factors.

Interferon

Interferons are divided into three subgroups on the basis of their different antigenic, chemical, and biological properties: virus-induced interferon-α (produced by leukocytes), interferon-β (produced by fibroblasts), and interferon-y (produced by T lymphocytes) after antigenic or mitogenic stimulation. Interferons show immunomodulatory properties of varying potency. These include the activation of macrophages, NK and T cells, as well as an enhanced expression of antigens and receptors on effector cells, indication of certain enzymatic cell processes, extension of the phases of the cell cycle, and inhibition of proto-oncogenes. This range of effects eventually led to the use of interferons in the treatment of tumors. According to current data, however, the systemic treatment of breast cancer by interferon is fairly ineffective.

Interleukins

Interleukins are polypeptides that establish communication between various cell types. They are released by the producing cell into its environment and act on the target cell through a receptor. So far, twenty interleukins have been identified. However, only the first three are available as recombinant interleukins for trials.

Interleukin-1 is produced by antigen-presenting cells (macrophages) in case of antigen-specific binding of T lymphocytes. It induces production of IL-2 by T cells. IL-1 obviously has a variety of other immunological effects, whose influence on the various cellular components of the immune system has not yet been completely clarified. IL-1's direct action on malignant tumors is currently being investigated in the first clinical trials. There are no results as yet.

Interleukin-2, a glycolysed polypeptide, was first described in 1976 as T cell growth factor in a culture supernatant of mitogen-stimulated lymphocytes. In humans, helper cells, suppressor cells, and NK cells can be stimulated to produce supressor cells, as well as IL-2. IL-2 seems to be required as a growth hormone for all T cell sub-populations. Mature T cells produce IL-2 only under the condition that there are antigen-presenting cells in addition to the specific antigen. IL-2 induces proliferation of T cells with interleukin-2 receptors and supplies the effector cells with the proper cellular immune response. Independently of proliferation, IL-2 also enhances the cytotoxic activity of NK cells, differentiation of thymocytes into cytotoxic T cells, and the production of interferon-y. This wide range of functions confers interleukin-2 a central role in the generation of cellular immune response. An attempt has been made to use IL-2 directly for in situ activation of effector cells, such as macrophages or NK cells for in vivo antitumor treatment. However, the first clinical trials have shown that systematic treatment with IL-2 did not yield any measurable antitumor effect in patients with advanced disease. Therefore, systemic use of IL-2 alone for immunotherapy of malignant tumors was abandoned.

Interleukin-3 and the growth factor granulocyte/macrophage colony stimulating factor (GM-CSF), influence hematopoiesis through their capacity to induce growth and differentiation of hematopoietic precursor cells. Generally, therapeutic indications for using IL-3 and GM-CSF are acceleration of bone marrow regeneration after intensive chemotherapy, containment of autonomous growth in certain types of leukemia, and activation of granulocytes and monocytes for nonspecific immune response. They are currently being investigated in clinical trials. Again, clinically relevant results are not yet available.

Tumor necrosis factors (TNF) are proteins that can be demonstrated in the serum during endotoxic shock, and may produce specific toxic effects on certain types of tumors. At present, two tumor necrosis factors are known; TNF-α, which is produced by macrophages, and TNF-β (lymphotoxin), which is produced by lymphocytes. The optimum dosage, mode of application, and the clinical value of TNF in immunotherapy for cancer, are currently being investigated and cannot yet be evaluated.

Enrichment of Autologous Stimulated Lymphocytes for Immunotherapy

The newly available lymphokines (in particular IL-2 with its capacity to activate effector cells in vitro) have led to a renaissance of immunotherapeutic approaches with autologous-stimulated lymphocytes.

One approach is specific immunotherapy of carcinoma. There are no sufficient data on the therapeutic success of this treatment in breast cancer as yet. Therefore, the effectiveness of this type of treatment with breast-cancer patients cannot be evaluated.

Another treatment concept uses "tumor-infiltrating lymphocytes" (TIL cells). Lymphocytes are isolated from the tumor by mechanical or enzymatic means, or through density gradient centrifugation, and are then stimulated in vitro, using high IL-2 dosages. Lymphocytes that are cultivated in this way may develop lytic activity on tumor cells that is several times greater than the one of LAK cells isolated from peripheral blood. The possibility of allowing such cells from patient tumors to mature by adding IL-2, led to the first clinical trials in melanoma, which seem to be promising, but has not been successfully applied to other tumors.

Two further procedures will be presented that are still in an experimental stage, but seem to be promising. One is specific immunotherapy with autologous virus-modified tumor cells. The other is a particularly interesting treatment approach that uses activated cytotoxic T lymphocytes (CTL therapy).

Specific immunotherapy with autologous virus-modified tumor cells (reactivated and modified by Shirrmacher) assumes that vaccination use can strengthen a weak-tumor antigen through nonspecific immune stimulation. This immunological tumor therapy has been successfully used in animal experiments and in some clinical trials. The vaccine consists of irradiated (200 Gy), but still metabolizing tumor cells, secondarily infected with the avirulent Newcastle disease virus (NDV). The vaccine is injected intradermally. The delayed-type hypersensitivity skin reaction is evaluated after 48 hours. Injections have been given at weekly intervals. For this immunotherapy scheme, positive skin reactions and some promising clinical improvements (in small patient populations) have been demonstrated, which indicates that this therapeutic approach might be promising for the treatment of breast cancer.

The fourth and most complex, but possibly also the most interesting immunotherapeutic approach to tumor therapy using autologous-stimulated lymphocytes in humans, is based on the observation that specific cytoxic T lymphocytes can be induced in vitro in a mixed lymphocyte/tumor cell culture under certain conditions. It is known from murine and human experimental tumor systems, that low-dose IL-2 application (e.g., 25 U/mL, as compared to 100 U/mL for TIL) in combination with antigen stimulation by autologous tumor cells induces specific and appreciably more active effector cell populations than does high-dose IL-2 application. The first clinical studies on melanoma show the high effectiveness of these specific, activated cytotoxic T cell clones (CTL). It is unknown if this concept, which has so far been largely experimental, is also applicable to breast cancer.

References

1. Aaltomaa S et al. Mitotic indices as prognostic predictors in female breast cancer. J Cancer Res Clin Oncol. 1992; 118:75–81.
2. Ahlert T, Bastert G, Schirrmacher V. Mamma- und Ovarialkarzinom mit autologen, virusmodifizierten Tumorzellen. Gynäkologie. 1989; 2:359.
3. Alpert S, Ghossein NA, Stacey P et al. Primary management of operable breast cancer by minimal surgery and radiotherapy. Cancer. 1978; 42:2054.
4. Anchini A, Fossati G, Parmiani G. Clonal analysis of the cytotoxic T-cell response to human tumors. Immunol Today. 1987; 8:385.
5. Andersen JA. Lobular carcinoma in situ of the breast. An approach to rational treatment. Cancer. 1977; 39:2597–2602.
6. Angell M. Breast implants–protection or paternalism? N Engl J Med. 1992; 326:1695–1696.
7. Apostolikas N, Petraki C, Agnantis NJ. The reliability of histologically negative axillary lymph nodes in breast cancer: Preliminary report. Path Res Pract. 1989; 184:35–38.
8. Ashikari R, Hajdu SI, Robbins GF. Intraductal carcinoma of the breast (1960–1969). Cancer. 1971; 28:1182–1187.
9. Ashikari R, Park K, Huvos AG, Urban JA. Paget's disease of the breast. Cancer. 1970: 26:680–685.
10. Aspegren K, Holmberg L, Adami HO. Standardization of the surgical technique in breast-conserving treatment of mammary cancer. Br J Surg. 1988; 75:807–810.
11. Auer G, Caspersson TO, Wallgren AS. DNA content and survival in mammary carcinoma. Analyt Quant Cytol. 1980; 2:161–165.
12. Barnard NJ, Hall PA, Lemoind NR, Kadar N. Proliferative index in breast carcinoma determined in situ by Ki-67 immunostaining and its relationship to clinical and pathological variables. J Pathol. 1987; 152:287–295.
13. Barr LC, Brunt AM, Goodman AG et al. Uncontrolled local recurrence after treatment of breast cancer conservation. Cancer. 1989; 64:1203–1207.
14. Bartlett K, Eremin O, Hutcheon A et al. Adjuvant tamoxifen in the management of operable breast cancer: The Scottish trial. Lancet. 1987; 2:171–175.
15. Bedwinek JM, Fineberg B, Lee J et al. Analysis of failures following treatment of isolated local regional recurrence of breast cancer. Int J Radiat Oncol Biol Phys. 1981; 7:581–585.
16. Berger MS, Locher GW, Saurer S et al. Correlation of c-erbB-2 gene amplification and protein expression in human breast carcinoma with nodal status and nuclear grading. Cancer Res. 1988; 48:1238–1243.
17. Berkel H, Birdsell DC, Jenkins H. Breast augmentation: A risk factor for breast cancer? N Engl J Med. 1992; 326:1649–1653.
18. Betsill WL, Rosen PP, Lieberman PH et al. Intraductal carcinoma: Long-term follow-up after treatment by biopsy alone. JAMA. 1978; 239:1863–1867.
19. Bishop HM, Blamey RW, Morris AH. Bone scanning: Its lack of value in the follow-up of patients with breast cancer. Brit J Surg. 1979; 66:752.
20. Black MM, Barclay THC, Hankey BF. Prognosis in breast cancer utilising histologic characteristics of the primary tumor. Cancer. 1975; 36:2048.
21. Bloom HJG. Prognosis in carcinoma of the breast. Br J Cancer. 1950; 4:259–288.
22. Bloom HJG. Survival of women with untreated breast cancer–past and present. In: Forrest APM, Kumkler PB. eds. Prognostic Factors in Breast Cancer. Baltimore: Williams and Williams; 1968.
23. Bloom HJG, Richardson WW. Histologic grading and prognosis in breast cancer. A study of 1409 cases of which 359 have been followed fifteen years. Br J Cancer. 1957; 11:359.
24. Böcking A, Chatelain R, Biesterfeld S et al. DNA grading of malignancy in breast cancer: Prognostic validity, reproducibility and comparison with other classifications. Analyt Quant Cytol Histol. 1989; 11:73–80.
25. Bohmert H, Leis HP, Jackson IT. Breast cancer: concervative and reconstructive surgery. Stuttgart: Thieme; 1989.
26. Bonadonna G, Valagussa P. Current status of adjuvant chemotherapy for breast cancer. Semin Oncol. 1981; 14:8–22.
27. Bonadonna G, Zambetti M, Valagussa P. Adjuvant chemotherapy for node negative breast cancer. In. Senn HJ, Goldbush A, Gelber RD, Osterwalder B. eds. Adjuvant therapy of primary breast cancer: recent results in cancer research. Heidelberg: Springer; 1989:175–179.

28. Boova RS, Roseann B, Rosato F. Patterns of axillary nodal involvement in breast cancer. Predictability of level one dissection. Ann Surg. 1982; 196:642–644.

29. Borg A, Tandon AK, Sigurdsson H et al. HER-2/neu oncogen amplification predicts poor survival in node positive breast cancer. Cancer Res. 1990; 50:4332–4337.

30. Bostwick J. Aesthetic and reconstructive breast surgery. St. Louis: Mosby; 1983.

31. Bostwick J, Vasconez LO, Jurkiewica MJ. Breast reconstruction after a radical mastectomy. Plast Reconstr Surg. 1978; 61:682.

32. Breasted JH. The Edwin Smith surgical papyrus, Volume 1. Chicago: University of Chicago Press; 1930:463.

33. Brown PW, Silverman J, Owens E et al. Intraductal "noninfiltrating" carcinoma of the breast. Arch Surg. 1976; 111:1063–1067.

34. Bruneton JN, Caramella E, Héry M et al. Axillary lymph node metastases in breast cancer: Preoperative detection with ultrasound. Radiology. 1986; 158:325–326.

35. Buzdar AU, Montague ED, Barker JL et al. Management of inflammatory carcinoma of breast with combined modality approach–an update. Cancer. 1981; 47:2537–2542.

36. Canellos GP, Hellmann S, Veronesi U. The management of early breast cancer. N Engl J Med. 1982; 306:1430–1432.

37. Cantwell B, Fennelly JJ, Jones M. Evaluation of follow-up methods to detect relapse after mastectomy in breast cancer patients. Ir J Med Sci. 1982; 151:1–5.

38. Cassel WA, Murray DR, Phillips HS. A phase II study on the postsurgical management of stage II malignant melanoma with Newcastle Disease Virus oncolysate. Cancer. 1983; 52:856.

39. Castiglione M, Goldhirsch A. Die adjuvante Behandlung des Mammakarzinoms. In: Becker R, Höffken K, eds. Die Systemtherapie des Mammakarzinoms. München: W. Zuckschwerdt; 1989: 51–64.

40. Cavalli F, Goldhirsch A, Jungi F et al. Randomized trial of low versus high dose medroxyprogesterone acetate in the induction treatment of postmenopausal patients with advanced breast cancer. J Clin Oncol. 1984; 2:414.

41. Champion HR, Wallace IWJ. Breast cancer grading. Cancer. 1971; 25:441–448.

42. Chaudary MM, Maisey MN, Shaw PJ et al. Sequential bone scans and chest radiographs in the postoperative management of early breast cancer. Br J Surg. 1983; 70(9):517–518.

43. Chen KK-Y, Montague ED, Oswald MJ. Results of irradiation in the treatment of locoregional breast cancer recurrence. Cancer. 1985; 56:1269–1273.

44. Ciatto S, Herd-Smith A. The role of chest X-ray in the follow-up of primary breast cancer. Tumori. 1983; 69:151–154.

45. Ciatto S, Rosselli del Turco M, Pacini P et al. Early detection of local recurrences in the follow-up of primary breast cancer. Tumori. 1984; 70: 179–18340.

46. Clark DH, Le MG, Sarrazin D et al. Analysis of local regional relapses in patients with early breast cancer treated by excision and radiotherapy: experience of the Institute Gustave Roussy. Int J Radiat Oncol Biol Phys. 1985; 11:137.

47. Clark GM, Dressler LG, Owens MA et al. Prediction of relapse or survival in patients with node-negative breast cancer by DNA flow cytometry. N Engl J Med. 1989; 320:627–633.

48. Clark RM, Wilkinson RH, Mahoney LJ et al. Breast cancer: A 21-year experience with conservative surgery and radiation. Int J Radiat Oncol Biol Phys. 1982; 8:967.

49. Clayton F, Wu J. The lability of estrogen receptor: Correlations of estrogen binding and immunoreactivity. Clin Chem. 1986; 32:1774–1777.

50. Consensus Development Conference. Therapy of advanced breast cancer depending on hormone receptor status. National Institute of Health. Bethesda, Washington; 1979.

51. Consensus Development Conference NIH. Bethesda, Washington. J Am Med Assoc. 1985; 254:3461–3463.

52. Consensus Development Conference. Therapeutic management of metastatic breast cancer. Munich; July 1988.

53. Consensus Development Conference NIH. Bethesda, Washington. June 1990.

54. Coombes RC, Dowsett M, Goss P et al. 4-Hydroxyandrostenedione in treatment of postmenopausal patients with advanced breast cancer. Lancet i. 1984; 1237–1239.

55. Cooper RG. Combination chemotherapy in hormone resistant breast cancer. Am Ass Cancer Res. 1969; 10:15–20.

56. Coulson PB, Thornthwaite JT, Wolley TW et al. Prognostic indicators including DNA histogram type, receptor content and staging related to human breast cancer patient survival. Cancer Res. 1984; 44:4187–4196.

57. Cronin TD, Upton J, McDonough JM. Reconstruction of the breast after mastectomy. Plast Reconstr Srug. 1977; 59:1.

58. Cuzick J, Stewart H, Peto R et al. Overview of randomized trials of post-operative adjuvant radiotherapy in breast cancer. Cancer Treat Rep. [In press].

59. Davis BW, Gelber RD, Goldhirsch A et al. Prognostic significance of tumor grade in clinical trials of adjuvant therapy for breast cancer with axillary lymph node metastases. Cancer. 1986; 58:2662–2670.

60. Dearlaney DP, Sloane JP, Ormerod MG et al. Increased detection of mammary carcinoma cells in marrow smears using antisera to epithelial membrane antigen. Br J Cancer. 1981; 44:85–90.

61. DeLellis RA, Sternberger LA, Mann RB et al. Immunoperoxidase technics in diagnostic pathology: report of a workshop sponsored by the National Cancer Institute. Am J Clin Pathol. 1979; 71:483–488.

62. DeLena M, Marzullo F, Somone G et al. Correlation between ERICA and DCC assay in hormone receptor assessment of human breast cancer. Oncology. 1988; 45:308–312.

63. DeLena M, Zucali R, Viganotti G et al. Combined chemotherapy-radiotherapy approach in locally advanced (T_{3b}-T_4) breast cancer. Cancer Chemother Pharmacol. 1978; 1:53–59.

64. Delides GS, Garas G, Georgouli G et al. Intra-laboratory variations in the grading of breast carcinoma. Arch Pathol Lab Med. 1982; 106:126–128.

65. DeSombre ER, Carbone PP, Jensen EV et al. Steroid receptors in breast cancer. N Engl J Med. 1979; 301:1011–1012.

66. DeSouza LJ, Shinde SR. The value of laparoscopic liver examination in the management of breast cancer. J Surg Oncol. 1980; 14:97–103.

67. Dewar JA, Kerr GR. Value of routine follow up of women treated for early carcinoma of the breast. Br Med J. 1985; 291:1464–1467.

68. Donegan WL, Perez-Mesa CM, Watson FR. A biostatistical study of locally recurrent breast carcinoma. Surg Gynecol Obstet. 1966; 122:529–540.

69. Dressler LG, Seamer LC, Owens MA et al. DNA flow cytometry and prognostic factors in 1331 frozen breast cancer specimens. Cancer. 1988; 61:420–427.

70. Early Breast Cancers Trialist's Collaborative Group. Effects of adjuvant tamoxifen and of cytotoxic therapy on mortality in early breast cancer. New Engl J Med. 1988; 319:1681–1692.

71. Early Breast Cancers Trialist's Collaborative Group. Treatment of early breast cancer. New York: Oxford University Press; 1990:83–87.

72. Early Breast Cancers Trialist's Collaborative Group. Systematic treatment of early breast cancer by hormonal cytotoxic, or immune therapy. Lancet. 1992; 339:8784, 1–15 (part 1). Lancet. 1992; 339:8785, 71–84 (part 2).

73. Ellis DL, Teitelbaum SL. Inflammatory carcinoma of the breast: A pathologic definition. Cancer. 1974; 33:1045–1047.

74. Ennis JT. Diagnostic radiological imaging for breast diseases. In: Bland KJ, Copeland EM III eds. The Breast. Philadelphia: W.B. Saunders; 1991:426–468.

75. Epstein AH, Connolly JL, Gelman R et al. The predictors of distant relapse following conservative surgery and radiotherapy for early breast cancer are similar to those following mastectomy. Int J Rad Oncol Biol Phys. 1989; 17:755–760.

76. Fastenberg NA, Buzdar AU, Montague ED et al. Management of inflammatory carcinoma of the breast. A combined modality approach. Am J Clin Oncol. 1985; 8:134–141.

77. Fechner RE, Histologic variants of infiltrating lobular carcinoma of the breast. Human Pathol. 1975; 6:373–378.

78. Fentiman IS, Matthews PN, Davison OW et al. Survival following local skin recurrence after mastectomy. Br J Surg. 1985; 72:14–16.

79. Ferguson DJ. The actual extent of mastectomy: a key to survival. Perspect Biol Med. 1987; 30:311–323.

80. Fisher B. Alternatives to radical mastectomy. N Engl J Med. 1979; 301:326.

81. Fisher B, Bauer M, Margolese R et al. Five-year results of a randomized clinical trial comparing total mastectomy and segmental mastectomy with or without radiation in the treatment of breast cancer. N Engl J Med. 1985; 312:665–673.

82. Fisher B, Fischer ER, Redmond C et al. Tumor nuclear grade, estrogen receptor, and progesterone receptor: Their value alone or in combination as indicators of outcome following adjuvant therapy for breast cancer. Breast Cancer Res Treat. 1986; 7:147–160.

83. Fisher B, Montague E, Redmond C et al. Comparison of radical mastectomy with alternative treatments for primary breast cancer. Cancer. 1977; 39:2827–2839.

84. Fisher B, Redmond C, Dimitrov NV et al. A randomized clinical trial evaluating sequential methotrexate and fluorouracil in the treatment of patients wtih node-negative breast cancer who have estrogen-receptor-negative tumors. N Engl J Med. 1989; 320:473–478.

85. Fisher B, Redmond C, Fisher ER. The contribution of recent NSABP clinical trials of primary breast cancer therapy to an understanding of tumor biology—An overview of findings. Cancer. 1980; 46:1009.

86. Fisher B, Redmond C, Fisher ER et al. Ten-year results of a randomized clinical trial comparing radical mastectomy and total mastectomy with or without radiation. N Engl J Med. 1985; 312:674–714.

87. Fisher B, Redmond C, Poisson R et al. Eight-year results of a randomized clinical trial comparing total mastectomy and lumpectomy with or without irradiation in the treatment of breast cancer. N Engl J Med. 1989; 320:822–828.

88. Fisher B, Redmond C, Wolmark N, Wieand HS. Disease-free survival at intervals during and following completion of adjuvant chemotherapy. The NSABP experience from three breast cancer protocols. Cancer. 1981; 48:1273–1280.

89. Fisher B, Rockette H, Fischer ER et al. Leukemia in breast cancer patients following adjuvant chemotherapy or post-operative radiation. The NSABP exprience. J Clin Oncol. 1985; 3:1640–1658.

90. Fisher B, Slack NH. Number of lymph nodes examined and prognosis of breast carcinoma. Surg Gynecol Obstet. 1970; 131:79–88.

91. Fisher B, Slack NH, Bross IDJ et al. Cancer of the breast: Size of neoplasm and prognosis. Cancer. 1969; 24:1071–1080.

92. Fisher B, Slack NH, Cavanaugh PJ et al. Postoperative radiotherapy in the treatment of breast cancer: results of the National Surgical Adjuvant Breast Project Clinical Trial. Ann Surg. 1970; 172:711–732.

93. Fisher B, Wolmark N. Conservative surgery: The American experience. Semin Oncol. 1986; 13:425.

94. Fisher B, Wolmark N, Bauer M et al. The accuracy of clinical nodal staging and of limited axillary dissection as a determinant of histologic nodal status in carcinoma of the breast. Surg Gynecol Obstet. 1981; 152:765–772.

95. Fisher E, Sass R, Fisher B et al. Pathological findings from the National Surgical Adjuvant Breast Project (Protoal 6). II. Relation of local breast recurrence to multicentricity. Cancer. 1986; 57:1717–1724.

96. Fisher ER, Gregorio RM, Fisher B. The pathology of invasive breast cancer: A syllabus derived from the findings of the National Surgical Adjuvant Breast Project (Protocol No. 4). Cancer. 1975; 36:1–85.

97. Fisher ER, Sass R, Fisher B et al. Pathologic findings from the National Surgical Adjuvant Breast Project (Protocol 6) I. Intraductal carcinoma (DCIS). Cancer. 1986; 57:197–208.

98. Fisher ER, Swamidoss S, Lee CH et al. Detection and significance of occult axillary node metastases in patients with invasive breast cancer. Cancer. 1978; 42:2025–2031.

99. Fisher JC. The silicone controversy–when will science prevail? N Engl J Med. 1992; 326:1696–1698.

100. Flowers JL, Burton GV, Cox EB et al. Use of monoclonal antiestrogen receptor antibody to evaluate estrogen receptor content in fine-needle aspiration breast biopsies. Ann Surg. 1986; 203:250–254.

101. Fourquet A, Campana F, Zafrani B et al. Prognostic factors of breast recurrence in the conservative management of early breast cancer: A 25-year follow-up. Int J Rad Oncol Biol Phys. 1989; 17:719–725.

102. Fowble B, Solin LJ, Schultz DJ, Goodman RL. Frequency, sites of relapse, and outcome of regional node failures following conservative surgery and radiation for early breast cancer. Int J Rad Oncol Biol Phys. 1989; 17:703–710.

103. Franklin WA, Bibbo M, Doria MI et al. Quantitation of estrogen receptor content and Ki-67 staining in breast carcinoma by the micro TICAS image analysis system. Analyt Quant Cytol Histol. 1987; 9:279–286.

104. Franzen S, Zajicek J. Aspiration biopsy in diagnosis of palpable lesions of the breast. Acta Radiol. 1968; 7:241.

105. Gelber R, Goldhirsch A, Senn HJ. 4th International Conference of Adjuvant Therapy of Primary Breast Cancer. Feb. 1992. St. Gallen, Switzerland. [In print].

106. Gerdes J, Lelle RJ, Pickarts H et al. Growth fractions in breast cancers determined in situ with monoclonal antibody Ki-67. J Clin Pathol. 1986; 39:977–980.

107. Gerdes J, Schwab U, Lemke H, Stein H. Production of a mouse monoclonal antibody reactive with a human nuclear antigen associated with cell proliferation. Int J Cancer. 1983; 31:1–20.

108. Gilliland MD, Barton RM, Copeland EM III. The implications of local recurrence of breast cancer as the first site of therapeutic failure. Ann Surg. 1983; 197:284–287.

109. Goldhirsch A, Gelber RD. Randomized perioperative therapy in operable breast cancer. In: Senn HJ, Goldhirsch A, Gelber RD, Osterwalder B. eds. Adjuvant therapy of primary breast cancer: recent results in cancer research. Heidelberg: Springer; 1989:43.

110. Greene CL, Nolan C, Engler JP, Jensen EV. Monoclonal antibodies to human estrogen receptor. Proc Natl Acad Sci USA. 1980; 77:5115–5119.

111. Greenough RB. Varying degrees of malignancy in cancer of the breast. J Cancer Res. 1925; 9:453–462.

112. Haagensen CD. Diseases of the breast. 2nd ed. Philadelphia: Saunders; 1971:576–584.

113. Haagensen CD. Treatment of curable carcinoma of the breast. Int J Radiat Oncol Biol Phys. 1977; 2:975–980.

114. Haagensen CD. Diseases of the breast. 3rd ed. Philadelphia: Saunders; 1986:808–814.

115. Haagensen CD, Bodran C, Haagensen DE Jr. Breast carcinoma: risk and detection. Philadelphia: Saunders; 1981:238.

116. Haffty BG, Goldberg NB, Fischer D et al. Conservative surgery and radiation therapy in breast carcinoma: Local recurrence and prognostic implications. Int J Rad Oncol Biol Phys. 1989; 17:727–732.

117. Hagelberg RS, Jolly PC, Anderson RP. Role of surgery in the treatment of inflammatory breast carcinoma. Am J Surg. 1984; 148:125–131.

118. Halsted WS. The results of operations for the cure of cancer of the breast performed at Johns Hopkins Hospital from June 1889 to January 1894. Johns Hopkins Hosp Rep. 1894; 4:297–350.

119. Halsted WS. The results of radical operations for the cure of carcinoma of the breast. Ann Surg. 1907; 46:1–19.

120. Hanna MG, Peters LC. Specific immunotherapy of established visceral micrometastases by BCG-tumor cell vaccine alone or as an adjuvant surgery. Cancer. 1978; 42:2613.

121. Harris JR, Hellman S. The results of primary radiation therapy for early breast cancer at the Joint Center for radiation therapy. In: Harris JR, Hellman S, Silen W, eds. Conservative management of breast cancer. Philadelphia: Lippincott; 1983: 47–52.

122. Harris JR, Hellman S, Henderson IC, Kinne DW. Breast Diseases. Philadelphia: Lippincott; 1987:1–75.

123. Harris JR, Hellman S, Kinne DW. Limited surgery and radiotherapy for early breast cancer. N Engl J Med. 1985; 313:1365–1368.

124. Harris JR, Recht A, Amalric R et al. Time course and prognosis of local recurrence following primary radiation therapy for early breast cancer. J Clin Oncol. 1984; 2:37.

125. Hartrampf CR, Scheflan M, Black PO. Breast reconstruction with a transverse abdominal island flap. Plast Reconstr Surg. 1982; 69:216.

126. Henderson C, Gelman R. Second malignancies from adjuvant chemotherapy? Too soon to tell. J Clin Oncol. 1987; 5:1135–1137.

127. Henderson IC, Canellos GP. Cancer of the breast. N Engl J Med. 1980; 302: 17–30.

128. Henderson IC, Harris JR, Klune DU et al. Cancer of the breast. In: De Vita VT, Hellman S, Rosenberg SA eds. Cancer: principles and practice of oncology. 3rd ed. Philadelphia: Lippincott; 1989: 1197–1268.

129. Henderson IC, Hayes DF, Come S et al. New agents and new medical treatments for advanced breast cancer. Semin Oncol. 1987; 14: 34–64.

130. Hoogstraten B, Osborne CK. Adjuvant therapy of breast cancer. In: Hoogstraten B, Burn I, Bloom HJG eds. Current Treatment of Cancer (UICC): Breast Cancer. New York: Springer; 1989: 199–210.

131. Hoover HC Jr, Peters LC, Brandhurst JS, Hanna MG Jr. Therapy of spontaneous metastases with an autologous tumor vaccine in a guinea pig model. J Surg Res. 1981; 30: 409.

132. Hoover HC, Surdyke MG, Dangel RB et al. Prospectively randomized trial of adjuvant active-specific immunotherapy for human colorectal cancer. Cancer. 1985; 55: 1236.

133. Howat JMT, Barnes DM, Harris M, Swindell R. The association of cytosol estrogen and progesterone receptors with histological features of breast cancer and early recurrence of disease. Br J Cancer. 1983; 629–640.

134. Hughes LP. Follow-up of patients with breast cancer. Br Med J. 1985; 290: 1229.

135. Jakesz R, Reiner G, Schemper M et al. Significant survival benefit of node negative breast cancer patients treated with adjuvant chemotherapy: Seven-year result. In: Senn JH, Goldhirsch A, Gelber RD, Osterwalder B. eds. Adjuvant therapy of primary breast cancer: recent results in cancer research. Berlin, Heidelberg, New York: Springer Verlag; 1989: 180–185.

136. Janjan NA, McNeese MD, Buzdar AU et al. Management of locoregional recurrent breast cancer. Cancer. 1986; 58: 1552–1556.

137. Kaufmann M, Jonat W, Kleeberg U et al. Zoladex (ICI 118630) a depot GnRH agonist in the treatment of premenopausal patients with metastatic breast cancer. J Clin Oncol. 1989; 7: 1113–1119.

138. Keffer BJH. Hormone-receptor assays and cancer of the breast: The pathologist's role. Am J Clin Pathol. 1978; 719–720.

139. Kennedy JC, El-Badawy N, DeRose PB et al. Comparison of cell proliferation in breast carcinoma using image analysis (Ki-67) and flow cytometric systems. Analyt Quant Cytol Hist. 1991; 14: 304–311.

140. Kessler DA. The basis for the FDA's decision on breast implants. N Engl J Med. 1992; 326: 1713–1715.

141. King WJ, DeSombre ER, Jensen EV, Greene GL. Comparison of immunocytochemical and steroid-binding assays for estrogen receptors in human breast tumors. Cancer Res. 1985; 45: 293–304.

142. King WJ, Greene GL. Monoclonal antibodies localize oestrogen receptor in the nuclei of target cells. Nature. 1984; 308: 745–747.

143. Knuth A, Danowski B, Oettgen HF, Old LJ. T-cell mediated cytotoxicity against autologous malignant melanoma: analysis with interleukin 2-dependent T-cell cultures. Proc Natl Acad Sci USA. 1984; 81: 3511.

144. Knuth A, Wölfel T, Keelmann E et al. Cytolytic T-cellclones against an autologous human melanoma: Specificity study and definition of three antigens by immunoselection. Proc Natl Acad Sci USA. 1984; 88: 2804.

145. Knuth A, Wölfel T, Meyer zum Büschenfelde K-H. Immunologische Melanomtherapie mit tumorinfiltrierenden Lymphozyten und Interleukin-2. Dtsch med Wschr. 1989; 46: 1815.

146. Kreienberg R. Wie frühzeitig sollte eine adjuvante Therapie beginnen—Prä-, intra- oder postoperativ? In: Kadack U, Kaufmann M, Kubli F, eds. Hormone, Antihormone, Zytostatika zur adjuvanten Therapie des Mammakarzinoms. Aktuelle Onkologie 27. München: Zuckerschwerdt; 1985: 121–131.

147. Kreienberg R. Allgemeine und spezifische Laborparameter im Rahmen der Tumornachsorge bei gynäkologischen Malignomen und beim Mammacarcinom. Gynäkologe. 1989; 22: 55–62.

148. Kreienberg R. Immundiagnostik und ihre Relevanz bei Tumorerkrankungen, Immuntherapie bei Tumorerkrankungen. Gynäkologe. 1990; 23: 122–129.

149. Kreienberg R. Adjuvante Chemotherapie des Mamma- und Ovarialcarcinomas. Gynäkologe. 1991; 24: 208–214.

150. Kreienberg R. Derzeitige Möglichkeiten der Immuntherapie bei gynäkologischen Malignomen und beim Mammacarcinom. In: Bender HG, ed. Gynäkologische Onkologie. 2. Aufl. Stuttgart: Thieme; 1991: 77–98.

151. Kurtz JM, Almaric R, Delouche G et al. The second ten years: Long-term risks of breast conservation in early breast cancer. Int J Radiat Oncol Biol Phys. 1987; 13: 1327–1332.

152. Kurtz JM. Local recurrence after breast conserving surgery and radiotherapy: frequency, time course and prognosis. Cancer. 1989; 63: 1912–1917.

153. Lacour J, Le M, Caceres E et al. Radical mastectomy plus internal mammary dissection. Ten-year results of an international cooperative trial in breast cancer. Cancer. 1983; 51: 1941–1943.

154. Lacour J, Le MG, Hill C et al. Is it useful to remove internal mammary nodes in operable breast cancer? Eur J Surg Oncol. 1987; 13: 309–314.

155. Lagios MD, Westdahl PR, Margolin FR et al. Duct carcinoma in situ: Relationship of extent of non-invasive disease to the frequency of occult invasion, multicentricity, lymph node metastases, and short-term treatment failures. Cancer. 1982; 50: 1309–1314.

156. Lagios MD, Westdahl PR, Rose MR. The concept and implications of multicentricity in breast carcinoma. Pathol Annu. 1981; 16(2): 83–102.

157. Lagios MD, Westdahl PR, Rose MR et al. Paget's disease of the nipple. Cancer. 1984; 54: 545–551.

158. Layfield LJ, Glasgow BJ, Cramer H. Fine-needle aspiration in the management of breast masses. Pathol Annu. 1989; 24(2):23–62.

159. Lee YTN. Breast carcinoma pattern of recurrence and metastasis after mastectomy. Am J Clin Oncol. 1984; 7:443–449.

160. Leggett CAC. Local recurrence of carcinoma of the breast. Aust NZ. J Surg. 1980; 50:298–300.

161. Lelle RJ, Heidenreich W, Stauch G, Gerdes J. The correlation of growth fractions with histologic grading and lymph node status in human mammary carcinoma. Cancer. 1987; 59:83–88.

162. Levine PH, Steinhorn SC, Ries LG, Aaaron JL. Inflammatory breast cancer: the experience of the surveillance, eidemiology, and end results (SEER) Program. J Natl Cancer Inst. 1985; 74:291–297.

163. Ludwig Breast Cancer Study Group. Prolonged disease-free survival after one course of perioperative adjuvant chemotherapy for node-negative breast cancer. N Engl J Med. 1989; 320:491–496.

164. Lynch HT, Marcus JN, Watson P, Lynch J. Familial breast cancer, family cancer syndromes and predisposition to breast neoplasia. In: Bland KJ, Copeland EM III, eds. The Breast. Philadelphia: Saunders; 1991:262–291.

165. Maddox WA, Carpenter JT, Laws HL et al. Does radical mastectomy still have a place in the treatment of breast cancer? Arch Surg. 1987; 122:1317–1320.

166. Mansi JL, Berger U, Easton D, McDonell T et al. Micrometastases in bone marrow in patients with primary breast cancer: Evaluation as an early predictor of bone metastases. Br Med J. 1987; 295:1093–1096.

167. Mansour EG, Gray R, Shatila AH et al. Efficacy of adjuvant chemotherapy in high-risk node negative breast cancer. N Engl J Med. 1989; 320:485–490.

168. Margolese R, Poisson R, Shibata H et al. The technique of segmental mastectomy (lumpectomy) and axillary dissection: A syllabus from the National Surgical Adjuvant Breast Project workshops. Surgery. 1987; 102:828–834.

169. Marrazzo A, Solina G, Pocosa V et al. Evaluation of routine follow-up after surgery for breast carcinoma. J Surg Oncol. 1986; 32:179–181.

170. McCarthy KS Jr, Miller LS, Cox EB et al. Estrogen receptor analysis. Correlation of biochemical and immunohistochemical methods using monoclonal antireceptor antibodies. Arch Pathol Lab Med. 1985; 109:716–721.

171. McDivitt RW, Stewart FW, Berg JW. Tumors of the Breast. Atlas of Tumor Pathology. 2nd Series, Fascicle 2. Washington DC: Armed Forces Institute of Pathology; 1968.

172. McGuire WL, Tandon AK, Allred DC et al. How to use prognostic factors in axillary node-negative breast cancer patients. J Natl Cancer Inst. 1990; 82:1006–1015.

173. McGurrin JF, Doria MI Jr, Dawson PJ et al. Assessment of tumor cell kinetics by immunohistochemistry in carcinoma of breast cancer. Cancer. 1987; 1744–1750.

174. Meier P, Ferguson DJ, Karrison T. A controlled trial of extended radical mastectomy. Cancer. 1985; 55:880–891.

175. Mendelsohn ML. The growth fraction: a new concept applied to tumors. Science. 1960; 132:1496.

176. Mendenhall NP. Palliative radiation therapy for disseminated breast cancer. In: Bland KI, Copeland EM III, eds. The Breast. Philadelphia: Saunders; 1991:957–973.

177. Mendenhall NP, Devine JW, Mendenhall WM et al. Isolated local-regional recurrence following mastectomy for adenocarcinoma of the breast treated with radiation therapy alone or combined with surgery and/or chemotherapy. Radiother Oncol. 1988; 12:177–185.

178. Mertelsmann R. Interleukin-2: Physiologie, Pathophysiologie und klinische Möglichkeiten. Münch Med Wschr. 1986; 128:11.

179. Mertelsmann R, Lindemann A, Henneman F. Hämatopoetische Wachstumsfaktoren in der Klinik. Münch Med Wschr. 1989; 131:123.

180. Meyer JS, Friedman E, McCrate M, Bauer WC. Prediction of early course of breast carcinoma by thymidine labelling. Cancer. 1983; 51:1879–1886.

181. Meyer JS, McDivitt RW, Stone KR et al. Practical breast cancer kinetics: Review and update. Breast Cancer Res Treat. 1984; 4:79.

182. Möbus V, Krienberg R, Schirrmacher V. Erfahrungen mit der aktiv-spezifischen Immuntherapie bei gynäkologischen Malignomen. Aktuel Onkol. [In print].

183. Montague D, Tapley NduV, Spanos WJ. Treatment techniques depending on tumor extent in cancer of the breast. In: Levitt SH, Tapley NduV, eds. Technological Basis of Radiation Therapy: practical clinical applications. Philadelphia: Lea and Febiger; 1984:228–243.

184. Mouridsen HT. Critical review of adjuvant therapy in premenopausal patients. In: Senn HJ, Goldhirsch A, Gelber RD, Osterwalder B, eds. Adjuvant Therapy of Primary Breast Cancer: recent results in cancer research. Heidelberg: Springer; 1989: 132–135.

185. Mouridsen HT, Palshof T, Brahm M, Rahlseck J. Evaluation of single drug versus multi drug chemotherapy in the treatment of advanced breast cancer. Cancer Treat Rep. 1977; 61:47–50.

186. Mouridsen HT, Palshof T, Pattersen J, Baltersby L. Tamoxifen in advanced breast cancer. Cancer Treat Rep. 1978; 5:131–141.

187. Muss HB, McNamara MCJ, Connelly RA. Follow-up after stage II breast cancer. A comparative study of relapsed versus non-relapsed patients . Am J Clin Oncol. 1988; 11:451–455.

188. National Cancer Institute. Standardized management of breast specimens: Recommended by pathology working group, breast cancer task force. Am J Clin Pathol. 1973; 60:789–798.

189. Nordenström B, Ryden H, Svane G. Stereotaxic breast biopsy. In: Zornoza J. ed. Percutaneus Needle Biopsies: a radiological approach. Baltimore: Williams + Wilkins; 1980.

190. Olivari N. The latissimus flap. Brit J Plast Surg. 1976; 29:126.

191. Page DL, Dupont WD, Rogers LW et al. Intraductal carcinoma of the breast: Follow-up after biopsy only. Cancer. 1982; 49:751–758.

192. Paik S, Hazan R, Fisher ER et al. Pathologic findings from the National Surgical Adjuvant Breast and Bowel Project: prognostic significance of erbB-2 protein overexpression in primary breast cancer. J Clin Oncol. 1990; 8:103–112.

193. Palshof T, Mouridsen HT, Daehnfelt JL. Adjuvant endocrine therapy of breast cancer–A controlled clinical trial of estrogen and anti-estrogen: Preliminary results of the Copenhagen breast cancer trials. In: Henningsen B, Linder F, Steichele C. eds. Endocrine Treatment of Breast Cancer: A New Approach. New York: Springer; 1980:185–189.

194. Pamilo M, Soiva M, Lavast E-M. Real-time ultrasound, axillary mammography, and clinial examination in the detection of axillary lymph node metastases in breast cancer patients. J Ultrasound Med. 1989; 8:115–120.

195. Pandya KJ, McFadden ET, Kalish LA et al. A retrospective study of earliest indicators of recurrence in patients on Eastern Cooperative Oncology Group Adjuvant Chemotherapy Trials for Breast Cancer. Cancer. 1985; 55:202–205.

196. Patey DH, Dyson WH. The prognosis of carcinoma of the breast in relation to the type of mastectomy performed. Cancer. 1948; 2:7–13.

197. Patterson JS, Balterby LA, Edwards. Review of the clinical pharmacology and international experience with Tamoxifen in advanced breast cancer. In: Jacobelli et al. eds. The Role of Tamoxifen in Breast Cancer. Raven, New York: Raven; 1982; 17–53.

198. Pedrazzini A, Gelber R, Isley M, Castiglione M, Goldhirsch A. First repeated bone scan in the observation of patients with operable breast cancer. J Clin Oncol. 1986; 4:389–394.

199. Perez CA, Fields JN. Role of radiation therapy for locally advanced and inflammatory carcinoma of the breast. Oncology. 1987; 1:81–93.

200. Pollock RE, Stephen KS, Balch CM. Surgical procedures for advanced local and regional malignancies of the breast. In: Bland KI, Copeland EM III, eds. The Breast. Philadelphia: Saunders; 1991:948–956.

201. Pollow K, Kreienberg R, Grill HJ. Pharmakokinetische und klinische Untersuchungen zur hochdosierten oralen Medroxyprogesteronacetat (MPA) Therapie beim fortgeschrittenen metastasierenden Mammakarzinom. Tumordiag Ther. 1988; 9:7–13.

202. Possinger K, Sauer HJ, Wilmanns W. Chemotherapie metastasierender Mammakarzinome. Deutsch Med Wschr. 1988; 113:224–230.

203. Possinger K, Wagner H, Langecker P, Wilmanns W. Treatment toxicity reduction: breast cancer. Cancer Treat Rev. 1987; 14:263.

204. Prichard KL, Thomson DB, Myers RE et al. Tamoxifen therapy in premenopausal patients with metastatic breast cancer. Cancer Trat Rep. 1980; 64:787–792.

205. Reiner A, Spona J, Reiner G et al. Estrogen receptor analysis on biopsies and fine-needle aspirates from human breast carcinoma. Correlation of biochemical and immunohistochemical methods using monoclonal antireceptor antibodies. Am J Pathol. 1986; 125:443–449.

206. Ridolphi RL, Rosen PP, Port A et al. Medullary carcinoma of the breast: A clinicopathologic study with 10 year follow-up. Cancer. 197; 40:1365–1385.

207. Rissanen PM, Holsti P. Paget's disease of the breast: The influence of the presence or absence of an underlying palpable tumor on the prognosis and on the choice of treatment. Oncology. 1969; 23:209–216.

208. Rose MA, Henderson C, Gelman R et al. Premenopausal breast cancer patients treated with conservative surgery, radiotherapy and adjuvant chemotherapy have a low risk of local failure. Int J Rad Oncol Biol Phys. 1989; 17:711–717.

209. Rosen PP. The pathology of breast cancers with intramammary lymphatic tumor emboli. Am J Surg Pathol. 1987; 7:639–641.

210. Rosen PP, Braun DW, Kinne DE. The clinical significance of preinvasive carcinoma. Cancer. 1980; 46:919–925.

211. Rosen PP, Braun DW, Lyngholm B et al. Lobular carcinoma in situ of the breast: Preliminary results of treatment by ipsilateral mastectomy and contralateral breast biopsy. Cancer. 1981; 47:813–819.

212. Rosenberg SA. Adoptice immunotherapy of cancer. accomplishments and prospects. Cancer Treat Rep. 1984; 68:233.

213. Rosenberg SA. Adoptive immunotherapy of cancer using lymphokine activated killer cells and recombinant interleukin-2. In: De Vita VT, Hellmann S, Rosenberg SA eds. Important Advanced in Oncology. Lippincott, Philadelphia: Lippincott; 1986; 55.

214. Rosenberg SA, Lotze MT, Muul LM et al. A progress report of the treatment of 157 patients with advanced cancer using lymphokine-activated killer cells and interleukin-2 or high dose interleukin alone. N Engl J Med. 1987; 31:789.

215. Rosenberg SA, Packard BS, Aebersold PM et al. Use of tumor infiltrating lymphocytes and Interleukin-2 in the immunotherapy of patients with metastatic melanoma. N Engl J Med. 1988; 319:1676.

216. Rouesse S, Sarrazin D, Mouriesse H et al. Primary chemotherapy in the treatment of inflammatory breast carcinoma: a study of 230 cases from the Institut Gustave-Roussy. J Clin Oncol. 1986; 4:1765–1771.

217. Rubin P, Bunyagidy S, Poulter C. Internal mammary lymph node metastases in breast cancer: detection and management. Am J Roentgenol Radium Ther Nucl Med. 1971; 111:588–598.

218. Sainsbury JRC, Farndon JR, Needham GK et al. Epidermal-growth-factor receptor status as a predictor of early relapse and death from breast cancer. Lancet. 1987; 1:1398–1402.

219. Santen JR, Demers LM, Adlercreutz H et al. Inhibition of aromatase with CGS 16949 A in postmenopausal women. J Clin Endocrinol. 1989; 68:90–106.

220. Sarrazin D, Le M, Rouesse J et al. Conservative treatment versus mastectomy in breast cancer tumors with macroscopic diameter of 20 millimeters or less: the experience of the Institute Gustave-Roussy. Cancer. 1984; 53:1209–1213.

221. Sarrazin D, Le MG, Arriagada R et al. Ten-year results of a randomized trial comparing a conservative treatment to mastectomy in early breast cancer. Rad Oncol. 1989; 14:177–184.

222. Sarrazin D, Le MG, Fontaine MF, Ariaginda R. Conservative treatment versus mastectomy in T1 or small T2 breast cancer—a randomized clinical trial. In: Harris JR, Hellman S, Silen W, eds. Conservative Management of Breast Cancer. Philadelphia: Lippincott; 1983:101–111.

223. Scanlon EF, Oviedo MA, Cunningham MP et al. Preoperative and follow-up procedures on patients with breast cancer. Cancer. 1989; 46:977–979.

224. Schafer P, Alberto P, Forni M et al. Surgery as part of a combined modality approach for inflammatory breast cancer. Cancer. 1987; 29:1063–1067.

225. Schirrmacher V. Immunology and immunotherapy of cancer metastases. Ten year studies in an animal model resulting in the design of an immunotherapy procedure now under clinical testing. Interdis Sci Rev. 1989; 14:291.

226. Schlom J. Future prospects in breast cancer research and management. In: Lippman ME, Lichter AS, Danfort DN Jr eds. Diagnosis and Management of Breast Cancer. Philadelphia: Saunders; 1988:549.

227. Schnitt SJ, Connolly JL, Recht A et al. Influence of infiltrating lobular histology and local tumor control in breast cancer patients treated with conservative surgery and radiotherapy. Cancer. 1989; 64:448–454.

228. Schnitt SJ, Silen W, Sadowsky NL et al. Current concepts: Ductal carcinoma in situ (intraductal carcinoma) of the breast. N Engl J Med. 1988; 318:898–903.

229. Schnürch HG. Medikamentöse Therapie bei Mammakarzinomerkrankungen. In: Bender HG ed. Gynäkologische Onkologie. Stuttgart: Thieme; 1991:377–423.

230. Senowsky GM, Wanebo HJ, Wilhelm MC et al. Has monitoring of the contralateral breast improved prognosis in patients treated for primary breast cancer? Cancer. 1986; 57:597.

231. Shah JP, Urban JA. Full thickness chest wall resection for recurrent breast carcinoma involving the bony chest wall. Cancer. 1975; 35:567–573.

232. Silvestrini R, Diadone MG, DiFronzo G et al. Prognostic implication of labeling index versus estrogen receptors and tumor size in node-negative breast cancer. Breast Cancer Res Treat. 1986; 7:161–169.

233. Skipper HT. Kinetics of mammary tumor cell growth and implications for therapy. Cancer. 1970; 28:1479–1499.

234. Slamon DJ, Clark GM, Wong SG et al. Human breast cancer: correlation of relapse and survival with amplification of the HER-2/neu oncogene. Science. 1987; 235:177–181.

235. Solin LJ, Fowble BL, Troupin RH, Goodman RL. Biopsy results of new calcifications in the postirradiated breast. Cancer. 1989; 63:1956–1961.

236. Stat O, Klinyenberg C, Franzen G et al. A comparison of static cytofluorometry and flow cytometry for the estimation of ploidy and DNA replication in human breast cancer. Breast Cancer Res Treat. 1986; 7:15.

237. Stenkvist B, Bengtsson E, Eriksson O et al. Histopathologic systems of breast cancer classification: reproducibility and clinical significance. J Clin Pathol. 1989; 36:392–398.

238. Stenkvist B, Westman-Naeser S, Vegelius J et al. Analysis of reproducibility of subjective grading systems for breast carcinoma. J Clin Pathol. 1979; 32:979–983.

239. Stuart-Harris RC, Smith IE. Aminoglutethimide in the treatment of advanced breast cancer. Cancer Treat Rev. 1984; 11:189–204.

240. Symposium on estrogen receptor determination with monoclonal antibodies. Cancer Res (Suppl). 1986; 46:4231s–4313s.

241. Tandon AK, Clark GM, Chamness GC et al. Cathespin D and prognosis in breast cancer. N Engl J Med. 1990; 322:297–302.

242. Tate JJT, Lewis V, Archer LT et al. Ultrasound detection of axillary lymph node metastases in breast cancer. Eur J Surg Oncol. 1989; 15:139–141.

243. Tchekymedyian NS, Tait N, Hisner J. High dose megestrol acetate in the treatment of postmenopausal women with advanced breast cancer. Semin Oncol (Suppl. 4). 1986; 13:20–25.

244. TNM Atlas. Thrid Ed. 2nd revision. Berlin: Springer; 1992.

245. Tomin R, Donegan WL. Screening for recurrent breast cancer. Its effectiveness and prognostic value. J Clin Oncol. 1987; 5:62–67.

246. Topalian SL, Muul LM, Solomon D, Rosenberg SA. Expansion of human tumor infiltrating lymphocytes for use in immunotherapy trial. J Immunol Meth. 1987; 102:127.

247. Tormey D, Carbone P, Band P. Breast cancer survival in simple and combination chemotherapy trials since 1968. Proc Am Ass Cancer Res. 1977; 18:64–68.

248. Treves N. The inoperability of inflammatory carcinoma of the breast. Surg Gynecol Obstet. 1959; 109:240–242.

249. Valagussa P, Bonadonna G, Veronesi U. Patterns of relapse and survival following radical mastectomy: Analysis of 716 consecutive patients. Cancer. 1978; 41:1170–1179.

250. Valagussa P, Tess T, Rossi A et al. Adjuvant CMF effect on site of first recurrence, and appropriate follow-up intervals, in operable breast cancer with

positive axillary nodes. Breast Cancer Res Treat. 1981; 1 : 349 – 356.

251. Veronesi U, Valagussa P. Inefficacy of internal mammary node dissection in breast cancer surgery. Cancer. 1981; 47 : 170 – 175.

252. Veronesi U, del Vecchio M, Greco et al. Results of quadrantectomy, axillary dissection, and radiotherapy (QUART) in T1N0 patients. In: Harris JR, Hellman S, Silen W, eds. Conservative Management of Breast Cancer. Philadelphia: Lippincott; 1983 : 90 – 91.

253. Veronesi U, Saccozzi R, Del Vecchio M et al. Comparing radical mastectomy with quadrantectomy, axillary dissection, and radiotherapy in patients with small cancers of the breast. N Engl J Med. 1981; 305 : 6 – 11.

254. Veronesi U, Zingo L, Cantù G. Extended mastectomy for cancer of the breast. Cancer. 1967; 20 : 677 – 680.

255. Veronesi U, Zucali R, Luini A. Local control and survival in early breast cancer: The Milan trial. Int J Radiat Oncol Biol Phys. 1986; 12 : 717 – 720.

256. The World Health Organization histological typing of breast tumor. 2nd Editon. Am J Clin Pathol. 1982; 78 : 806 – 816.

257. Wallgren A, Arner O, Bergström J et al. The value of preoperative radiotherapy in operable mammary carcinoma. Int J Radiat Oncol Biol Phys. 1980; 6 : 287 – 290.

258. Wallgren A, Arner O, Bergström J et al. Radiation therapy in operable breast cancer: Results from the Stockholm trial on adjuvant radiotherapy. Int J Radiat Oncol Biol Phys. 1986; 12 : 533 – 537.

259. Wickerham L, Fisher B, Cronin W et al. The efficacy of bone scanning in the follow-up of patients with operable breast cancer. Breast Cancer Res Treat. 1984; 4 : 303 – 307.

260. Williams MR, Walertz KJ, Turhas A et al. The use of an LH-RH agonist ICI 118630 Zoladex in advanced premenopausal breast cancer. Br J Cancer. 1986; 53 : 629 – 636.

261. Wilson RE. Recommendations for the surgical management of advanced breast cancer. Oncology. 1987; 1 : 21 – 26.

262. Winchester DP, Sener SF, Khandekar JD et al. Symptomatology as an indicator of recurrence or metastatic breast cancer. Cancer. 1979; 43 : 956 – 960.

263. Wölfel R, Klehmann E, Müller C et al. Lysis of human melanoma cells by autologous cytolytic T cell clones. J Exp Med. 1989; 130 : 397.

264. Wong SY, King G, Angus et al. Quality control of estrogen receptor assays using frozen breast tumors. J Clin Pathol. 1986; 39 : 690 – 691.

265. Zhou D, Battifora H, Yokota J et al. Association of multiple copies of the c-erbB-2 oncogene with the spread of breast cancer. Cancer Res. 1987; 47 : 6123 – 6125.

Index